MIND, BRAIN, AND SCHIZOPHRENIA

MIND, BRAIN, AND SCHIZOPHRENIA

Peter Williamson, MD, FRCP(C)

Tanna Schulich Chair in Neuroscience and Mental Health
Schulich School of Medicine
University of Western Ontario
Canada

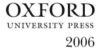

OXFORD
UNIVERSITY PRESS
2006

OXFORD
UNIVERSITY PRESS

Oxford University Press, Inc., publishes works that further
Oxford University's objective of excellence
in research, scholarship, and education.

Oxford   New York
Auckland   Cape Town   Dar es Salaam   Hong Kong   Karachi
Kuala Lumpur   Madrid   Melbourne   Mexico City   Nairobi
New Delhi   Shanghai   Taipei   Toronto

With offices in
Argentina   Austria   Brazil   Chile   Czech Republic   France   Greece
Guatemala   Hungary   Italy   Japan   Poland   Portugal   Singapore
South Korea   Switzerland   Thailand   Turkey   Ukraine   Vietnam

Copyright © 2006 by Oxford University Press, Inc.

Published by Oxford University Press, Inc.
198 Madison Avenue, New York, New York 10016
www.oup.com

Oxford is a registered trademark of Oxford University Press

Library of Congress Cataloging-in-Publication Data
Williamson, Peter, 1953–
Mind, brain, and schizophrenia / Peter Williamson.
p. ; cm.
Includes bibliographical references and index.
ISBN-13 978-0-19-517637-7
ISBN 0-19-517637-5
1. Schizophrenia. 2. Neuropsychiatry.
[DNLM: 1. Schizophrenia—diagnosis. 2. Schizophrenia—etiology. 3. Brain—physiopathology.
4. Brain Chemistry. 5. Diagnostic Imaging—methods. 6. Models, Neurological. 7. Nerve Degenera-
tion. WM 203 W732m 2005] I. Title.
RC514.W48 2005
616.89′8—dc22   2004029471

The science of medicine is a rapidly changing field. As new research and clinical experience
broaden our knowledge, changes in treatment and drug therapy do occur. The author and
publisher of this work have checked with sources believed to be reliable in their efforts to
provide information that is accurate and complete, and in accordance with the standards accepted at the time of publication. However, in light of the possibility of human error or
changes in the practice of medicine, neither the author, nor the publisher, nor any other
party who has been involved in the preparation or publication of this work warrants that the
information contained herein is in every respect accurate or complete. Readers are encouraged to confirm the information contained herein with other reliable sources, and are
strongly advised to check the product information sheet provided by the pharmaceutical
company for each drug they plan to administer.

1 2 3 4 5 6 7 8 9
Printed in the United States of America
on acid-free paper

This volume is dedicated to Judy Reidy,
Doug Leiper,
John Livesley,
and Bob Cleghorn
—great teachers who made a difference.

Preface

....

During my psychiatry residency, the study of schizophrenia was not
seen as an attractive option. Most residents preferred Freud and the
mysteries of psychoanalysis. At the time there was good reason for
the reluctance to take on this puzzling condition. Postmortem studies had not been very successful and there were few ways to study
what was going on in the brains of these patients. A lot has changed
over the 20 years since I have become a psychiatrist.

We are living in a very exciting period of psychiatry. Remarkable technical advances have come along that have allowed us to examine brain structure, function, and chemistry in living patients. We
have also seen incredible progress with molecular genetics in many
conditions. However, I fear that many of my students and colleagues
fail to recognize the potential for understanding the conditions that
we treat. Part of the problem may be the technical nature of the information that makes this work inaccessible. One of the reasons for
writing this book is to give some of the background knowledge of
neuroanatomy, neurochemistry, and neuronal circuitry necessary to
understand recent findings in schizophrenia.

The second purpose is to provide a clinician's perspective on
the pathophysiology of schizophrenia. I have spent most of my ca-

reer trying to understand what goes wrong in this condition. My own work has moved through neuropsychological tests and quantitative electroencephalography, to computerized tomography scans and magnetic resonance imaging, and finally to magnetic resonance spectroscopy and functional magnetic resonance imaging. With each new window it has become clear to me that we are looking at a failure of several brain circuits that may be damaged for a variety of reasons. This book is about the early attempts to define these final common pathways. My apologies, in advance, to the basic scientists who may think that I have oversimplified their ideas.

I would like to express my appreciation to the Schulich family for their generous support of a Chair in Neuroscience and Mental Health; my wife, Elizabeth, for her patience and editorial assistance; Dick Drost, my friend and medical biophysics collaborator over many years; Nic Russell for his sage advice; Ruth Lanius and Walter Rushlow for their suggestions on the manuscript, Sheri Bradshaw for her assistance with the research; and the wonderful teachers along the way who have given me the encouragement to continue this work.

Contents

....

MIND, BRAIN,
AND SCHIZOPHRENIA

The Evolving Concept of Schizophrenia

S chizophrenia is a uniquely human disorder. Many other psychiatric disorders have their counterpart in the animal world. Dogs suffer from acral lick dermatitis, which bears some resemblance to obsessive-compulsive disorders in humans (Stein et al., 1992). Learned-helplessness models in animals also closely approximate depression in humans (Maier and Seligman, 1976). However, no naturally occurring animal model captures the collection of symptoms that we have come to know as schizophrenia (Overall, 2000).

The disorder is common. It occurs in all races and cultures at about the same lifetime prevalence of just under 1%. For the most part, men and women are affected equally, although some hospital-based studies have shown a higher incidence in males. This discrepancy may be related to a later onset and better outcome in females (Seeman, 1982; Tamminga, 1997). Although some investigators have suggested that the incidence of schizophrenia has been declining in recent years, this is probably due to a number of factors such as changing diagnostic habits and the decreasing availability of hospital beds (Munk-Jorgensen, 1995).

Mesopotamian literature suggests that schizophrenia has been with us as least as long as civilization (Jeste et al., 1985). While not often described in literature, Shakespeare was apparently "fond of visiting Elizabethan madhouses." Hamlet shows many characteristics of manic-depressive illness whereas the behavior of Ophelia suggests a schizoaffective disorder (Andreasen, 1976). In the Middle Ages, sufferers of this disorder were likely viewed as eccentric or possessed by demons. It is only in the last century-and-a-half that schizophrenia has been seen as a medical condition, although many early physicians recognized that madness was not related to moral or religious shortcomings (Hunter and MacAlpine, 1982).

Emil Kraepelin, Father of Modern Psychiatry

The first comprehensive description of the condition was provided by Kraepelin, who described a condition he called *dementia praecox,* around the end of the nineteenth century. These patients were differentiated from those with manic-depressive insanity and paranoia by virtue of the fact that most of them never recovered. His description of these patients (Kraepelin, 1919) is remarkable, even when viewed after a century has passed.

Kraepelin observed that "patients perceive in general what goes on around them often much better than one would expect from their behavior" but they "do not take any notice of what they may perceive quite well, nor do they try to understand it; they do not follow what happens in their surroundings even though it may happen to be of great importance for them." Patients were found to be emotionally dull with a loss of interest and singular indifference toward others. They had "no real joy in life," "no human feelings"; to them "nothing matters," "everything is the same," and they feel "no grief and no joy."

The same patients were haunted by auditory hallucinations, which Kraepelin (1919, pp. 7–8) described:

> Sometimes it is only a whispering, "as if it concerned me" as the patient says, a secret language, "taunting the captive"; sometimes the voices are loud or suppressed, as from a ventriloquist, or the call of a telephone, "childrens' voices"; a patient heard "gnats speak." Sometimes they shout as a chorus or all confusedly; a patient spoke of "drumming in the ear"; another heard, "729,000 girls." Sometimes the voices appear to have a metallic sound, they are "resonant voices," "organ voices," or as of a tun-

ing fork. At other times they do not appear to the patients as sense perceptions at all. . . . There is an "inner feeling in the soul," an "inward voice in the thoughts"; "it is thought inwardly in me"; yet "sounded as if thought."

Visual, olfactory, and somatoform hallucinations were described by Kraepelin (1919, p. 29) with equal clarity, as well as delusions of persecution and grandiose delusions:

The patient is "something better," born to a higher place, the "glory of Israel," an inventer, a great singer, can do what he will. He is noble, of royal blood, an officer of dragoons, heir to the Throne of Bulgaria; Willhelm Rex, the Kaiser's son, the greatest man in Germany, more than king or kaiser. Or he is the chosen one, the prophet, influenced by the Holy Ghost, guardian angel, second Messiah, Saviour of the world, the little God who distributes grace and love, more than the Holy Ghost, the Almighty.

Kraepelin went on to point out that even more characteristic of the disorder was the sense that "one's thoughts are being influenced" and the perception of knowing the thoughts of other people. His patients reported that they were frequently watched through the telephone or "connected up by wireless telegraphy or by Tesla currents"; a comment now ironic with the advent of magnetic resonance imaging.

A generalized "constraint of thought" was described as well as "incoherence of the train of thought," resulting in marked disturbances in behavior and judgment. Kraepelin (1919, p. 56) noted:

The most different ideas follow one another with most bewildering want of connection, even when the patients are quite quiet. A patient said, "Life is a dessert-spoon," another, "We are already standing in the spiral under a hammer," a third, "Death will be awakened by the golden dagger," a fourth, "The consecrated discourse cannot be over split in any movement."

Kraepelin felt that memory was little affected but he did observe that mental efficiency and intention were affected. Although neuropsychological testing had yet to be developed, he asked patients to perform calculation tasks and observed that they performed poorly even after a rest period, a pattern which seemed to differ from that of alcoholic patients and healthy volunteers. It is not certain that we have learned a lot more with modern neuropsychological batteries.

The term *dementia praecox* implied a progressively deteriorating illness but Kraepelin realized that the course of dementia praecox was extremely variable. Some patients followed a malignant downward course while others had periodic exacerbations with some degree of recovery in between. In the time before antipsychotic medication, the periods of improvement rarely lasted longer than 3 years. More recent follow-up studies of up to 30 years have shown that antipsychotic medication improves outcome (Ciompi, 1980; Hogarty et al., 1974; Huber et al., 1980; May et al., 1981; Tsuang et al., 1979). Yet at the same time, schizophrenia is not a benign illness. Antipsychotic medications help the majority of patients to control hallucinations and delusions but are less effective with lack of motivation and flattened affect. Patients have difficulty handling critical comments from family members and often break down under stress (Norman and Malla, 1993). Very few patients recover enough to return to full-time work, get married, or raise a family. Most are left with lifelong disability, leading the World Health Organization to place it on the list of the 10 most disabling medical illnesses (Murray and Lopez, 1996).

Although Kraepelin recognized variability in course of illness, he thought that it should have a characteristic neuropathology, just like another form of dementia described by his colleague, Alzheimer. The English translation of *dementia praecox* and *paraphrenia* comes with detailed diagrams from microscopic examination of neuropathological specimens showing "sclerotic nerve-cells" and "nerve-cells diseased in high degree filled with lipoid products of disintegration" (Kraepelin, 1919). Unfortunately, the idea that schizophrenia is a brain disorder never really took hold, in part because of the rise of psychoanalysis but also because very few, if any, neuropathological changes could be replicated. Before long, schizophrenia became known as the "graveyard of neuropathologists."

Modern Use of the Term *Schizophrenia*

Although the term *schizophrenia* was coined later by Bleuler, there can be no doubt that modern ideas about schizophrenia owe their origin to Kraepelin (Shorter, 1997). Indeed, the *Diagnostic and Sta-*

tistical Manual of Mental Disorders, fourth edition, text revision (DSM-IV) criteria (American Psychiatric Association, 2000) currently in use to make the diagnosis of schizophrenia has drawn heavily on Kraeplin's descriptions of dementia praecox.

DSM-IV criteria

The DSM-IV requires two or more of the following to be present for a significant portion of a 1-month period: delusions, hallucinations, disorganized speech, grossly disorganized or catatonic behavior, and negative symptoms. Only one of these is required if the delusions are bizarre like those described by Kraepelin, if the hallucinations consist of a voice making a running commentary on the person's behavior or thoughts, or two or more voices converse with each other. Consistent with dementia praecox, one or more areas of functioning such as work, interpersonal relations, or self-care must be markedly below the level of functioning before the onset of the disorder. Symptoms must also last at least 6 months and not be better accounted for by other diagnoses such as mood disorders and drug abuse.

Subtypes

The current DSM-IV criteria include several subtypes described by Kraepelin. Of these, the most prevalent and stable one appears to be the *paranoid* type, characterized by a preoccupation with one or more delusions or frequent hallucinations. A *disorganized* type is recognized that best corresponds to Kraepelin's hebephrenic subtype. These patients show prominent disorganized speech, disorganized behavior, and flat or inappropriate behavior. The DSM-IV *catatonic* type, also described by Kraepelin, is defined by two or more of motor immobility, excessive motor activity, extreme negativism, peculiarities of movement as evidenced by posturing, and echolalia or echopraxia. *Undifferentiated* and *residual* subtypes are included to cover cases that do not fit easily into a category and patients with chronic negative symptoms, respectively. It is curious that hebephrenic and catatonic types are seen much less frequently than in Kraepelin's time (Mahendra, 1981; Morrison, 1974). The reason for this is not known, although positive effects of pharmacotherapy and rehabilitation have been suggested.

Other approaches to heterogeneity

Although the standard subtypes of schizophrenia are still used, most clinicians agree that they are not very useful in predicting outcome or planning treatment. In response to these concerns, there have been several attempts to surmount heterogeneity with dichotomous constructs such as positive–negative, type I–type II, and deficit–nondeficit (Andreasen, 1982; Crow, 1989; Tamminga et al., 1992). While these constructs are useful, the most enduring approach has been to attempt to determine which symptoms tend to go with others. Using this approach, Liddle (1987) defined three clinical syndromes. The first is *psychomotor poverty,* characterized by such features as poverty of speech, decreased spontaneous movements, slowness, and blunted affect. The other two are *disorganization syndrome,* including incongruous affect, poverty of content of speech, incoherence, tangentiality, distractibility, and self-neglect, and *reality distortion,* which includes auditory hallucinations and delusions of persecution and reference. These syndromes are probably best viewed as dimensions, as they overlap extensively in individual patients.

Schizophrenia as a Neurodevelopmental Disorder

Interest in schizophrenia began to increase again with the chance discovery of chlorpromazine. With the development of other antipsychotic agents, it became clear that all affected dopamine levels, which resulted in speculation about the role of dopamine in schizophrenia. Other studies began to examine neuropsychological and electrophysiological changes associated with the disorder. It soon became clear that many deficits were present long before the onset of delusions and hallucinations, leading to the idea that schizophrenia may be a neurodevelopmental disorder.

Lesion studies in animals seemed to suggest that at least some of the behavioral and physiological studies seen in schizophrenia could be replicated by lesioning parts of the brain, such as the hippocampus. While animals with these lesions were obviously not schizophrenic, it did raise the possibility that the brain could be damaged in some way early in development, lie dormant until maturity, and then express itself in the symptoms of schizophrenia. Although the nature of this damage has remained elusive, genetic factors, viral illnesses, and obstetric complications have all been implicated.

Technological Advances

The last two decades have seen two important technological advances that have the potential to lead to important new insights into the nature of schizophrenia: molecular genetics and brain imaging.

Molecular genetics

It has been known for some time that there is a strong genetic basis to schizophrenia. First-degree relatives of schizophrenic patients have an almost 10-fold increased risk of developing schizophrenia, whereas identical twins have an almost 50-fold increase in risk compared to the general population. Despite the obvious importance of this factor, several genome scan studies in schizophrenic pedigrees have revealed only a few modest linkages that are usually not replicated in other pedigrees. For many investigators working in the field, it is becoming increasingly clear that there are many genes implicated in the development of schizophrenia and that we are not likely to find major genes that account for the majority of cases. It is also clear that schizophrenia can be caused by factors other than genetic inheritance. The fact that identical twins have roughly a 50% concordance suggests that there are other factors. These may include the effects of viral illnesses early in brain development and obstetric complications.

Brain imaging

Neuropathological studies have always been limited by the effects of aging, other diseases, medication, and deterioration after death. With brain imaging, it is now possible to examine the brain in living patients. Brain structure can be examined with high resolution with techniques such as computerized tomography (CT) and magnetic resonance imaging (MRI). The response of the brain to neuropsychological tasks can be examined with positron emission tomography (PET) and functional magnetic resonance imaging (fMRI). Neurotransmitters and other aspects of brain chemistry can also be examined with PET and magnetic resonance spectroscopy (MRS).

　　As with the genetic studies, preliminary structural findings have been somewhat disappointing. The most consistent structural finding has been larger lateral ventricles and reduced gray matter throughout the association cortex. These findings are not present in all patients and are sometimes found in other conditions. Although these changes seem to be present at the beginning of the illness, recent studies have suggested progressive enlargement of ventricles and loss of gray matter, rekindling the ideas about neuronal degeneration first introduced by Kraepelin.

When functional imaging techniques such as PET were introduced about 20 years ago, there was a sense that schizophrenia would soon be understood. This has turned out not to be the case, although several replicated observations have been made. The first of these is the finding that many patients show dopaminergic hyperresponsivity on PET, in keeping with the dopamine models. Another finding that seems to be fairly widely replicated is a failure of frontal activation during frontal lobe tasks on both PET and fMRI. To some extent, these activation deficits correlate with volume deficits, particularly in the temporal lobes. More recent studies of functional connectivity have demonstrated many deficits involving several parts of the brain, but not all of these findings have been replicated.

Final Common Pathway

Schizophrenia is a very complicated disorder. No two patients seem to share exactly the same combination of symptoms or findings. Yet all seem to have a syndrome that we can recognize as schizophrenia. Findings in these patients are scattered throughout the brain but seem to involve the frontal and temporal cortices as well as the basal ganglia and thalamus more than other regions. Most investigators would accept that these regions seem to be damaged at least in some patients early on and that at least some patients show a progressive increase in ventricles and loss of gray matter.

Many investigators in the field have been implicitly assuming that schizophrenia is a disease. As such, it must have a cause. This could be a gene involved in brain development, a viral infection in utero, obstetrical complications, or any number of other factors. What seems to be emerging from more recent work is that the cause is unlikely to be one gene or even several genes. Brain development is dependent upon thousands of different genes, all of which interact with several other factors including nutrition, stress, viral illnesses in utero, and obstetric complications, making the search for the cause of schizophrenia in a particular patient a very frustrating task.

In some ways, psychiatry is at the same crossroads that medicine was almost 400 years ago when William Harvey was about to discover the circulatory system (Ackerknecht, 1968). Patients with heart failure presented with characteristic symptoms such as edema and shortness of breath. Their livers were found to be distended and their jugular venous pulses elevated. There was some variability in symptoms in that some patients would have more edema and others had both edema and shortness of breath, depending on whether it was left-sided heart failure or left- and right-sided heart failure. The best knowledge at the time suggested that the problem was an "imbalance of humors." There was no knowledge of the circulatory system and, indeed, most physicians believed that blood flowed away from the liver.

Modern medicine was born when William Harvey trained with a man named Fabricius in Italy who described venous valves. This observation led Harvey to question the prevailing view at the time that the blood flowed away from the liver. With venous valves, it could flow only one way and that was back to the heart. From there, he constructed the idea of a circulatory system in which blood is pumped from the body to the heart to the lungs, back to the heart, and to the body. When the pump breaks down, symptoms such as edema, shortness of breath, an enlarged liver, and an elevated jugular venous pulse become understandable. It is of note that this occurs no matter what the cause. Any number of genetic abnormalities can affect the heart, as well as atherosclerosis and kidney disease, among other disorders. No matter what the cause, the characteristic symptoms result.

Schizophrenia may be a similar problem. With schizophrenia, the characteristic symptoms are not edema and shortness of breath but rather flattened affect, hallucinations, delusions, and thought disorder. Like heart failure, schizophrenia probably has a number of causes that are unlikely to be fully elucidated in any one patient. After all, we do not fully understand all the causes of heart failure even after 400 years.

Should We Set Aside the Search for the Cause of Schizophrenia?

The purpose of this volume is to suggest that it may be time to set aside the search for the *cause* of schizophrenia and focus on the *final common pathway*. Although we may not be able to fully understand how the multitude of causative factors interact to lead to schizophrenia in any one patient, it seems likely that all of these factors affect a final common pathway, the equivalent of the circulatory system in the explanation of heart failure. Understanding the nature of this pathway is not going to be easy. However, with brain imaging techniques there has been incredible progress in the last decade. We have learned much about language processing, memory, attention, and learning. The next chapter will review some of the neuro-anatomy and neuronal circuitry relevant to these functions.

Subsequent chapters will examine the *clues*. While it is clear that we do not have any venous valves, we do have some very important clues arising from observations in patients before the illness begins. In many cases, patients are perfectly normal before they develop schizophrenia. Others perform more poorly than expected in school and demonstate subtle neurological and behavioral findings suggestive of an early neurodevelopmental problem. The tendency of drugs such as amphetamines to cause positive symptoms such as hallucinations and delusions suggests a role for dopamine. Other drugs that block a type of glutamate receptor seem to cause both positive symptoms and negative symptoms, such as flat affect and lack of motivation. Many of the brain regions involved in thinking, perception, and affect are regulated by dopamine while glutamate is the most common neurotransmitter used in the connections between these brain regions.

As Kraepelin astutely observed, schizophrenic patients have difficulty performing psychological tasks. The nature of these deficits and those seen with physiological probes provide some insight into the brain regions involved. However, far more information can be obtained from imaging brain structure and function. The findings from these studies are not yet clear, but they do point to structures that might be involved in a final common pathway. They also seem to suggest that there could be progressive structural and metabolic changes in the early years of illness compatible with, but not necessarily related to, neurodegeneration.

We are a long way from understanding anything like the equivalent of the circulatory system as it applies to schizophrenia, but there have been several attempts to sketch this out. The evidence for key areas will be surveyed. Models that try to put together the pieces will then be examined from a perspective of what we already know about schizophrenia. Some of this knowledge has treatment implications, and the preliminary efforts to design better drugs and novel, non-pharmacological interventions will be highlighted. Finally, some thought will be given to what is missing in our current models and how a better understanding of the final common pathway of schizophrenia might relate to understanding consciousness.

2

Candidate Neuronal Circuits

Although schizophrenia and other neuropsychiatric disorders are now clearly viewed as brain disorders, psychiatrists do not spend a lot of time thinking about the brain in the same way that neurologists think about the brain or cardiologists think about the heart. This is understandable to some extent in that we have not understood much about the brain until recent decades.

At first, the sheer complexity of the brain appears to be overwhelming. There are over 100 billion individual nerve cells of two principal types, designated neurons and glial cells. *Neurons* make up the signaling pathways in the brain by virtue of their ability to form synapses, where chemicals called *neurotransmitters* are released to pass the message on to the next neuron—a process sometimes referred to as *signaling*. Some of the neurotransmitters involved in schizophrenia include dopamine, glutamate, and serotonin. *Glial cells* are the supporting cells of the brain, although they can also participate in signaling.

Functions such as attention, memory, and language depend on complex interactions between cells and different parts of the brain. Specific processing can be specialized to one area but the overall function depends on the coordination of several different brain areas. Any one neuron can receive input from up to 150,000 other neurons. These connections form in a very systematic way as the brain develops.

Brain Development

The brain develops from a neural plate that folds onto itself to form the neural tube. In the beginning there are three vesicles: the prosencephalon (forebrain), the mesencephalon (midbrain), and the rhombencephalon (hindbrain). The prosencephalon goes on to develop into the telencephalon and the diencephalon. The telencephalon in turn goes on to form the cerebral cortex, the basal ganglia, the hippocampus, the amygdala, and the olfactory bulb. The diencephalon goes on to form the thalamus, the hypothalamus, the retina, and the optic nerves. The mesencephalon and rhombencephalon form the brain stem, the cerebellum, and the spinal cord. Some of these stages are illustrated in Figure 2–1.

Most cognitive processes are dependent upon the cerebral cortex, which begins to form around the second trimester of pregnancy with the migration of six cell layers from the subplate. Neurons in the cortex are highly topographically organized. There are specific regions in the brain that are responsible for particular types and locations of sensation as well as movement. The connections that al-

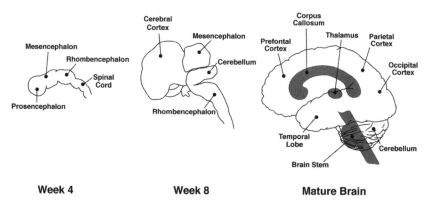

| Week 4 | Week 8 | Mature Brain |

Figure 2–1. Brain development at 4 weeks and 8 weeks, and mature brain. Used with permission, adapted in part from O'Rahilly, R., Müller, F., and Bossy, J. (1986). Atlas des stades du développement des formes extérieures de l'encéphale chez l'embryon humain. *Archives D'anatomie, D'histolgie, et D'embryologie Normales* **69**, 3–39.

low this cortical specificity are highly dependent upon neurons arising from the thalamus and projecting up to the subplate (O'Leary
et al., 1994). For example, in rats, barrel fields that are very specific
to sensation from a certain part of the rat's body develop in the somatosensory cortex (Schlaggar and O'Leary, 1993). These barrel
fields do not seem to be a property of the cortical neurons themselves, as cells from the occipital cortex can be transplanted into the
somatosensory cortex and they will also form barrel fields, providing
there are thalamocortical afferents. It is not known for sure if the
same process applies to other parts of the cortex, such as the frontal
cortex, but the role of thalamocortical neurons in cortical specificity
in these regions is suspected to be important as well.

The brain unfolds in a highly predictable sequence dependent
upon the activation of various genes and proteins. Much of the cell
migration involved in the formation of cortical layers and cortical
specificity occurs in the second trimester of pregnancy, but brain development does not stop at birth. In fact, myelinization goes on well
into adolescence and early adulthood (Benes et al., 1994). There is
also ongoing cortical pruning that proceeds throughout childhood
and is more or less complete by adulthood. Generally speaking, higher-
order association cortices mature after lower-order somatosensory and
visual cortices. Phylogenetically older brain areas mature earlier than
newer ones (Gogtay et al., 2004a). Almost 60% of corticocortical connections involving associative regions such as the prefrontal and auditory cortices are lost in this way (Huttenlocher and Dabholkar, 1997).

Curiously, human brains are surprisingly like those of apes.
While the human brain has a much larger association cortex, there
is not much evidence to indicate that humans have new cortical areas. Many of the regions involved in speech also have homologs in
nonhuman primates. Nonhuman primates also possess at least some
degree of cortical asymmetry. However, humans are capable of complex behaviors not possible in apes. Let us examine some of the brain
regions involved in these behaviors.

Critical Brain Regions

Essentially, the brain is organized to filter and unify sensory information so that a coherent behavioral response can be made, ensur-
ing survival. There are several brain regions participating in com-

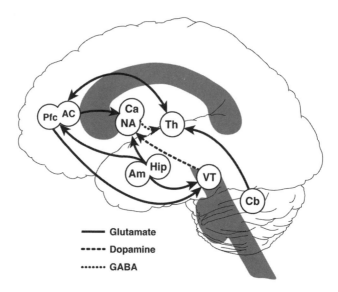

Figure 2–2. Critical brain regions. AC, anterior cingulate; Am, amygdala; Ca, caudate; Cb, cerebellum; Hip, hippocampus; NA, nucleus accumbens; Pfc, prefrontal cortex; Th, thalamus; VT, ventral tegmentum.

plex behaviors that could be related to schizophrenia. Some of these regions are illustrated in Figure 2–2.

Prefrontal region

Probably the most important of the regions involved in complex behavior is the prefrontal cortex (Fuster, 1998; Stuss and Knight, 2002). The prefrontal cortex is very prominent in primates and small in mammals such as rats that have been used for most of the animal models of schizophrenia. The prefrontal cortex can be divided into the *dorsolateral region,* which roughly underlies the forehead, and the *orbitofrontal region,* which lies medially and at the base of the brain. The dorsolateral region is primarily involved in working memory. This part of the brain receives input from almost all regions including the hippocampus, which provides information about the context of current stimuli on the basis of previous experience. Through this process, an action plan is made and implemented with connections to the motor regions of the brain.

The medial and orbitofrontal parts of the prefrontal cortex have much different functions, although they also receive multiple inputs from other parts of the brain. The orbitofrontal cortex appears to be important in evaluating the reward value of stimuli (Rolls, 1999). Damage to the orbitofrontal cortex can impair learning of stimulus–reinforcement associations. One of the most famous examples of this is Phineas Gage, who was setting explosives with an iron bar while working on a railway over a century ago. When the explosives prematurely ignited, the bar severely damaged his medial prefrontal cortex. Surprisingly, his working memory was intact and he appeared to be more or less normal, apart from the fact that he could not inhibit socially inappropriate behaviors. Whereas he had been an upstanding and hard-working citizen before, he was no longer interested in work and took to abusing alcohol and gambling. Therefore, the orbitofrontal cortex appears to be associated with emotional aspects of behavior and the inhibition of inappropriate behavior.

The prefrontal cortex also plays an important role in shaping the temporal flow of information. Using simultaneous single-cell recordings in primates, Constantinidis et al. (2002) showed that there are inbitory interactions between neurons active at different time points relative to the cue presentation, delay interval, and response in a working-memory task. Thus, the prefrontal cortex not only holds information on-line in working memory but also shapes the temporal sequence of response.

Temporal region

The temporal cortex is also well developed in humans—particularly the *superior temporal gyrus,* which is involved in language processing. Within the superior temporal gyrus is the *Heschl gyrus,* which is the primary auditory cortex that plays an important role in auditory perception. Just posterior to the Heschl gyrus is the *planum temporale,* which has close connections with the Heschl gyrus and overlaps Wernicke's language association cortex. Both the Heschl gyrus and planum temporale are critical to language processing. This role perhaps explains why the planum temporale shows the most left–right asymmetry in the human brain (Mesulam, 2000).

The temporal lobe also includes the hippocampus and amygdala. The *hippocampus* is recognized as being important in facilitating long-term memory via its extensive connections with almost every part of the cortex. The *amygdala* is also closely connected with other cortical regions, particularly the obitofrontal cortex. It facilitates emotional memories and fear conditioning (Aggleton, 1992; Mesu-lam, 1990; Squire, 1992). Both the hippocampus and amygdala are older parts of the brain, seen in all mammals. These brain regions have three layers, in contrast to the six layers seen in other parts of the cortex involved in processing multiple sensations, referred to as *heteromodal* cortex.

A structure closely related but generally considered to be sepa-rate from the four main lobes of the hemisphere is the *insula*, which lies between the stiatum and the temporal lobe along the lateral fis-sure. The insula is closely connected to the parts of the brain that monitor internal states of the body. It is also important in speech ar-ticulation and pain perception, and is often activated when subjects are asked to produce well-learned category-specific knowledge (Mar-tin et al., 1996).

Anterior cingulate

The *cingulate cortex* winds around the *corpus callosum*, which joins the left and right sides of the brain. The *anterior cingulate* is closely con-nected with the hippocampus and prefrontal cortex. It is also part of an attentional network involving the prefrontal, parietal, and tempo-ral regions (Devinsky and Luciano, 1993). The upper part of the an-terior cingulate participates in error detection and is often activated when subjects are asked to do a complex task in a brain-imaging ex-periment. The middle part of the anterior cingulate participates in salience or the determination of whether a stimulus is important. The inferior part of the anterior cingulate below the genu of the corpus callosum is important in processing emotion, with some of the infe-rior regions of the prefrontal cortex referred to as *area 25* and the *amygdala* in the temporal lobe. Damage to the anterior cingulate of-ten results in affective flatness and even mutism in severe cases.

Thalamus

The *thalamus*, which lies just above the brain stem at the center of the brain, is essentially the central switchboard of the brain. Neu-rons carrying information about all senses, with the exception of ol-faction, synapse in the thalamus on their way to conveying informa-tion to various parts of the cortex. Visual information is sent first to the occipital cortex and then through different pathways involving the parietal cortex and temporal lobes, eventually to the prefrontal cortex. Auditory information is mostly processed through the temporal lobe on its way to the prefrontal cortex. Olfaction follows a different pathway from the olfactory bulb to the olfactory tubercle, piriform cortex, amygdala, entrorhinal cortex, and orbitofrontal cortex.

Dorsal and ventral striatum

Immediately anterior and somewhat superior to the thalamus is the corpus striatum. The striatum is made up of a dorsal tier including the putamen, globus pallidus, and caudate nucleus, which is directly connected with the amygdala, and a ventral tier, which includes the nucleus accumbens. The dorsal tier is closely connected with the prefrontal cortex and motor areas. The ventral tier is also connected with the prefrontal cortex but receives input from the amygdala and hippocampus as well. The corpus striatum and other subcortical structures such as the subthalamic nucleus and the substantia nigra comprise the *basal ganglia.* Appetitive behavior and reinforcement are most closely associated with the ventral striatum, whereas the dorsolateral straitum mediates procedural or stimulus–response learning. Spatial learning has been associated with both the dorsomedial and ventral striatum (Voorn et al., 2004).

One of the structures in the ventral striatum, the nucleus accumbens, deserves further comment. This tiny nucleus at the base of the brain is the gateway between the limbic system and motor system—the link between motivation and action (Mogenson et al., 1980). The shell of this structure is likely a component of the extended amygdala whereas the core has more in common with the dorsal striatum. Covergence of input from prefrontal and limbic regions results in groups of cells firing together in an ensemble which in turn influences activity in the thalamus and prefrontal regions (Heimer, 2000; O'Donnell et al., 1999).

Limbic system

Certain parts of the cerebral hemispheres and diencephalon are often referred to as the *limbic system.* Originally described by Papez (1937) and modified and popularized by MacLean, the limbic system includes the cingulate and parahippocampal gyri, the hippocampal formation, a large part of the amygdala, parts of the hypothalamus, and the anterior nucleus of the thalamus (MacLean, 1978). This system is present in all mammals and is felt to play a special role in the emotional aspects of behavior and memory. Since the original description, the nucleus accumbens and medioorbital prefrontal cortex have come to be considered by many investigators as part of the extended limbic system because of their close interconnections with the principal components of the system.

Cerebellum

The cerebellum lies between the brain stem and occipital cortex. It is also a phylogenetically old part of the brain that was felt to be mostly involved in the coordination of motor movements. More recently, it has been recognized that it may also play a role in cognition. One of the models discussed in Chapter 11 draws heavily on the role of the cerebellum in cognition.

Many of these brain regions are interconnected in functional circuits used in learning new behaviors. Probably the best known are the basal ganglia–thalamocortical neuronal circuits.

Basal Ganglia–Thalamocortical Neuronal Circuits

The basal ganglia are part of the extrapyramidal motor system, which contributes to a variety of skeletomotor, occulomotor, cognitive, and emotional processes. The heterogenous nature of basal ganglia activity may be due in part because to their unique position within the brain. The basal ganglia receive projections from the prefrontal cortex then project via the thalamus back to these same regions, allowing highly specific and coordinated control of neuronal activity. Originally there were five basal ganglia–thalamocortical neuronal circuits, characterized by Alexander and colleagues (1990). The mapping has become somewhat more complicated since then (Middleton and Strick, 2001), but most of the circuits still hold up reasonably well, so they will be described below in some detail.

Motor, cognitive, and affective circuits

The motor circuit begins in the supplementary motor area and motor cortex and projects via glutamatergic neurons to the putamen where it follows a direct and indirect γ-aminobutyric acid (GABA) pathway to the thalamus. The indirect pathway goes through the subthalamic nucleus, allowing an extra synapse, and because GABAergic neurons are inhibitory, this pathway has an opposite effect compared to the direct pathway. Both of these pathways converge on the thalamus, which in turn is reciprocally connected with the supplementary motor area and motor cortex, forming a loop circuit. Occular movements are controlled by a similar pathway beginning in the frontal eye fields and supplementary eye fields, projecting to the caudate by excitatory glutamatergic neurons, and then, as with the motor circuit, projecting directly and indirectly to the thalamus, where reciprocal connections are made with the sites of origin in the cortex.

There are three basal ganglia–thalamocortical neuronal circuits that participate in cognition and emotion. The first two of these follow very similar pathways and are referred to as the *prefrontal circuits.* One originates in the dorsolateral prefrontal cortex and the other in the lateral orbital prefrontal cortex. These circuits are shown in Figure 2–3. Both project via excitatory glutamatergic neurons to the caudate and directly and indirectly through the subthalamic nucleus via GABAergic neurons to the thalamus, which in turn is reciprocally connected with the sites of origin in the cortex.

The *limbic* basal ganglia–thalamocortical neuronal circuit follows a different route, beginning in the anterior cingulate and medioorbital prefrontal cortex, and projects via glutamatergic neurons to the ventral striatum, including the nucleus accumbens. From the ventral striatum there are direct and indirect GABAergic pathways similar to the other circuits ending in the thalamus, which is reciprocally connected with the anterior and medioorbital prefrontal cortex. This pathway is unique in that it receives substantial input from other parts of the limbic system, including the amygdala and hippocampus.

The arrangement of the direct and indirect pathways allows for opposing input back to the cortex either inhibiting or stimulating certain pathways. Dopamine plays an important role in modulating these circuits by facilitating conduction through the direct pathway. This has an excitatory effect on the thalamus. Dopamine also suppresses conduction through the indirect pathway, which has an inhibitory effect on the thalamus. This input has a number of implications for both motor disorders and neuropsychiatric disorders such as schizophrenia.

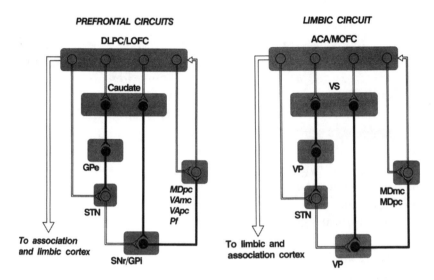

Figure 2–3. Prefrontal and limbic basal ganglia–thalamocortical neuronal circuits. ACA, anterior cingulate area; DLPC, dorsolateral prefrontal cortex; GPe, external segment of globus pallidus; GPi, internal segment of globus pallidus; LOFC, lateral orbitofrontal cortex; MDmc, nucleus medialis dorsalis pars magnocellularis; MDpc, nucleus medialis dorsalis pars parvicellularis; MOFC, medial orbitofrontal cortex; Pf, nucleus parafascicularis; STN, subthalamic nucleus; SNr, substantia nigra pars reticulate; VAmc, nucleus ventralis anterior pars magnocellularis; VApc, nucleus ventralis anterior pars parvocellularis; VP, ventral pallidum; VS, ventral striatum. Used with permission, from Alexander et al. (1990).

Regulation by dopamine, amygdala, and hippocampus

Dopamine input from the ventral tegmental area to the nucleus accumbens is regulated by the prefrontal cortex (Taber et al., 1995) and the neurotransmitter serotonin (Dewey et al., 1995; Kapur and Remington, 1996). The nucleus accumbens also sends a projection back to the ventral tegmental area, which provides further regulation of dopamine output. More recent work has demonstrated that hippocampal and amygdala glutamatergic inputs to the nucleus accumbens *gate* activity within the basal ganglia–thalamocortical circuits. This allows behavior to be influenced by past experience presumably arising from information made accessible by the hippocampus. It also allows for past emotional experience to influence behavior via input from the amygdala. This input is able to override past experiential input from the hippocampus in certain circumstances. This finding has led to one of the recent models of schizo-phrenia, which will be discussed in Chapter 12. A simplified diagram illustrating some of these connections is shown in Figure 2–2.

Role in response learning

There are several theories of how the frontal lobe and basal ganglia lead to response learning (Alexander et al., 1990; Graybiel, 1995). The frontal cortex seems to act when new rules need to be learned or older ones rejected. The basal ganglia, by contrast, potentiate pre-viously learned rules on the basis of current context and reinforce-ment history. Wise et al. (1996) have presented a plausible model as to how this comes about. They suggest that direct pathway neurons recognize the pattern of corticostriatal inputs promoting a rule through positive-feedback loops. Dopaminergic neurons originating in the midbrain increase activity during learning and enhance gene expression within the direct pathway and at the same time suppress neurons of the indirect pathway. Thus, dopamine increases activity in loops triggered by a recognized context and activates context-dependent activity within these modules. Dopamine seems to po-tentiate direct-pathway activity through its effect on a subtype of dopamine receptors called D_1 *receptors* and suppresses the indirect pathway through another subtype of dopamine receptors called D_2 *receptors.*

While basal ganglia–thalamocortical neuronal circuits are likely essential for learning most new behaviors, they are not the only cir-cuits that might be related to conscious awareness. In the following section we will consider some structures that might be involved in consciousness.

Consciousness

We are at a very early stage of understanding the brain circuits that mediate consciousness. In fact, there is still a lot of debate as to what consciousness is (Chalmers, 1996; Damasio, 1999; Metzinger, 2000). A basic subjective awareness of surroundings is likely maintained via brain-stem nuclei, the hypothalamus, and somatosensory cortex. Self-awareness extends this network to the medioprefrontal cortex, cin-gulate, thalamus, and superior colliculi.

Brain imaging studies of self-awareness

In a recent functional magnetic resonance imaging (fMRI) study (Gusnard et al., 2001), subjects were asked to make two judgements, one self-referential and the other not, in response to affectively normed pictures. The self-referential tasks were accompanied by activation of the medioprefrontal cortex, in keeping with the role of this part of the brain in self-referential mental activity and emotional processing. In another fMRI study by Johnson et al. (2002), subjects were asked to respond to self-referential statements or statements requiring semantic knowledge. As in the earlier study, medioprefrontal regions were activated as well as posterior cingulate regions. These findings were consistent with the inability of patients with medioprefrontal damage to infer mental states in others (Damasio et al., 1990; Stuss et al., 2001). Damage to either the right or left prefrontal cortex can lead to deficits in the ability to understand or predict other peoples' behavior (Rowe et al., 2001).

40 Hz oscillations

Specific aspects of conscious experience can correlate with changes in activity in specific brain regions in association with specific stimuli, memories, or even dreams, but conscious experience as a whole involves activation or deactivation of widespread brain regions. Subjects who are comatose or in slow-wave sleep show severely reduced activity in both the cerebral cortex and thalamus. Conversely, mental activity seems to be associated with temporal binding of 40 Hz oscillations, which reflect synchronous activity of reentrant corticothalamic loops (Llinás and Pare, 1991; Tononi and Edelman, 1998a, 1998b). Activity within the loops can be focused by an attentional network involving the dorsolateral prefrontal cortex, anterior cingulate, right inferior parietal lobe, and some temporal lobe structures. Comparison of the current experience with past experiences and their emotional valence is accomplished via input from the hippocampus and amygdala, respectively.

The binding problem

One of the perennial problems in brain research is explaining how such a complex collection of sights, sounds, smells, and physical sensations is integrated into a unitary experience, with a subjective sense of self and an objective sense of self, in an external, ever-changing world. This is referred to as the *binding problem*. There have been several proposals to elucidate how consciousness becomes a unitary experience (Cleeremans, 2003; Crick, 1984; Gray, 1995, 2004; Jones, 2001; Laberge, 1995; Llinás and Pare, 1991; Llinás et al. 1994; Newman 1997a, 1997b; Newman and Grace, 1999; Posner, 1994; Tononi and Edelman, 1998a, 1998b). All of these investigators recognize the importance of thalamocortical connections and fast activity generated by these connections simultaneously at multiple cortical locations in the maintenance of consciousness. There is also some concensus that attention involves many brain regions, such as the prefrontal cortex, anterior cingulate, and parietal cortex. However, there are differing ideas as to how attention is shifted and how current experience is compared to past experience.

Gray (1995) proposed that a hippocampal *comparator* generates the contents of consciousness—that is, on a moment-to-moment basis, the current state of an organism's perceptual world is compared with a predicted state. However, there are some problems with this model, not the least of which is the fact that patients with damage to the hippocampus have full consciousness, albeit in a somewhat chaotic and altered form (Gray, 2004). Newman and Grace (1999) took a different approach to the problem. They saw the comparative function to be mediated hippocampal inputs to the nucleus accumbens, which in turn influences the nucleus reticularis, a thin shell covering the thalamus, the likely basis of selective awareness. This model has a number of strengths in that it integrates the role of the reticular activating system, known to be involved in sleep-wake cycles. It also integrates known information about gating from the hippocampus, which is important in memory and context. At the same time, it is consistent with the idea that consciousness is based on thalamocorical loops synchronized by fast activity.

The binding problem has some relevance for schizophrenia, as the symptoms of the disorder would seem to involve deficits in the binding of experience. Often schizophrenic patients complain that their thoughts and feelings are controlled by an outside force. Could this phenomenon be related to the dysfunction of regions such as the medial prefrontal cortex known to be activated when self-attributions are made? Patients incorrectly attribute malevolent feelings to others or develop grandiose ideas about their own powers. Could this thought process be related to the dysfunction of brain regions known to process affect, such as the amygdala, anterior cingulate, and ventral prefrontal cortex? Many schizophrenic patients suffer from internal voices tormenting them with comments and commands. Are these comments and commands mislabeled thoughts arising from brain regions involved in speech processing, such as the temporal lobes? It is time to review some of the clues.

3

When Does Schizophrenia Begin?

While the hallucinations, delusions, and other symptoms of schizo-phrenia begin in most patients by the end of adolescence or early adulthood, there is evidence to suggest that the illness actually begins long before this. This chapter will review some of the observations leading us to believe that schizophrenia arises from defects in early brain development in the womb or in later brain development–perhaps involving cortical pruning at adolescence. Some of the ar-guments for an early neurodevelopmental origin will be reviewed, followed by a discussion of likely locations for the defect and some of the possible causes.

Signs Before the Onset of Illness

Physical abnormalities

Minor physical anomalies such as differences in head circumference, an enlarged gap between the first and second toes, or hyperteliorism can suggest a disruption of normal development in early embryonic life. Such anomalies are common in Down syndrome, childhood hy-perkinesias, and autism, but they can also be seen in schizophrenia.

Gualtieri et al. (1982) studied 64 hospitalized, chronic schizo-phrenic patients; 38 alcoholic patients; 50 children with attention-deficit disorder with hyperactivity; 39 children with autism; and healthy volunteers, with a standardized rating scale for minor phys-ical anomalies. Not surprisingly, both the autistic and hyperkinetic children had increased ratings of minor physical anomalies but schizo-phrenic patients had even higher ratings of minor physical anomalies; the alcoholic patients fell within the normal range. Higher scores for minor physical anomalies in schizophrenic patients have been associated with impaired cognitive flexibility, family his-tory of schizophrenia in a first-degree relative, maternal history of obstetric complications, and male gender. However, on the whole, minor physical anomalies appear to be more reliably associated with genetic rather than obstetric factors (O'Callaghan et al., 1991a).

Another physical feature that has received considerable atten-tion in schizophrenia is the study of fingerprints, or dermatoglyph-ics. Although dermatoglyphic patterns are largely genetically deter-mined, in utero viral infections such as rubella and cytomegalovirus in the first 6 months of pregnancy can also alter them. There have been many studies involving more than 4000 schizophrenic patients; the overwhelming majority have shown abnormalities. However, there is not a specific pattern of dermatoglyphic abnormality in schizo-phrenia, nor is this abnormality specific to schizophrenia. Dermato-glyhic abnormalities can be seen in Down syndrome, phenylke-tonuria, Huntington disease, epilepsy, and other disorders (Torrey and Kaufmann, 1986).

Soft neurological signs

Schizophrenic patients often have a number of neurological soft signs as well. Although some of these can be attributed to medica-tion that affects motor function, many of these abnormalities, such as disorders of equilibrium, tremor, and adiadochokinesia, were de-scribed by Kraepelin (1919) long before medications were discov-ered. Soft signs seem to be more common in schizophrenia than in other psychiatric conditions and can be seen before onset of the dis-order and in neuroleptic-naïve patients (Boks et al., 2004; Gupta et al., 1995). Soft signs can be related to genetic and environmental factors, and studies of discordant monozygotic twins suggest that both factors may be important. One such study of monozygotic twins showed that the well twin had neurological impairment intermediate between that of the ill twin and normal comparison twins, and this impairment was related to a history of obstetric complications (Cantor-Graae et al., 1994a). Therefore, neurological signs in schizophrenia may be related to a subtle gene-environment interaction.

Social and intellectual deficits

Abnormalities before the onset of the illness are not limited to appearance and soft neurological signs. Schizophrenic patients often show a variety of social and intellectual deficits in childhood prior to the onset of the disorder. Typically, scholastic test scores are nonsignificantly below average in primary grades but drop significantly between ages 13 and 16, perhaps as a precursor to the cognitive impairment seen early in the illness (Fuller et al., 2002). Other more subtle differences were shown in a study of more than 500 schizophrenic patients and a matched control group who had been assessed by the Israeli Draft Board as adolescents, prior to the patients developing schizophrenia. Interestingly, the strongest predictors for the development of schizophrenia were deficits in social and intellectual functioning and in organizational skills (Davidson et al., 1999a).

One of the more creative approaches to looking at deficits before the onset of psychotic symptoms comes from a study of home movies of patients who later developed schizophrenia. Both graduate students and experienced clinicians were told that they would be viewing home movies of children who later developed schizophrenia, but they were not told how to determine which children would develop schizophrenia. Amazingly, the raters were able to identify the preschizophrenic children fairly accurately on the basis of the perception that these children manifested atypical emotional expressions and movements (Walker and Lewine, 1990).

Thus before the onset of psychotic symptoms, schizophrenic patients show a number of physical, intellectual, and social anomalies from the same characteristics measured in other children. Although both males and females are affected, poor school performance and soft neurological signs have been noted more frequently in males than in females who later develop schizophrenia (Jones et al., 1994). Because males also tend to have more obstetric complications, it is possible that differences may be associated with early hypoxia (Kirov et al., 1996). Other neurodevelopmental anomalies are also possible. Evidence from postmortem studies offers a different perspective on what is going wrong in the brains of these patients.

Evidence from Postmortem Studies

Since Kraepelin's description of "sclerotic nerve-cells" there have been many attempts to define a neuropathology of schizophrenia. Unfortunately, none of the observations proved to be very useful until studies of the hippocampus and entorhinal cortex suggested cytoarchitectural differences consistent with early neurodevelopmental abnormalities (Falkai and Bogerts, 1993). In the hippocampus, generalized atrophy, neuronal loss, reduced neuronal size, and pyramidal cell disarray have been reported (Benes et al., 1991b; Bogerts et al., 1985; Falkai and Bogerts, 1986; Kovelman and Scheibel, 1984), whereas in the entorhinal cortex a loss of normal clustering has been found (Jacob and Beckmann, 1986). Other studies report a reduction of neuron number and volume reductions in the mediodorsal thalamus and nucleus accumbens, but these changes could have occurred after the onset of the illness (Pakkenberg, 1990, 1992; Stevens, 1982).

Several studies have suggested abnormalities in cell migration early in brain development (Falkai and Bogerts, 1993). Cortical cell migration is heavily dependent upon the subplate, particularly for the ingrowth of thalamic neurons. Using a marker for neurons involved in subplate migration, nicotinamide-adenine dinucleotide phosphate-diaphorase, Akbarian et al. (1993a, 1993b) found that these neurons were more deeply distributed in frontal and temporal cortex white matter in schizophrenic patients than in controls. This finding could indicate difficulties with the formation of connections at the subplate that are critical for the development of basal ganglia–thalamocortical neuronal circuits and cortical specificity, as indicated in Chapter 2.

Not necessarily related to cell migration but perhaps in keeping with early neurodevelopmental abnormalities is the finding of decreased inhibitory GABAergic interneurons in the anterior cingulate cortex (Benes et al., 1991a). Other findings point to abnormalities in brain connectivity. In widely cited studies, Selemon et al. (1995, 1998) found elevated neuronal density in the dorsolateral pre-

OXFORD UNIVERSITY PRESS ORDER FORM

CREDIT CARD: ☐ AMEX ☐ VISA ☐ MasterCard

4020 4900 0028 2518

SUZANNE BARBIER   09/08 ✓

Promotion Code: _____ Rep _____ Date _____

☐ Taken
☐ Cash/Check/Travelers Check

☐ Ship
☐ Ship/Bill

Your Address _____
_____
_____

Signature, phone#, and email required

Phone/email _____

Sign here _____

Qty	Author/Editor: Title	ISBN	Price
1	W. Allerman	517-6375-	55.30

Tukan

SPECIAL INSTRUCTIONS

Domestic Orders: Please allow 2-3 weeks for delivery.
International Orders: Please allow 2-4 weeks for delivery. Extra shipping charge applies.
In compliance with state & local laws, sales tax will be applied where applicable, GST tax will be added to Canadian orders.

3

Subtotal _____
Shipping _____
Each add'l book _____
Tax _55.30_
Total _____

CUSTOMER SERVICE
2001 Evans Road
Cary,NC 27513
1-800-451-7556
Fax: (919) 677-1303

NEW YORK OFFICE
198 Madison Avenue
New York, NY 10016
1-212-726-6000

Visit our website at *www.oup.com/us*

Thank You for your order!

frontal cortex (areas 9 and 46) in schizophrenic patients by means of stereological methods. In the 1995 study, 16 brains from patients with schizophrenia were compared with 19 brains from normal subjects, 6 from patients with schizoaffective disorder, and 9 from patients with Huntington disease. Figure 3–1 shows the markedly increased neuronal density in layers III to VI. There is a slight loss of cortical thickness in a schizophrenic patient, in contrast to a more

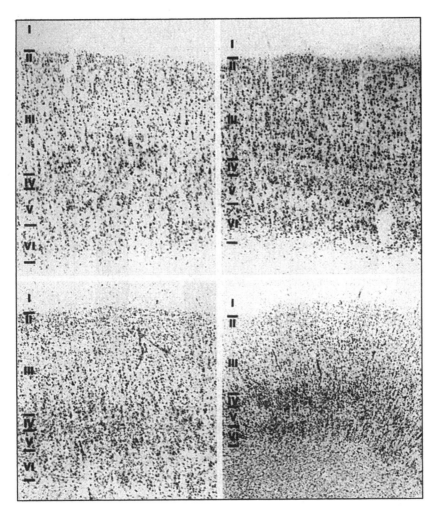

Figure 3–1. Nissl-stained coronal sections of area 9 in normal brain (*top left*), a schizophrenic brain (*top right*), a schizoaffective brain (*bottom left*), and a patient with Huntington disease (*bottom right*). Used with permission, from Selemon et al. (1995).

localized loss in a Huntington patient, leading to markedly increased glial density and drastically reduced cortical thickness. These observations were interpreted as evidence of reduced neuropil in schizophrenia, a phenomenon possibly related to fewer cortical and/or thalamic excitatory inputs to these neurons (Glantz and Lewis, 2000).

The finding of reduced neuropil could also be interpreted to suggest abnormal cortical pruning. Synaptic density reaches a maximum at age 2. From that point until age 16 there is a loss of approximately 50% of mostly corticocortical connections due to normal pruning (Huttenlocher, 1979). A fault in programmed synaptic elimination during adolescence has been suggested to underlie cases of schizophrenia that emerge around this age (Feinberg, 1982/1983). Therefore, neuropathological abnormalities could reflect anomalies in brain development that continue to occur throughout childhood and adolescence.

All of these studies failed to observe gliosis, a finding taken as evidence that schizophrenia must be a neurodevelopmental disorder, since other degenerative conditions such as Alzheimer disease are associated with evidence of active inflammation or repair reflected in gliosis. However, it has been been pointed out that gliosis is not always demonstrable after neural injury, nor is it always associated with apoptosis, a type of programmed cell death that might be related to schizophrenia (Harrison, 1999).

It is necessary to bear in mind that very few postmortem findings have been reliably replicated, for reasons mostly related to the nature of postmortem work. Often, older, medicated patients are studied who may have other diseases. There are also many limitations related to the collection of specimens and the small numbers of patients studied. In fact, the most reliable findings seem to be structural changes, such as enlarged ventricles, decreased cortical and hippocampal volume, and alterations in normal cerebral assymetries. The probable explanation for decreased cortical volume is reduced neuropil rather than a loss of neurons, with the possible exception of thalamic neurons (Harrison, 1999). Whether the loss of neuropil occurs in the womb or during adolescence is unknown, but other postmortem findings would seem to indicate that there must also be some abnormalities in early brain development. We will now look at some of the possible causes of these changes in brain structure and histochemistry.

Possible Causes of Early Neurodevelopmental Abnormalities

If there are early neurodevelopmental anomalies in schizophrenic patients, what could cause them? A few possibilities will be considered: obstetric, viral, nutritional, and genetic.

Obstetric causes

Pasamanick et al. (1956) were the first to suggest a relationship between pregnancy and obstetric complications and schizophrenia. Since their study, there have been dozens of case-control studies of the association between prenatal and perinatal complications and the development of schizophrenia. Although there is still some controversy about selection factors and other biases, the general consensus seems to be that subjects exposed to obstetric complications are twice as likely to develop schizophrenia (Geddes and Lawrie, 1995).

The exact nature of these complications has been difficult to define; nonetheless, three types of complications seem to be more frequent in schizophrenia (Cannon et al., 2002). The first includes complications of pregnancy such as bleeding, diabetes, rhesus incompatibility, and preeclampsia. The second group includes signs of abnormal fetal growth and development such as low birth weight, congenital malformations, and reduced head circumference. The third type includes complications of delivery such as uterine atony, asphyxia, and emergency cesarean section.

Obstetric complications seem to be more common in schizophrenic patients who become ill at an early age, but there is little relationship with a family history of schizophrenia or gender (Verdoux et al., 1997). Pregnancy or delivery complications have been linked to minor physical anomalies (Cantor-Graae et al., 1994b) and structural changes on magnetic resonance imaging (McNeil et al., 2000) in discordant monozygotic twins. However, these anomalies are not necessarily specific to schizophrenia, as several studies have found a link between bipolar disorders and prenatal and perinatal complications (Buka and Fan, 1999). This finding would not be a surprise to Pasamanick (1956) who saw schizophrenia as just one disorder in a spectrum of possible conditions related to obstetrical complications.

Viral infections in the womb

It has long been known that schizophrenic patients are more likely to have been born in the winter months. However, not until Mednick et al. (1988) examined the incidence of schizophrenia in Helsinki, Finland, after the 1957 A2 influenza epidemic was the possibility of an association between this disorder and maternal infections suggested. Individuals who were in their second trimester of fetal development during the epidemic had a much higher risk of developing schizophrenia in later life. A later analysis revealed that this risk was elevated 86.7% by exposure in the second trimester, whereas exposure in the first or third trimesters led to a 20% increased risk (Mednick et al., 1994).

Subsequent studies of the 1957 A2 influenza epidemic and other maternal infections have both replicated and failed to replicate the original findings. Some of these difficulties may be related to a failure to establish whether the mothers actually contracted an infection. A more recent study has collected blood samples from mothers at the end of pregnancy for class-specific immunoglobins and antibodies. The offspring of mothers with elevated levels of total IgG IgM immunoglobins and antibodies to herpes simplex virus type 2 were at increased risk for the development of schizophrenia and other psychotic illnesses (Buka et al., 2001). The mechanism of increased risk is not known, but prenatal exposure to infection could release inflammatory cytokines, which have been shown to significantly reduce dendritic development in animal models (Gilmore et al., 2004).

A further problem with subsequent studies has been whether exposure occurred in the second trimester. When this factor and the effects of seasonal variation (which could be due to other factors) were controlled for, Barr et al. (1990) were able to replicate the earlier findings from Helsinki in a large, well-defined population in Denmark. It is instructive to note, however, that only 4% of the variance is accounted for by the association between influenza and schizophrenia. Clearly, other factors are involved.

Nutritional deficiencies

Another factor that could lead to neurodevelopmental abnormalities in the womb is maternal malnutrition. A unique natural opportunity to study this factor occurred during the course of World War II, when Dutch railroad workers went on strike to aid the Allies. The Nazis retaliated by attempting to starve the inhabitants of Dutch cities. A famine resulted between November 1944 and May 1945. Because the Dutch kept excellent medical records, it was possible to examine the effects of this famine on the subsequent incidence of schizophrenia.

Susser and Lin (1992) found that women, but not men, whose mothers were in the first trimester of pregnancy during the famine had an elevated risk of developing schizophrenia. A subsequent study (Susser et al., 1996), using refined criteria, found an approximately twofold increased risk for schizophrenia in both men and women. Males whose mothers were exposed in the second trimester also had an increased risk of affective disorders (Brown et al., 1995).

Genetic factors

Of all possible etiologies of schizophrenia, there is no doubt that genetic factors are the strongest. Most investigators would estimate heritability to be in the range of 60%–90%, based on overwhelming evidence from family, twin, and adoption studies (Cardno and Gottesman, 2000; Ingraham and Kety, 2000; Kendler et al., 1993). Whereas the risk in the general population is on the order of 1%, the risk in a first-degree relative is 10 times that, and in identical twins the concordance rate is around 50% in most studies. In those patients with a family history of schizophrenia, the age of of onset tends to be earlier (Suvisaari et al., 1998).

With advances in molecular genetic techniques, it has been possible to examine linkage in large-scale studies often involving thousands of patients and their families. Results from these studies make it clear that familial clustering cannot be explained by a major gene or even a few genes; a large number of genes are likely involved. Making the task of finding the gene more difficult is the fact that carriers of genes involved in schizophrenia do not necessarily express the disease but may have abnormal behaviors or psychobiological markers related to schizophrenia, such as abnormal eye tracking. Even clinical subtypes are not necessarily transmitted according to a Mendelian pattern.

Of the 15 published genome scan studies on schizophrenia, only 5 have calculated power to detect differences and only 2 have accounted for heterogeneity (Waterworth et al., 2002). Despite this, there is some replication of linkages at chromosomes 1q, 6, 8, 13, 15, and 22 and some of the linkages are interesting (Owen et al., 2004). For example, a candidate gene that links to 1q21 may modulate dopaminergic neurons in nigrostriatal and mesolimbic pathways (Dror et al., 1999). Linkages on chromosome 15 might be related to a nicotinic receptor involved in gating deficits seen in many schizophrenic patients (Leonard et al., 2002), while linkages on chromosome 22 could be related to catechol-*O*-methyltransferase (COMT), an enzyme that inactivates dopamine (Egan et al., 2001).

It should also be pointed out that there have been many failures to replicate these linkages, which suggests that the genes related to these linkages are associated with risk in only a subgroup of patients. Whether these linkages relate to brain development is unclear. As noted above, there are some familial correlates of minor physical abnormalities and soft neurological signs. There are a few unconfirmed reports of abnormalities in neurodevelopmental gene expression in postmortem samples from schizophrenic patients (Arnold and Rioux, 2001; Guidotti et al., 2000). Abnormalities in genes involved in neurodevelopment and glutamatergic transmission are beginning to emerge in some population-based studies, but none seem to account for a large amount of the variance, nor are they necessarily specific to schizophrenia (Harrison and Owen, 2003; Harrison and Weinberger, 2005; Perlman et al., 2004).

Neurodevelopmental Models

The widespread nature of postmortem findings, nonspecific premorbid social and intellectual deficits, and lack of a major gene for schizophrenia do not offer many clues as to where the brain may be damaged early in schizophrenia. One of the ways to understand and determine the parts of the brain that could be involved in schizophrenia is to examine the delayed effects of early lesions in animals. As far as we know, animals do not develop auditory hallucinations or paranoid delusions, but they do show some findings associated with schizophrenia. The best known is the early ventral hippocampal lesion model, although this is by no means the only lesion that leads to delayed effects that resemble schizophrenia. Early subplate lesions and even generalized lesions with hypoxia, stress, and drugs that prevent cell division can have similar effects in animals if the damage occurs at critical points of development. Some of these studies warrant a closer look.

Ventral hippocampal lesions

Lipska et al. (1992, 1993) studied the effects of neonatal excitotoxic ventral hippocampal damage on behavior related to dopaminergic transmission in rats. Lesioned animals appeared normal until maturity, when they manifested hyperresponsivity to apomorphine, compared to sham rats. The results were interpreted as neonatal excitotoxic hippocampal lesions causing enhanced dopaminergic sensitivity in the nucleus accumbens by the effects of these lesions on the medial prefrontal cortex. This is not unlike the mesolimbic dopaminergic hyperresponsivity found in schizophrenic patients, as we will see in the next chapter.

Rats with neonatal ventral hippocampal lesions show a number of other characteristics in common with schizophrenic patients. For example, changes were found in postpubertal prepulse inhibition of startle in rats with ventral hippocampal lesions (Lipska et al., 1995). Rats with early ventral hippocampal lesions have shown a delayed, attenuated c-fos response to amphetamine in several cortical and subcortical regions, indicating an effect on dopamine signal transduction as well (Lillrank et al., 1996). These effects can to some extent be attenuated by neuroleptic medication (Lipska, 2004).

Subplate lesions

Neonatal rats with lesions to the subplate show many of the same delayed behavioral abnormalities. Rajakumar et al. (2004) showed that rats with subplate lesions induced by subplate injections of p75 antibody in the first few days of life (equivalent to second-trimester pregnancy in humans) showed significantly increased amphetamine-induced locomotion and rearing and impairment of prepulse inhibition of acoustic startle at 10 weeks but not at 5 weeks. A related study using subplate lesions induced by brain-derived neurotrphic factor demonstrated similar dopaminergic hyperresponsivity that could be reversed by antipsychotic medication. Postmortem examination showed that these animals had GABAergic abnormalities like those of schizophrenic patients. Furthermore, neuronal number did not change in the prefrontal cortex but was reduced in the thalamus, as in schizophrenic patients (Rajakumar and Rajakumar, 2003).

Hypoxia and stress

While both of these models provide very specific targeted lesions leading to the development of dopaminergic hyperresponsivity at maturity, it is also possible to create dopaminergic hyperresponsivity with perinatal hypoxia and prenatal stress in animals (Boksa and El-Khodor, 2003; Brake et al., 1997; Henry et al., 1995). For example, cesarean-sectioned male rats develop a number of signs of increased dopaminergic activity. When under stress as adults, they develop dopaminergic hyperresponsivity not unlike that seen with the hippocampal- and subplate-lesioned rats. For some reason, female rats seem to be less vulnerable to this. The regions damaged by these models are widespread but likely involve many parts of the limbic system, including the hippocampus.

Effects of methylazoxymethanol acetate

Methylazoxymethanol acetate (MAM) is an antimitotic compound that prevents cell division. If given at gestation day 17, it has been shown to disrupt the development of corticolimbic pathways including the hippocampus, enthorinal cortex, and thalamus. Rats exposed to MAM at gestational day 17 are hyperresponsive to mild stress and amphetamine (Flagstad et al., 2004). The effect on dopamine appears to be greater in the nucleus accumbens than in the medial prefrontal cortex. Animals were also observed to engage in less frequent social interaction than controls, a finding suggesting that the behavioral changes associated with MAM may mimic both positive and negative symptoms.

The Case for an Early Insult in Schizophrenia

According to the studies discussed above, hippocampal, subplate, and a variety of perinatal insults early in brain development can lead to behavioral and postmortem changes similar to those seen in schizophrenic patients. It is noteworthy that both the hippocampus and subplate are vulnerable to early insults. The hippocampus is particularly vulnerable to hypoxia, which could be associated with prenatal and obstetric complications. As we saw in Chapter 2, the subplate plays a very important role in the development of cortical specificity. There is reason to believe that a large number of genes are involved in activating and deactivating neuronal function at critical times during cortical development (Rubenstein and Rakic, 1999). It is also worth remembering that genes continue to regulate cortical development until well into adolescence. An anomaly in any of these genes could disrupt necessary connections between brain regions leading to the later development of schizophrenia. Many of these connections are glutamatergic and dopaminergic. The next chapter will examine the role of these and other neurotransmitters.

4

Clues from Drugs That Affect Dopamine, Glutamate, and Other Neurotransmitters

Although it is difficult to imagine a time when dopamine was not associated with schizophrenia, our understanding of dopamine's role in the disorder is relatively new. Most of the fundamental work on the metabolism of norepinephrine and dopamine was done in the 1950s. About this time, the first amino acid neurotransmitter, GABA, was discovered, followed by glutamate. But it was not until 1976 that it was demonstrated that the relative potencies antipsychotic medication were directly related to their ability to block dopamine receptors (Snyder, 2002).

The dopamine hypothesis of schizophrenia arose not only from the effects of conventional antipsychotic medications on dopamine receptors (Carlsson, 1988; Seeman, 1987) but also from the tendency of dopamine agonists to lead to hallucinations and delusions that looked a lot like schizophrenia. Unfortunately, the story was not so simple because it was soon recognized that clozapine was effective despite low dopamine receptor occupancy. This raised the possibility that other transmitters could be involved.

Probably the strongest case for the involvement of other neurotransmitters in schizophrenia can be made for glutamate. Drugs that block N-methyl-D-aspartate (NMDA) glutamate receptors cause not only positive symptoms such as paranoia and thought disorder but also many negative symptoms, such as amotivation and blunted affect and inattention, when given to normal volunteers and schizophrenic patients (Krystal et al., 1994; Lahti et al., 1995b). However, a case can be made for the involvement of serotonin by virtue of its effects on dopaminergic neurotransmission and the fact that many new atypical antipsychotic agents affect serotonin. The importance of GABA is highlighted by postmortem studies and its effect on glutamatergic neurotransmission. This chapter will examine some of this evidence.

Dopamine

Dopamine pathways

Dopamine is an important modulating neurotransmitter in the brain. There are three main pathways in the brain. The first arises from the ventral tegmental area of the brain stem (A10) and projects to the nucleus accumbens in the ventral striatum, the medial prefrontal cortex, and several other parts of the mesolimbic system. Because of the involvement of limbic structures, this pathway is probably the most relevant to schizophrenia. The second pathway arises in the substantia nigra (A9) and projects to the dorsal striatum. This pathway is primarily involved in movement. A third tuberoinfundibular pathway runs from the hypothalamus to the pituitary gland, suggesting an endocrine role. However, more recent work has suggested that this classical view may not be entirely accurate. The dorsal regions of the prefrontal cortex in primates appear to receive dopamine projections originating in not just the brain stem but in the substantia nigra as well (Williams and Goldman-Rakic, 1998).

There are several types of dopamine receptors, falling into two families: D_1 like (D_1 and D_5) and D_2 like (D_2, D_3, and D_4). D_1 receptors tend to be distributed more to cortical regions while D_2 receptors are primarily subcortical. Antipsychotic medications are thought to act mostly on the D_2 receptor type in the A10 pathway (Jones and Pilowski, 2002). It is of note that dopamine regulates many of the basal ganglia–thalamacortical pathways involved in affect and in learning new behaviors, discussed in Chapter 2.

Dopamine release in the nucleus accumbens has both a tonic and a phasic component that is controlled in large part by glutamatergic projections from the hippocampus and amygdala (Grace, 1991; Moore et al., 1999). However, regulation of dopamine release is complex. Glutamatergic projections from the prefrontal cortex influence dopamine release in the nucleus accumbens as well. This effect is likely mediated by metabotropic glutamate receptors (Taber and Fibiger, 1995; Verma and Moghaddam, 1998).

Abnormalities in schizophrenia

While the correlation between D_2 receptor occupancy and neuroleptic clinical potency provides strong evidence for the involvement of dopamine in schizophrenia, it has been very difficult to demonstrate abnormalities in the dopamine receptor in postmortem and in vivo studies. The original dopamine theory of schizophrenia suggested that hyperactivity of dopamine transmission was responsible for the symptoms of the disorder. With the work of Pycock et al. (1980), which demonstrated that destruction of frontal cortical dopamine afferents in rats lead to up-regulation of subcortical dopamine transmission, some modifications to the dopamine hypothesis were made. Weinberger (1987) suggested that a developmental-specific dysfunction of dopaminergic innervation to the prefrontal cortex could lead to enhanced subcortical dopamine tone.

Although Pycock's work was not completely replicated (Deutch, 1993), some aspects of the theory have remained. The first is that decreased dopamine in the prefrontal cortex is the basis of negative symptoms whereas positive symptoms are related to increased subcortical dopamine activity (Davis et al., 1991; Swerdlow and Koop, 1987; Weinberger 1987). Grace (1993) supported the suggestion that low levels of dopamine cause negative symptoms but argued that these low levels lead to excessive phasic or burst firing of dopaminergic neurons, which results in positive symptoms. What is the evidence for these assertions?

Postmortem studies. Most D_1 postmortem studies in schizophrenia have not shown differences from controls. In contrast, the majority of postmortem investigations have demonstrated striatal increases in D_2 receptors in chronic patients (Soares and Innes, 1999). However, the issue of effects of medication invariably arises, as treatment with neuroleptic medication is usually associated with a compensatory increase in the number of receptors. Some deficits in dopaminergic innervation of the prefrontal cortex have been reported but suffer from the same limitation with regard to the effects of medication (Akil et al., 1999).

Genetic linkage. Early studies failed to find direct links to D_2 receptor abnormalities but other genes associated with schizophrenia have shown some promise. A candidate gene that links to 1q21 is a potassium channel gene that may modulate dopaminergic neurons in nigrostriatal and mesolimbic pathways (Dror et al., 1999). Linkages related to catechol-O-methyltransferase (COMT), an enzyme that inactivates dopamine, have also been found on chromosome 22 in schizophrenic pedigrees (Egan et al., 2001).

Positron emission tomography and single photon emission computed tomography studies. One of the ways around the problem of medication was to study untreated patients in vivo with either positron emission tomography (PET) or single-photon emission computed tomography (SPECT). Through these techniques, a radioactive label is attached to a drug that binds to a dopamine receptor. Density of receptors can be estimated by measuring the resulting ionizing radiation emitted around the head by a ring of detectors.

Early PET studies showing decreases in D_1 receptor availability have not been replicated (Karlsson et al., 2002). In fact, increased binding of D_1 receptors in the dorsolateral prefrontal cortex has been found with a more sensitive ligand (Abi-Dargham et al., 2002). This may not necessarily indicate decreased stimulation, as chronic dopamine depletion could be associated with up-regulation. So the in vivo evidence for decreased D_1 receptor availability in schizophrenia is not yet clear.

The evidence for increased D_2 receptor binding in the striatum is much stronger. However, early PET studies found conflicting results. Investigations using ^{11}C raclopride showed an increase in D_2 receptors in these patients, but other investigators, using somewhat different techniques, did not (Farde et al., 1990; Martinot et al., 1990; Pilowsky et al., 1994). Two meta-analyses of postmortem and brain imaging studies found evidence for increased D_2 density in the striatum but there was considerable overlap with healthy subjects (Laruelle, 1998; Zakzanis and Hansen, 1998).

Recent PET studies have examined presynaptic dopamine activity. McGowan et al. (2004) found increased ^{18}F fluorodopa uptake in the ventral striatum of medicated chronic schizophrenic patients. Because ^{18}F fluorodopa is taken up in presynaptic monoaminergic neurons and metabolized to dopamine, increased uptake was interpreted to suggest increased dopaminergic activity in the ventral striatum, which had been found in five of seven previous studies using comparable methods (Dao-Castellana et al., 1997; Elkashef et al., 2000; Hietala et al., 1995, 1999; Lindström et al., 1999; Meyer-Lindenberg et al., 2002; Reith et al., 1994). Other studies with dopamine transporter ligands have not revealed overall differences in the striatum but have found a lack of asymmetry in schizophrenic patients (Hsiao et al., 2003; Laasko et al., 2000). As might be expected, subchronic haloperidol has been found to down-regulate dopamine synthesis in a PET study of schizophrenic patients (Gründer et al., 2003b).

McGowen et al. (2004) used a second-generation, highly sensitive PET camera that allowed them to look at prefrontal dopaminergic activity. Surprisingly, they did not find the predicted decrease in cortical dopamine activity that would be expected from the revised dopamine hypothesis. More revealing is the dopamine response to pharmacological stimulation. When schizophrenic patients were given amphetamine, the occupancy of striatal dopamine receptors was twice the level of normal subjects (Abi-Dargham et al., 1998; Laruelle et al., 1996). Similar findings were seen by another group using a different technique (Breier et al., 1997b). These studies suggest that the problem with dopamine in schizophrenia may be one of regulation. However, even in these studies, only about a third of patients showed abnormalities, a finding suggesting that dopamine cannot be the whole story in schizophrenia.

Animal models

Dopamine-releasing drugs such as amphetamines or dopamine receptor–stimulating drugs such as apomorhine when given chronically lead to some behaviors in animals related to schizophrenia (Robinson and Becker, 1986). Even a single exposure to amphetamines can lead to lasting changes in behavior and sensitization (Vanderschuren et al., 1999). Changes in sensorimotor gating and prepulse inhibition seen in many schizophrenic patients (discussed in the next chapter) are also seen in these animals (Swerdlow et al., 2000; Tenn et al., 2003). Most of these effects are reversed by antipsychotic drugs.

Behavioral correlates

Stress increases the release and turnover of dopamine, which may account for the frequent relapse of patients under stress (Deutch, 1993; Moghaddam, 2002). Dopamine is also essential for good performance on cognitive tasks. As we shall see in Chapter 6, schizophrenic patients have difficulty with a wide variety of cognitive tasks. Some of these difficulties may relate to attention, which is affected by dopamine release (Servan-Shreiber et al., 1998), whereas others relate to memory and executive problems.

D_1 receptors play an important role in working memory. Chronic blockade of dopamine receptors by antipsychotic drugs down-regulates D_1 receptors in the prefrontal cortex, resulting in working-memory impairments. These deficits were reversed in monkeys by short-term administration of a D_1 agonist (Castner et al., 2000). Therefore working-memory deficißts in schizophrenic patients could be related to D_1 receptor anomalies.

Glutamate

Glutamate pathways

Glutamate is found almost everywhere in the brain, but there are two pathways of particular relevance to schizophrenia. One is the ascending pathway arising from the hippocampus and extending to the basal ganglia and cingulate cortex. The other is a descending pathway from the neocortex down to the ventral and dorsal striatum (Greenamyre and Porter, 1994). It is of note that glutamate is the principal neurotransmitter involved in the cortical–subcortical connections of the basal ganglia–thalamocortical neuronal circuits involved in learning new behavior and integrating affect into behavior, described in Chapter 2. Glutamate has been implicated in brain growth and development and memory, and plays a role in neuroplasticity (Konradi and Heckers, 2003). There is also evidence to indicate that glutamate plays a role in neurotoxicity associated with hypoxic injury and apoptosis, in which cells are pruned during normal development without gliotic changes (Goff and Wine, 1997).

There are several types of glutamate receptors (Nakanishi, 1992). Three are ionotropic, which means that they open calcium channels. The most common of these is the mino-3-hydroxy-5-methyl-4-isoxazole-propionic acid (AMPA) receptor. Overactivity of AMPA and another ionotropic receptor, kainite, can lead to excitotoxic cell injury. NMDA receptors are also ionotropic and are concentrated in the hippocampus, anterior cingulate, and other parts of the limbic system. These receptors are blocked by phencyclidine (PCP) and ketamine, leading to both positive and negative symptoms in schizophrenic patients and normal controls (Tamminga, 1999). In addition to the ionotropic glutamate receptors, there are the metabotropic receptors, eight of which have been cloned. These receptors act via phospholipase C or by inhibiting adenyl cyclase (Tsai and Coyle, 2002).

As indicated in the previous section, glutamatergic projections from the hippocampus (and probably amygdala) play an important role in regulating dopamine in the nucleus accumbens—the target of A10 dopaminergic neurons, which are hyperpolarized by antipsychotic drugs (Moore et al., 1999). Glutamatergic neurons in the prefrontal cortex also regulate A10 dopaminergic neurons via projections to the ventral tegmentum (Taber and Fibiger, 1995).

Abnormalities in schizophrenia

Postmortem studies. Postmortem investigations in schizophrenia have produced seemingly contradictory findings (Krystal et al., 2000). Studies of the prefrontal region in schizophrenia have shown some evidence of an excess of glutamatergic receptors and uptake sites (Deakin et al., 1989; Ishimaru et al., 1994; Toru et al., 1988). However, a decrease in aspartate and glutamate and an increase in *N*-acetylaspartateglutamate, a neuropeptide concentrated in glutamatergic neurons, has also been reported (Tsai et al., 1995). The enzyme that breaks down *N*-acetylaspartateglutamate was also decreased so the results were interpreted to suggest glutamatergic hypofunction. Increased glutamate-immunoreactive axons have been found in the cingulate cortex of schizophrenic patients (Benes et al., 1992a). The finding of normal AMPA receptors (Healy et al., 1998; Longson et al., 1994) would argue against an increase in the number of glutamatergic synapses in this region.

A more consistent pattern emerges in temporal regions. Several studies have shown that the AMPA receptor is abnormally decreased in expression in the hippocampus. Subunit transcripts, protein levels, and binding sites all seem to be involved (Meador-Woodruff and Healy, 2000). Similar decreases can also be seen in the hippocampus in kainate receptor expression (Meador-Woodruff and Healey, 2000). The NMDA receptor studies have been inconsistent in their findings in this region, but a recent examination of subunit expression suggests that NR1 subunit of the NMDA receptor may be deficient in some schizophrenic patients (Gao et al., 2000).

The postmortem studies would seem to suggest that there are glutamatergic abnormalities in schizophrenia, but paradoxically both increases and decreases can be seen. Most of the evidence for increased glutamatergic receptors comes from the anterior cingulate and prefrontal/orbitofrontal regions, whereas deficits are seen in most glutamergic receptor types in hippocampal and temporal regions. This pattern would seem to argue against a generalized loss of glutamatergic synapses but could be in keeping with abnormal glutamatergic activity and/or a loss of synapses in specific neuronal circuits.

Genetic linkage. Genetic linkage studies have identified a number of candidate susceptibility genes for schizophrenia related to glutamate (Harrison and Owen, 2003; Moghaddam, 2003; Perlman et al., 2004). These include neuregulin, which regulates the expression of glutamate receptor subunits (Stefansson et al., 2002); RGS4 proteins, which inhibit metabotropic receptor signaling (Chowdari et al., 2002); dysbindin, which affects NMDA receptor activity (Straub et al., 2002); and a calcineurin subunit gene, which is involved in NMDA-mediated plasticity (Gerber et al., 2003). Most of these findings are not always specific to schizophrenia and have yet to be replicated, but they do point toward the importance of genes involved in glutamatergic neurotransmission in the genesis of schizophrenia.

Animal models

A few hours after mature (but not immature) rats are given an acute low dose of PCP, they begin to show a vacuole reaction in the posterior cingulate and retrosplenial cortex, followed by a heat shock protein reaction at 24 hours. At higher doses, a neuron-necrotizing reaction can be seen that spreads to other parts of the limbic system including the anterior cingulate, parietal, temporal, piriform, and entorhinal cortices, hippocampus, amygdala, and taenia tecta (Olney and Farber, 1995). Figure 4–1 shows some of these changes brought about by PCP in rat brains.

Because PCP blocks NMDA receptors, this kind of reaction might be difficult to understand. However, glutamatergic neurons

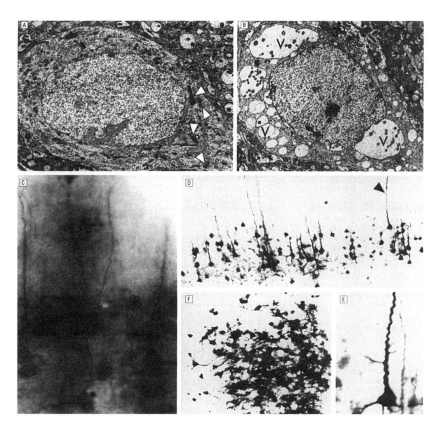

Figure 4–1. Electron micrograph of a normal pyramidal posterior cingulate cortical neuron with many normal-appearing mitochondria (arrowheads) (*A*), and after treatment with 5 mg/kg phencyclidine (PCP) 4 hours earlier leading to vacuoles (V; *B*). Pyramidal posterior cingulate neurons show heat shock protein with immunocytochemical labeling 24 hours after injection of an NMDA antagonist, MK-801 (*C*), and PCP (*D*). A magnified view of an injured neuron (see arrowhead in D) shows a corkscrew appearance suggesting cytoskeletal changes (*E*). A large cluster of injured neurons in the rat amygdala shows expression of heat shock protein 24 hours after injection with PCP (*F*). Used with permission, from Olney and Farber (1995).

likely maintain tonic inhibitory control over several pathways that converge on the posterior cingulate by their stimulation of inhibitory GABAergic neurons. When this stimulation is blocked, there is a paradoxical increase in activity in excitatory pathways, leading to the neuronal damage (Olney and Farber, 1995). Curiously, similar neurodegeneration is seen after intracerebroventricular kainic acid administration in rats (Csernansky et al., 1998). The effects of NMDA receptor antagonists can be blocked to some extent by pretreatment with some antipsychotic drugs, particularly clozapine, group II metabotropic agonists, and topiramate, which potentiate GABA and antagonize AMPA and kainate receptors (Deutsch et al., 2002; Farber et al., 1993; Moghaddam and Adams, 1998).

Acute administration of PCP or ketamine profoundly increases forebrain dopamine transmission, which might explain why some antipsychotic drugs can attenuate the effects of PCP on rats (Jentsch and Roth, 1999). However, chronic lower doses of PCP tend to decrease frontal dopamine transmission. Furthermore, subchronic treatment with PCP leads to increased responsivity in the mesolimbic dopamine pathway to D-amphetamine or mild stress, much like the PET findings in schizophrenic patients (Jentsch et al., 1998). Similar modulation of amphetamine-induced striatal dopamine release was reported with ketamine on PET (Kegeles et al., 2000a). Thus changes in glutamatergic activity are closely linked to dopamine transmission.

Behavioral correlates

NMDA receptor antagonists such as ketamine are capable of inducing the many cognitive deficits found in some schizophrenic patients. Neuropsychological abnormalities will be discussed in more detail in Chapter 6, but it is worth noting here that when given ketamine, healthy volunteers show deficits similar to those of schizophrenic patients on continuous-performance tasks (Umbricht et al., 2000). Long-term PCP administration in rats has been shown to lead to deficits in frontal function on tasks such as the delayed-response task, as seen in some schizophrenic patients. Single-dose PCP has also been shown to disrupt prepulse inhibition in rats, an effect similar to startle-gating deficits seen in schizophrenic patients (Jentsch and Roth, 1999). However, low-dose ketamine actually increases prepulse inhibition in healthy volunteers, so some of the animal studies may not be generalized to schizophrenic patients (Abel et al., 2003).

The effects of NMDA deficiency on frontal lobe function are complex. Two distinct mechanisms have been identified in rats: an increase in disorganized spike activity, which may enhance cortical noise, and a decrease in burst activity, which reduces transmission of cortical neurons (Jackson et al., 2004). It is not possible to assess glutamatergic receptors directly with PET in humans. Labels that are antagonists could cause psychosis whereas agonists are at risk of causing excitotoxic damage. However, there have been some small studies of the effects of ketamine on metabolic activity and blood flow, using PET in normal volunteers and schizophrenic patients. In normal individuals, ketamine leads to increased cerebral blood flow and metabolic activity in anterior cingulate and medial prefrontal regions, which correlates with the development of psychotic symptom formation in these subjects (Breier et al., 1997a; Holcomb et al., 2001; Vollenweider et al., 1997). In schizophrenic patients, cerebral blood flow was observed to increase in the anterior cingulate cortex and decrease in the hippocampus and primary visual cortex (Color Plate 4–1). The five medicated schizophrenic patients in this study developed not only psychotic symptoms with the ketamine but also the same individual pattern of symptoms that they had previously displayed (Lahti et al., 1995a).

Whereas the stress response involves activation of the hypothalamic–pituitary–adrenal (HPA) axis and dopamine neurotransmission, there is increasing evidence that this response may be modulated, and in some cases modulated by glutamate neurotransmission in the prefrontal cortex (Moghaddam, 2002). The initial response likely is mediated by a rapid efflux of glutamate in forebrain regions leading to increased dopamine release, which sustains immediate decision-making and goal-directed behaviors relevant to the stress. The longer-term adaptation to stress involves the HPA axis and continued release of glutamate and monoamines such as dopamine in limbic regions, including the hippocampus. Interestingly, stress can lead to a reversible loss of neuropil in the hippocampus that is sensitive to NMDA receptor agonists and not associated with gliosis (McEwen, 1999).

Other Neurotransmitters

Serotonin

The possible role of serotonin in schizophrenia has already been suggested by the effects of atypical neuroleptics on serotonin 5-HT$_{2A}$ receptors. Although this has been eclipsed to some extent by receptor dissociation rate theories, there are other reasons to believe that serotonin could be involved in schizophrenia. Serotonin modulates dopamine neurotransmission in several regions relevant to schizophrenia—the prefrontal cortex, the striatum, including the nucleus accumbens, and the ventral tegmentum (Kapur and Remington, 1996).

Seven of 11 postmortem studies reviewed by Soares and Innes (1999) found decreased 5-HT$_{2A/C}$ levels, particularly in cortical regions. However, two PET studies using ^{18}F-setoperone did not find any differences between schizophrenic patients and controls (Lewis et al., 1998; Trichard et al., 1998). Several postmortem studies have shown 5-HT$_{1A}$ receptors in prefrontal and some limbic regions in chronic schizophrenic patients (Burnett et al., 1996; Hashimoto et al., 1991; Joyce et al., 1993; Simpson et al., 1996). Earlier efforts to use PET to study serotonin receptors in schizophrenic patients were hampered by the fact that 5-HT$_{1A}$ receptors could be studied only in their high-affinity state. In a recent investigation (Tauscher et al., 2002), using this newer methodology, 5-HT$_{1A}$ receptor binding in drug-naïve patients was found to be increased in the medial temporal cortex bilaterally but not in the prefrontal regions, as suggested by the postmortem studies.

γ-aminobutyric acid

There has been increasing interest in the role of GABA in schizophrenia (Wassef et al., 2003). Probably the most convincing evidence comes from postmortem studies showing a deficit in small interneurons (which are GABAergic) in the prefrontal and cingulate cortices of schizophrenic patients (Benes et al., 1991a). In addition to these GABAergic interneurons in the cortex, glutamatergic neurons synapse on subcortical GABAergic neurons, which in turn synapse on neurons in the thalamus projecting back to the cortex. A deficit in these GABAergic neurons could result in a similar pattern of overactivity in limbic regions to the effects of NMDA antagonists, because NMDA potentiates activity in GABAergic neurons (Olney and Farber, 1995).

The synthesizing enzyme for GABA, glutamate decarboxylase (GAD), has been measured in a number of postmortem studies of schizophrenic patients. Messenger RNA expression of GAD was found to be decreased in the prefrontal region in two studies (Akbarian et al., 1995; Volk et al., 2000). However, another study found increased prefrontal GAD activity using a different methodology (Gluck et al., 2002), thus it is difficult to draw any conclusions from these studies. In vivo SPECT imaging studies using ^{123}I-iomazenil failed to find any differences in GABA activity between schizophrenic patients and controls (Abi-Dargham et al., 1995; Busatto et al., 1997).

Neurotransmitter Involvement in Schizophrenia

The balance of the evidence would seem to implicate GABA and serotonin in schizophrenia, but the case is not nearly as compelling as that for dopamine and glutamate. There is very good in vivo evidence for dopaminergic hyperresponsivity in schizophrenic patients, and thus far all of our antipsychotic drugs seem to act on D_2 receptors. The involvement of glutamate seems likely from postmortem studies. However, both an increase in the anterior cingulate and a decrease in the hippocampus in glutamatergic activity have been suggested. Animal models have shown that it is possible to have both an increase and a decrease in glutamergic activity, as drugs that block NMDA receptors can lead to a paradoxical increase in activity throughout the limbic system by virtue of their regulation of inhibitory GABAergic neurons.

Animal studies point out a close connection between glutamate and dopamine, for chronic administration of NMDA blockers can lead to dopaminergic hyperresponsivity. It is possible that a similar deficit in glutamatergic activity caused by genetic, hypoxic, or neurodevelopmental factors could lead to dopaminergic hyperresponsivity in schizophrenia. All of this may point to a very vulnerable brain in schizophrenia that tends to overreact to stress. But what are the other psychophysiological consequences of this vulnerability? The next chapter will examine some of the data relevant to addressing this question.

5

Some Clues from Psychophysiology

In the age of brain imaging, we sometimes forget the insights of investigators who carefully applied the technology of their day. Not long after Kraepelin described dementia praecox, Diefendorf and Dodge (1908) described eye movement abnormalities in these patients. This chapter will look at some findings from studies of eye movements, as well as studies of olfaction, electroencephalography (EEG), and event-related potentials (ERP). More recent innovations such as magnetoencephalography (MEG) will also be considered in this section because of the similarities to EEG.

Eye Movement Abnormalities in Schizophrenia

The observations of Diefendorf and Dodge (1908) were largely forgotten until they were rediscovered by Holzman et al. in 1973. What these investigators noticed was that when schizophrenic patients were asked to follow a target with their eyes, they were not able to do so in a smooth and efficient way (see Fig. 5–1). The finding was robust in that all eight nonparanoid, 6 of 10 paranoid schizophrenic patients, and 2 of 3 schizoaffective patients showed abnormal tracking whereas only 1 of 4 manic-depressive patients and 4 of 33 normal

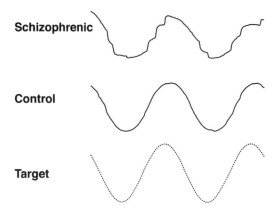

Figure 5–1. Illustrative tracings of smooth-pursuit eye movements of a schizophrenic patient (*top panel*) and a normal control (*middle panel*), following a 0.4 Hz sine wave target (*bottom panel,* dotted line). Used with permission, from Holzman (2000).

controls had an abnormal pattern. Subsequent studies have shown that schizophrenic patients typically fall behind the target (low gain), leading to increased saccades in an effort to catch up (Levy et al., 1994).

Eye-tracking abnormalities have been observed in schizophrenic patients on and off medication in numerous studies. However, eye-tracking abnormalities can also be seen in relatives of schizophrenic patients. In fact, about 45% of clinically well first-degree relatives have eye-tracking deficits (Levy et al., 1994). Thus, eye-tracking deficits are not necessarily markers for the development of schizophrenia, but they do represent the expression of a latent genetic trait leading to both schizophrenia and eye-tracking abnormalities (Holzman, 1996). There has been some debate as to whether eye-tracking abnormalities are specific to schizophrenia. Diefendorf and Dodge (1908) thought they differed from manic-depressive patients, but more recent work has shown some abnormalities in other psychiatric conditions (Levy et al., 1994).

Some investigators have suggested that patients with eye-movement abnormalities also have difficulties on frontal lobe tests (Litman et al., 1991) such as the Wisconsin Card Sorting Test (WCST), but pursuit abnormalities do not have any clear symptom correlates, with the possible exception of schizotypal symptoms in relatives. It is of interest that ketamine can produce similar eye-tracking abnormalities in healthy volunteers (Avila et al., 2002). Eye movements are controlled by one of the five basal ganglia–thalamocortical loops involved in learning new behaviors. The cerebellum may also play a role in coordinating movements.

Electrodermal Responses

Skin conductance is measured by passing a small, constant voltage across electrodes on the palmar surfaces of hands or fingers. An *orienting response* can be elicited by novel stimuli. If the same stimulus is repeatedly given, habituation tends to occur. Approximately 40%–60% of chronic schizophrenic patients fail to exhibit orienting responses, compared to 5%–10% of controls (Zahn et al., 1991). Subsequent work revealed that there was a lateralized response in some patients. A greater left than right asymmetry in orienting response was seen in patients with behavioral overactivity, pressure of speech, and manic grandiose and paranoid ideas. Patients with social and emotional withdrawl, blunted affect, poverty of speech, and motor retardation had greater right than left asymmetry in orienting response (Gruzelier, 1999). These observations led Gruzelier and others to propose that neuropsychophysiological asymmetry may be central to schizophrenia, a thought that we will return to in later chapters.

Olfactory Deficits

As noted in Chapter 2, olfaction is one of the more primitive senses that is not directly routed through the thalamus but involves structures such as the olfactory bulb, entorhinal cortex, amygdala, and mediofrontal cortex. Hurwitz et al. (1988) reported that chronic, medicated schizophrenic patients had olfactory deficits on a standardized test. Subsequent investigations have confirmed these findings, particularly in males, regardless of medication status (Moberg et al. 1999).

Olfactory deficits have been associated with impaired memory performance (Good et al., 2002). Interestingly, nonverbal memory impairment was found in patients with left and right microsmia but patients with verbal memory deficits had left nostril microsmia. Relatives of schizophrenic patients have been shown to have some olfactory impairment, but olfactory deficits do not appear to be specific to schizophrenia. Similar deficits have been observed in first-episode affective psychoses (Brewer et al., 2001) and a number of other conditions including Korsakoff syndrome, multiple sclerosis, and Alzheimer disease.

Electroencephalographic Studies

A psychiatrist, Hans Berger, was the first to show that an EEG could be recorded from the human head (Berger, 1929). The rhythms recorded reflect thalamocortical activity. The repetitive alpha frequency (8–12 Hz) seen in resting waking states is dependent upon a pacemaker in the reticular thalamic nucleus. Sensory information is transferred to the cortex from thalamic neurons during burst firing. Faster waves are associated with the waking state and may reflect sensory or remembered conscious experience, which is bound by 40 Hz oscillations (Llinas and Pare, 1991). Other repetitive patterns of firing are associated with slower waves (<8 Hz) seen in sleep (Steriade et al., 1990).

Some fascinating EEG studies have been done with implanted electrodes in patients with chronic schizophrenia (Hanley et al., 1972; Heath, 1954). Spike activity was recorded from the septal area at the base of the brain, which likely included the head of the caudate, lateral septal nuclei, nucleus accumbens, and olfactory tubercle. While these patients did not have epilepsy, the spikes suggested partial denervation from other structures (Stevens, 1973).

Some of the original surface EEG reports in schizophrenic patients described little alpha activity, with disorganized, very fast, random frequency described as "choppy." Other investigators noted a high incidence of sharp waves suggestive of epilepsy, reduced reactivity to external stimuli, and frontal slowing. More recent quantitative studies have confirmed frontal slowing and have also indicated posterior fast activity. However, these findings are not specific to schizophrenia, nor are they uniform across patients (Shagass, 1991).

With quantitative, computerized EEG, it is possible to assess coherence between brain regions. Coherence generally increases between regions involved in a task. For example, it has been shown that coherence increases in the right hemisphere when subjects are asked to do spatial tasks involving these regions. When schizophrenic patients are asked to do continuous calculation tasks like those used by Kraepelin, an interesting pattern of coherence emerges. Patients showed much less frontal and temporal coherence than matched controls, a result indicating that they may not be able to focally activate brain regions necessary for the task. However, they had no difficulty activating right posterior regions during spatial tasks. Medication tended to normalize but not completely alleviate the deficit that, on discriminant analysis, was found to correctly classify 81.4% of the subjects (Morrison-Stewart et al., 1991). As with many other physiological markers, EEG coherence abnormalities have been reported in most but not all studies of schizophrenic patients and their family members (Mann et al., 1997; Winterer et al., 2001, 2003).

The EEG has always been limited by the fact that recordings are from the scalp and likely reflect multiple brain processes. With evoked potential recordings it is possible to look at the response of the brain to various sensory stimuli, in a very short time frame, that is not visible with other techniques.

Event-Related Potentials Findings

The EEG contains very low–voltage changes within the first 400 milliseconds (ms) following a stimulus. By averaging hundreds of these responses to a stimulus, it is possible to record an ERP associated with the stimulus. Early components (<250 ms) vary with the physical properties of the stimulus whereas later components (particularly P300) reflect cognitive processes associated with the stimulus.

Early event-related potentials components

Many studies have found abnormalities in early ERP components suggesting impaired reticular filtering or subcortical monitoring (Holzman, 1987). In some cases, there was a reversal of normal lateral asymmetry in early ERP components (Gruzelier, 1999). However, findings were not specific to schizophrenia in that they could be seen in a number of other conditions such as depression (Friedman and Squires-Wheeler, 1994).

Mismatch negativity

In the mismatch negativity (MMN) paradigm, subjects are asked to pay attention to a stimulus as part of a task while ignoring other stimuli in the background that periodically change. Mismatch negativity occurs when the ignored stimulus changes to the infrequent form. Associated with this is a negative evoked potential with a peak around 200 ms. Several investigators have found reduced MMN in schizophrenia, which could be related to a deficiency of NMDA receptors (Javitt et al., 1993).

P50

One of the more interesting early ERP findings in schizophrenia was the P50, which is measured by presenting two auditory stimuli approximately 500 ms apart. Unlike normal subjects, schizophrenic patients fail to suppress the second tone; this failure has been interpreted to indicate defective gating at the subcortical level (Freedman et al., 1987). While other explanations are possible for the P50, such as abnormal refractory periods not involving filtering or gating, the defect can be genetically transmitted in association with a variant of the $\alpha7$ nicotinic acetylcholine receptor subunit gene (Leonard et al., 2002). Nicotine itself also reverses the defect, which perhaps explains why so many schizophrenic patients are hopelessly addicted to smoking.

Prepulse inhibition

Prepulse inhibition is very similar to the P50 paradigm. If a weak prepulse precedes a startling stimulus, the response to the startling stimulus is reduced in normal subjects. Studies that have used this paradigm suggest a widespread failure to suppress the startle response in schizophrenia (Braff and Geyer, 1990). Schizophrenic patients also have a deficit in the habituation of the startle reflex, which is remarkably reproducible and stable (Ludewig et al., 2002). Animal models have suggested that increased nucleus accumbens dopamine tone, similar to that found in schizophrenia, may cause the sensorimotor gating failure (Braff and Geyer, 1990). Unfortunately, like other ERP abnormalies, prepulse inhibition deficits can be found in a number of other conditions, such as obsessive-compulsive disorder, Huntington disease, attention-deficit disorder, and Tourette syndrome (Swerdlow and Geyer, 1998).

P300

Later ERP components are usually studied with an *oddball* paradigm in which a repeated tone is interspersed with a less frequent event to which the subject must respond in some way. The majority of these investigations have found a reduction in the amplitude of the P300 in schizophrenia. It has also been suggested that there is an abnormal topographic distribution of the P300 with a shift anteriorly to the right of the normal centroparietal distribution, but this has not been replicated by other investigators (Friedman and Squires-Wheeler, 1994).

Although Winterer et al. (2003) found differences in the connectivity of frontal P300 and temporoparietal P300 amplitude in schizophrenic patients and their unaffected siblings, most investigators have not found abnormalities in the schizotypal relatives of schizophrenic patients. However, P300 abnormalities are present in a number of other conditions, such as dementia, alcoholism, and major depression (Friedman and Squires-Wheeler, 1994).

Overall, ERP studies suggest that schizophrenic patients have difficulty attending to relevant stimuli and suppressing irrelevant stimuli. Although ERP findings are not specific to schizophrenia, they are robust. In a meta-analysis of 66 P50 and P300 studies in schizophrenic patients, differences from control groups were comparable to those found in neuropsychological and brain imaging studies (Bramon et al., 2004).

Magnetoencephalography

Magnetoencephalography is a newer psychophysiological tool that has been developed over the last decade. It measures extracranial magnetic fields produced by ionic current flow within cortical pyramidal cells. It has the advantage over EEG of being relatively unaffected by the intervening scalp, fluids, or air. The raw MEG looks much like the EEG and ERP when used in stimulation paradigms but requires no reference and can be quantified with the same computer techniques in much the same way.

Thus far, the findings from MEG are very similar to those found with EEG and ERP (Reite et al., 1999). During mental arithmetic, schizophrenic patients failed to show the expected increase in frontotemporal regions (Kissler et al., 2000). Reduced laterality has been found in schizophrenic patients during auditory stimulation (Heim et al., 2004; Teale et al., 2003) and the results with MMN paradigms are similar to those of ERP studies (Kasai et al., 2002). An increase in fast MEG activity in the left auditory cortex was reported in association with auditory hallucinations as well (Ropohl et al., 2004). However, investigations with MEG are at a much earlier stage than those with EEG or ERP. With MEG it should be possible to apply more relevant paradigms with much better source localization in the same time frame.

Psychophysiological Findings

The psychophysiological studies have produced some important information about schizophrenia. Eye movement studies have suggested problems with coordination. Electrodermal, EEG, and ERP studies have showed possible difficulties with attention, habituation, and information processing. Olfactory and ERP studies have also highlighted the asymmetrical nature of many findings in schizophrenia. However, there was always considerable overlap between patients and controls in these studies, and none of the findings were found to be specific to schizophrenia. Nevertheless, the psychophysiological studies have provided a firm base for neuropsychological investigations, which we will consider next.

6

Neuropsychological Studies

Kraepelin's astute observations about the difficulties that patients had with calculation tasks highlighted the presence of cognitive problems in schizophrenia. He speculated that this deficit went beyond the effects of fatigue. Either a "rapid yielding of will-tension" or a problem with attention seemed to be the cause. There have been countless studies since then devoted to trying to define the nature of this psychological deficit. Schizophrenic patients perform poorly on tests of general intelligence. Superimposed on this deficit are more specific deficits. Most of the tests used to assess specific deficits were developed by investigators at the Montreal Neurological Institute, who studied the performance of more than 1000 patients with intractable epilepsy, tumors, or vascular malformations before and after corrective surgery.

In an influential study, Kolb and Whishaw (1983) used a variety of tests developed at the Montreal Neurological Institute that were sensitive to left or right frontal temporal or parietal function. They also used a general intelligence test. Kolb and Whishaw looked at a group of 30 medicated schizophrenic patients fairly early in their illness and compared them to a group of 30 healthy controls of comparable age, gender, handedness, and educational level. Not surprisingly, the patients had a much lower performance IQ than that of controls, but there was no significant difference on the verbal scale, which suggests that there could have been some deterioration in functioning after the onset of the illness. On the temporal lobe tests, patients performed more poorly than controls on every test of verbal and nonverbal memory except digit span and block span. Similarly, patients did poorly on all four tests of frontal function but did much better on parietal lobe tests. It was concluded that schizophrenic patients show bilateral dysfunction of frontal and temporal lobe function. The studies that followed have by and large borne out these results.

Frontal Lobe Function

As we saw in Chapter 2, the frontal lobes play a critical role in language production, executive function, and working memory. All of these functions seem to be affected in schizophrenia.

Word fluency

When schizophrenic patients are asked to produce as many words as they can starting with a certain letter, they usually produce fewer words than would be expected (Gruzelier et al., 1988; Kolb and Whishaw, 1983). Whether this is due to a "rapid yielding of will-tension," as Kraepelin suggested, is not clear. However, the fact that they are able to perform well on many visuospatial tests, which involve posterior regions of the brain, suggests that deficits may affect frontal regions more than other parts of the brain (Morrison-Stewart et al., 1992). This deficit also appears to be independent of intellectual functioning (Crawford et al., 1993).

Performance on word fluency tasks can be influenced by dopamine. McGowan et al. (2004) found that there was a positive correlation with ^{18}F fluorodopa uptake on PET in the ventral striatum and performance on a word fluency test in healthy volunteers. However, schizophrenic patients showed just the opposite, which suggests that dopamine activity may improve neuropsychological performance up to a certain point. Beyond that, performance is hindered by too much dopamine activity, as in the schizophrenic patients.

Linkage studies are beginning to examine the behavioral correlates of candidate genes in schizophrenia. A recent family-based study (Egan et al., 2004) has linked a GRM3 (metabotropic glutamate receptor-modulating synaptic glutamate) haplotype with word-list learning abnormalities in both schizophrenic patients and family members. However, healthy controls demonstrated the similar abnormalities when they had the same haplotype.

Executive function

A test that is often used to assess executive reasoning ability is the WCST. During the WCST, subjects are given 128 cards on which are printed one or more figures, each of which is the same shape (circle, star, cross, triangle) and the same color (green, red, yellow, and blue). The subject must sort each card to one of four stimulus cards: one red triangle, two green stars, three yellow crosses, and four blue circles, according to a principal that the subject must deduce from the examiner's feedback of *right* and *wrong* as the subject lays down each card. After 10 consecutive correct placements according to the category of color, the category or rule changes to shape and number.

Schizophrenic patients have trouble doing the WCST. They complete fewer categories and also show tendencies to perseverate on the same category in much the same way as neurological patients who have had a frontal lobe injury (Van der Does and Van den Bosch, 1992). Similar deficits can be seen in schizophrenic patients on other executive function tasks, such as the Tower of Hanoi task (Goldberg et al., 1990).

Working memory

Tests such the WCST tap a number of functions. More recent investigations have suggested that the underlying deficit in WCST deficits may be in the speed of encoding information into working memory (Hartman et al., 2003). If so, it would join a wide range of tests on which working-memory deficits have been demonstrated in schizophrenic patients, including the Letter-Number Sequencing Test, and the N-back, delayed response, and delayed match-to-sample tasks (Carter et al., 1998; Gold et al.,1997; Keefe, 2000).

Working memory enables the holding of information after sensory input is ended so that a course of action can be planned. Most models of working memory include some sort of supervisory attentional system in the dorsolateral prefrontal cortex (Goldman-Rakic, 1994) and phonological and visuospatial components using more posterior motor and sensory systems (Baddeley, 1992). The difficulties experienced by schizophrenic patients on verbal working-memory tasks have been linked to problems with visual retention, visual orientation, simple motor function, and executive function whereas spatial working-memory deficits were correlated with visual retention, visual orientation, and memory for objects and faces but not attention, executive function, or visuomotor coordination. These findings could suggest that on-line storage may be related to many of the cognitive-performance deficits seen in schizophrenic patients (Silver et al., 2003).

There is some evidence that relatives of schizophrenic patients show significant deficits in working memory on oculomotor and visual manual delayed-response tasks (Park et al., 1995). It is also of note that patients with a polymorphism of the COMT gene implicated in schizophrenia (see Chapter 3) perform poorly on both the WCST and N-Back task (Egan et al., 2001; Goldberg et al., 2003). This observation could be explained by the COMT *Met* allele's association with reduced dopamine breakdown, leading to increased levels of tonic dopamine that would decrease flexibility of neural networks involved in memory and executive functions (Bilder et al., 2004).

Declarative Memory

Declarative memory includes episodic memory (memory for events) and semantic memory (memory for facts). Unlike declarative memory, nondeclarative memory can take place out of conscious awareness and includes classical conditioning, nonassociative learning, priming, and procedural memory.

Most patients with schizophrenia are well oriented and can recall a few words after a few minutes when asked to do so. However, schizophrenic patients generally perform poorly on short-term and long-term memory tasks in standard test batteries. The effect size in the majority of studies is in the moderate to large range, indicating that most but not all patients demonstrate some degree of impairment that does not seem to be related to medication or duration of illness (Aleman et al., 1999; Heinrichs and Zakzanis, 1998).

In a review of verbal declarative memory dysfunction in schizo-phrenia, Cirillo and Seidman (2003) pointed out that a problem with encoding accounted for most of the difficulties. *Encoding* refers to the stage of information processing in which the information is ini-tially learned. At this stage, information in its raw physical form is translated into a form more amenable to higher-order cognitive func-tions. In contrast, schizophrenic patients do not seem to have as much trouble with the storage or retrieval stages and findings are unlikely to be accounted for by intelligence, attention, medication, or symptom severity.

Other investigators have suggested that schizophrenic patients have impaired ability to process contextual information (Bazin et al., 2000; Rizzo et al., 1996; Servan-Schreiber et al., 1996). This deficit seems to be largely in binding together different pieces of contex-tual information to form a memory representation (Danion et al., 1999; Waters et al., 2004). This finding is interesting because the brain regions for content and context of memory may be different (Nyberg et al., 1996). The processes that bind different elements into a unified memory representation are just beginning to be under-stood (Chalfonte and Johnson, 1996).

Attention

McGhie and Chapman (1961) pointed out that schizophrenic pa-tients complain of being bombarded by stimuli that they are unable to filter out. Such an input overload could lead to disturbances in the control and direction of motility or willed action. With height-ened awareness of bodily sensations and volitional impulses usually outside of conscious awareness, distinguishing self from nonself could become increasingly difficult. While this is an appealing idea, attention and perception are complex contructs dependent upon many factors. One of the more straightforward ways of assessing at-tention is the Continuous Performance Test (CPT), in which the sub-ject observes a stimulus briefly flashing on a screen. If it is an *X*, the subject is required to press a lever. About 40% of chronic schizo-phrenic patients are markedly impaired on this test (Orzack and Kornetsky, 1966).

There have been well over 40 CPT studies of schizophrenic pa-tients. Cornblatt and Keilp (1994) have argued that, on the basis of these studies, impaired attention is evident in schizophrenic patients, independent of clinical state and even before the onset of illness. Thus the impaired attention is not a medication effect. They also point out that the pattern of impairment is different from that in other psychiatric disorders. Although there is some reason to believe that attentional deficits may be inheritable, the classic version of CPT is generally not sufficient to demonstrate abnormalities in first-degree relatives.

Even a task as simple as the CPT involves a number of functions. The stimulus is initially briefly stored and activates codes in long-term memory. Long-term memory is then searched for additional aspects of the context of a stimulus. The process depends on voluntary attention that places the stimulus in the focus of attention, enhancing the processing of the selected stimulus. Information processing in the task also depends on the formation of normal habituation in that stimuli not relevant to the task are not attended to. Manipulations of CPT and various backward masking paradigms seem to point to early perceptual processing abnormalities, possibly involving the executive use of active working memory, rather than attentional difficulties in schizophrenic patients (Neuchterlein et al., 1994).

Syndrome Correlates

While there are no widely accepted subtypes of schizophrenia, there have been many attempts to look at differences between paranoid and nonparanoid patients. Paranoid patients do not demonstrate higher intellectual functioning than nonparanoid patients and both groups perform about the same on verbal ability and visual–spatial functions. Many studies have found better performance on tests of executive functions, attention, and memory, but the results have been inconsistent and likely influenced by other factors such as chronicity and severity of illness and medication effects (Zalewski et al., 1998).

Strauss et al. (1974) distinguished two symptom profiles: *positive*, characterized by hallucinations, delusions, and disorganized thinking; and *negative*, characterized by blunted affect, emotional withdrawl, and cognitive deficiency. From these profiles, Crow (1980) suggested that there may be two processes of schizophrenia that could occur in the same individual. Type I was seen as a problem of increased dopamine receptors and type II was characterized by affective flattening, loss of drive, and structural changes leading to a poor prognosis. More recently, Carpenter et al. (1988) have argued that negative symptoms do not form a stable or unitary concept and should be replaced with *deficit syndrome,* incorporating many of the features of Crow's type II with intractable outcome.

Negative symptoms have been associated with a variety of global and specific cognitive impairments in schizophrenia, including slower information processing, but the relationship generally accounts for only a minor portion of the variance (Addington et al., 1991; Bilder et al., 1985; Green and Walker, 1985; Heydebrand et al., 2004; Neuchterlein et al., 1986; Pantelis et al., 2004). Patients with the deficit syndrome have been found to perform poorer on neuropsychological tests sensitive to frontal and parietal lobe functions (Buchanan et al., 1994). Deficit syndrome patients are also more likely to have smell identification deficits that have been linked to cognitive deficits involving the parietal cortex (Seckinger et al., 2004). Other investigators, however, have questioned the positive–negative dichotomy, noting that positive symptoms also correlate with deficits on frontal lobe and encoding memory tasks (Neufeld and Williamson, 1996).

In recent years, a three-factor model has become widely accepted as superior to earlier two-factor models (Liddle, 1987). On the basis of correlations between symptoms in patients who had been stable for at least 6 months, Liddle defined the three syndromes as *psychomotor poverty* (poverty of speech, blunted affect), *disorganized* (formal thought disorder, inappropriate affect), and *reality distortion* (delusions and hallucinations). Psychomotor poverty was found to be associated with reduced verbal fluency and slow free-choice guessing (Baxter and Liddle, 1998; Liddle and Morris, 1991). Disorganization was associated with intrusion of inappropriate words in word fluency tasks, errors on CPT, and difficulties in set-shifting (Frith et al., 1991; Pantelis et al., 2004). Reality distortion has been associated with widespread cognitive dysfunction (Baxter and Liddle, 1998).

Is There a Core Deficit on Neuropsychological Tests?

Performance impairments on neuropsychological tests in schizophrenia are widespread, involving both hemispheres. Although frontal and temporal regions seem to be affected most, it should be remembered that not all patients have deficits. In fact, the effect size for most findings is on the order of 1.0 (Heinrichs and Zakzanis, 1998). With this difference between patients and controls, in most cases only about 25% of patients would have scores outside the normal range if the data were normally distributed.

Another issue is whether neuropsychological deficits are specific to schizophrenia. Recent meta-analyses would suggest that they are not. Patients with major depression also perform poorly on frontal lobe tasks and some memory tasks. Although the effect sizes are somewhat smaller than in schizophrenia, the largest differences from controls were seen on measures of encoding and retrieval from episodic memory. Intermediate effect sizes were seen on tests of psychomotor speed and attention whereas minimal effect sizes were found on semantic and working-memory tasks (Veiel, 1997; Zakzanis et al., 1998). Patients with bipolar disorders also show some deficits in executive functions, attention, speed of information processing, learning, and memory similar to those of depressed patients but probably less than those of schizophrenic patients, particularly if patients are asymptomatic at the time of testing (Bearden et al., 2001).

Despite the lack of specificity and obvious overlap with controls, there have been many attempts to define a common denominator for neuropsychological findings in schizophrenia. One of the obvious common denominators would seem to be working memory, which is clearly impaired in schizophrenia (Goldman-Rakic, 1994; Silver et al., 2003). While working memory deficits may underlie many deficits, it is difficult to believe that it could account for all the deficits in declarative, attention, and executive function that are observed in these patients. Several investigators have commented on the difficulties with the encoding of information in schizophrenic patients (Carter and Neufeld, 1999). Difficulties at this stage can be related to working-memory capacity, but not exclusively. Rather, what seems to be missing in many patients is the ability to efficiently link the current stimulus with a cognitive set necessary for the task at hand.

Frith (1995) argued that the classical neuropsychological approach may not be appropriate for the study of schizophrenia because it is based on studies of neuropsychological patients with circumscribed lesions, whereas schizophrenic patients have widespread lesions. From this broader perspective, it was proposed (Frith, 1995; Frith and Done, 1988) that there is a *poverty of will* in schizophrenia that accounts for negative symptoms and difficulties on word fluency tasks. In addition, there is a *failure of self-monitoring* leading to positive symptoms such as thought insertion (failure to recognize one's own thoughts) and auditory hallucinations (attribution of internal speech to someone else). Failure of self-monitoring may reflect a more widespread failure of linking current stimuli with higher-order cognitive functions or action plans, i.e., encoding. There is support for Frith's theory, however, in that diminished recall is related to negative but not positive symptoms in schizophrenic patients (Torres et al., 2004).

Other failures in the linkage of information-processing systems have been proposed in schizophrenia. One of the more influential of these was proposed by Hemsley (1987), who suggested that there is a weakening of the influences of stored memories of the regularities of previous input on current perception. Information without context could be misinterpreted in a number of ways, perhaps explaining some positive symptoms and difficulties with tasks that require contextual information such as the WCST.

Gray et al. (1991) provided an interesting way of integrating Frith's failure of self-monitoring with Hemsley's weakening of the influences of stored memories. They pointed out that there may be a disruption in the input of the limbic system (in particular, the memory- and context-enabling structures of the temporal lobe) to the basal ganglia (in particular, the nucleus accumbens and structures involved in learning and monitoring behavior and affect). A failure of integration of information processing at this level could account for at least some of the problems that patients have with motivation, encoding, memory, and self-monitoring.

Some Emerging Themes

One could say that the findings from neuropsychological studies are both encouraging and discouraging. Discouraging because no finding differentiates all patients from controls, and what findings there are do not seem to be specific to schizophrenia. However, a few themes are starting to emerge from the data that are encouraging. First, there are abnormalities in a number of brain regions—the frontal, temporal, and basal ganlia regions being more common than others. Secondly, many of the abnormalities found are related to known functions of these areas—executive function, verbal fluency, memory, and encoding, among others. Finally, none of these regions could account for these abnormalities in isolation. They are linked in functional neuronal circuits that appear to be damaged in some way. But what and where is the damage? Clearly, neuropsychological tests do not allow us to look into the brain, but brain imaging techniques do. The next chapter will review findings from structural brain-imaging studies.

7

Imaging Brain *Structure* in Living Patients

It is usually assumed that structural brain-imaging studies began with the computerized tomography (CT) studies in the 1970s but this is not the case. Almost 50 years before this, pneumoencephalography was used to outline the ventricular system and cortex with X-rays of the head after air had been injected into the lumbar subarachnoid space (Dandy, 1919). These studies demonstrated enlarged lateral and third ventricles as well as cortical sulci atrophy, which to some extent correlated with poor outcome (Haug, 1962; Jacobi and Winkler, 1927). However, the technique was somewhat invasive and difficult to use in psychiatric patients, so it was not until the development of CT that brain structure was examined systematically in schizophrenia.

Although it was possible to measure the ventricular system fairly accurately with CT, it was not until magnetic resonance imaging (MRI) became available in the 1980s that gray matter and the volumes of specific brain structures could be examined. More than 200 MRI studies have now been completed in first-episode, drug-naïve, and chronic schizophrenic patients. The findings from these studies will be reviewed.

Computerized Tomography Studies

With CT it became possible to image the brain in three dimensions by projecting X-ray beams through axial sections of the brain at many angles. A back-projection computer algorithm is then used to construct images based on the attenuation values of the X-rays. Because CT allows visualization of fluid-filled spaces in the brain it is very good for assessing the ventricular system. There is not much gray-white contrast in the images, however, so it is difficult to decipher specific brain structures.

The first CT study in schizophrenic patients examined 17 chronically institutionalized schizophrenic patients. Compared to eight normal volunteers from the ancillary staff of Northwick Park Hospital and Clinical Research Centre matched for age and premorbid occupational attainment, the patients showed enlarged ventricles with very little overlap between groups. In fact, only one patient had a ventricular size in the normal range. Schizophrenic patients also demonstrated a highly significant negative correlation between ventricular enlargement and poor performance on cognitive tests such as serial sevens and delayed recall (Johnstone et al., 1976). Even though much of this had been known from the earlier pneumoencephalographic studies, the study was a landmark. It encouraged investigators from around the world to use the rapidly advancing brain-imaging techniques in schizophrenia research.

Lateral ventricular enlargement

The studies that followed Johnstone et al. (1976) by and large confirmed the original observation that ventricles are enlarged in a substantial number of schizophrenic patients. It also became clear that it was predominantly the lateral ventricles that were enlarged. This finding was of interest because the lateral ventricles are related to many subcortical structures such as the caudate, putamen, and globus pallidus as well as the thalamus, hippocampus, and corpus callosum, all of which have been implicated in schizophrenia. Changes in the volume of these structures could be reflected in larger lateral ventricles.

Of the 36 studies reviewed by Shelton and Weinberger (1986) comparing schizophrenic patients to a nonpsychiatric control population, 26 (about 75%) showed significantly enlarged ventricles in schizophrenic patients. However, this is not to say that enlarged ventricles occur in all schizophrenic patients. Even with this rather robust finding the effect size is only around 0.70, on the same order as neuropsychological findings reviewed in the previous chapter (Raz and Raz, 1990). Nevertheless, there is some consensus that lateral ventricular enlargement can be seen from the onset of the illness and is linked with poor premorbid adjustment and poor outcome with more frequent hospitalizations.

A number of studies have found an association between impaired performance on neuropsychological test batteries sensitive to brain damage and lateral ventricular enlargement (Golden et al., 1980; Weinberger et al., 1979). There also seems to be a familial component to ventricular enlargement. Weinberger et al. (1981) found larger ventricles in affected siblings compared to their unaffected siblings. However, the unaffected siblings had larger ventricles than those in an unrelated control group. Reveley et al. (1982) came to a similar conclusion in a study of eight pairs of monozygotic twins discordant for schizophrenia. In seven of the pairs, the schizophrenic twin had larger ventricles but there was also a trend toward increased ventricular size in the unaffected twin compared to that in other twins without schizophrenia.

Third ventricle enlargement

The third ventricle connects with the anterior horns of the lateral ventricles through the foramina of Monro and fourth ventricle through the aqueduct of Silvius. In very close proximity are the thalamus and the fornix, an extension of the hippocampus. Of the 12 studies reviewed by Shelton and Weinberger (1986), 10 (about 83%) showed increased third-ventricle size in schizophrenic patients compared to controls. The effect size in these and subsequent studies was on the same order as the lateral ventricular studies, i.e., 0.66 (Raz and Raz, 1990).

Some studies have found an association with third-ventricle enlargement and length of illness but others have not. In fact, there does not seem to be a correlation between third-ventricle enlargement and a variety of clinical variables, including age of onset, cumulative hospitalizations, prior treatment, premorbid adjustment, or subtype (Boronow et al., 1985).

Cerebellar pathology

As we shall see in the following chapters, the cerebellum has been implicated in schizophrenia by several investigators. Although it is somewhat difficult to quantify on CT, there have been a number of attempts to rate the degree of atrophy. Cerebellar atrophy seems to occur in about 10% of schizophrenic patients, which is more than the 1% expected from routinely interpreted CT scans (Shelton and Weinberger, 1986). However, Raz and Raz (1990) placed the effect size at 0.17, which is not significantly different from zero. There did not seem to be a relationship with age or duration of illness.

Cerebral asymmetry

Right-handed healthy volunteers tend to have larger right frontal and left occipital lobes, which may reflect lateralization of handedness and language. This normal pattern is often reversed in conditions such as autism and dyslexia. While Crow (1990b) argued that it is a *failure* to develop asymmetry, particularly in the temporal lobes, rather than *reversed* asymmetry that characterizes schizophrenia, the CT findings appear to be very mixed (Shelton and Weinberger, 1986).

     Although CT studies have provided some fairly strong evidence that several brain regions may be affected in schizophrenia, it is not possible to determine what these are with CT. Enlarged lateral and third ventricles would suggest that the thalamus, hippocampus, and other temporal structures could be involved. Magnetic resonance imaging techniques allows us to examine this possibility.

Magnetic Resonance Imaging Studies

Magnetic resonance imaging does not involve the use of ionizing radiation but depends on the excitation of protons with a radiofrequency transmitter in a coil surrounding the head of the patient. Because protons have an odd atomic number they spin like tops when excited by a specific frequency (Larmor frequency), producing a magnetic field oriented along the axis of rotation of the nucleus. The patient is in a large, super-cooled magnet that forces the spinning protons to orient with or against the magnetic field of the magnet. The radiofrequency forces a proportion of the protons into the

higher energy state against the magnetic field. When the radiofrequency is turned off, the protons decay to their equilibrium state before excitation with the Larmor frequency. As they do this they give
off a radiofrequency that can be detected by a radiofrequency re-
ceiver not unlike your radio at home. T_1 (spin-lattice) is the time
taken for protons to return to alignment with the magnetic field at
lower-energy state whereas T_2 (spin-spin) is the time taken to decay
in the transverse plane.

Magnetic resonance imaging machines have gradients in the
three orthogonal axes. The specific resonating frequency for protons is different in different field strengths, much like the pitch of
a guitar string under different tensions. By systematically manipu-
lating these gradients in the three axes, T_1 and T_2 values are generated in three-dimensional space by taking advantage of the difference in resonanting frequencies within the gradient. As it turns out,
T_1 is very different in gray and white matter and cerebrospinal fluid,
allowing high-resolution (about 1 mm^3) maps of brain structure to
be constructed. T_2 is not quite as good for looking at neuroanatomy
but is sensitive to tissue changes in some forms of neuropathology
such as brain tumors. With this technique it became possible to examine all brain structures in living patients with almost the same pre-
cision as gross postmortem samples. Not surprisingly, one of the first
places examined was the ventricular system.

Whole head size, cerebral spinal fluid, and ventricular enlargement

Whereas CT provides only rough estimates of ventricular size and atrophy, detailed measurements of brain size and the ventricular system can be made with MRI. Some investigators have suggested that
smaller brain size could reflect perinatal and/or neurodevelopmental abnormalities. In a comprehensive review of MRI findings in schizophrenia, Shenton et al. (2001) found 50 MRI studies that looked at
whole-brain volumes. Only 11 of these reported significant differences from controls, so it appears that schizophrenic patients do not
have smaller brains in most cases. Another review and meta-analysis
found a small, but statistically significant, reduction in brain and in-
tracranial size in schizophrenia but no evidence for a reduction of
extracranial size (Ward et al., 1996).

The evidence for increased cerebral spinal fluid in schizophrenic patients is a bit more convincing, with most studies finding

an increase in extracerebral (sulcal) cerebral spinal fluid space (Narr et al., 2003; Woods, 1998; Woods and Yurgelin-Todd, 1991; Woods et al., 1996). In the case of twins, the differences between well and affected twins can be quite striking (Fig. 7–1). This is an interesting finding because increased cerebral spinal fluid suggests that there was some loss of brain tissue after the the skull sutures fused. Such a loss would not be compatible with an early neurodevelopmental lesion but could be consistent with an abnormality of brain growth or neuronal degeneration.

Shenton et al. (2001) reviewed 55 studies that examined the ventricular system in first-episode and chronic schizophrenic patients. Lateral ventricular enlargement, more prominent on the left side, was found in 80% of these studies. In many studies the temporal horn of the lateral ventricle on the left side appeared to be particularly affected, a finding in keeping with observations from postmortem studies. However, a recent meta-analysis has suggested that the increases are relatively small. Assuming a comparison group volume of 100%, the body of the left lateral ventricle was 116% and the

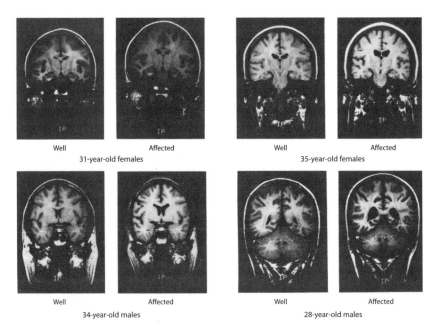

Figure 7–1. Magnetic resonance images from four pairs of monozygotic twins discordant for schizophrenia showing increased cerebrospinal fluid spaces in the affected twin. Used with permission, from Weinberger (1995).

left temporal horn was 110% in schizophrenic patients (Wright et al., 2000). As in the CT studies, the third ventricle was also enlarged in 73% of the 33 studies reviewed by Shenton et al. (2001), but only 20% of studies found fourth-ventricle enlargement in schizophrenic patients.

Total gray matter volume

One of the great advantages of MRI over CT is the ability of MRI to quantify gray-matter volumes overall and in specific structures. Zipursky et al. (1992) examined 22 right-handed male veterans of the United States Armed Services who met DSM-III-R criteria for schizophrenia and 20 male veterans recruited from the community who were of comparable age, handedness, and intelligence. Alcohol consumption was also similar between the groups. The main finding was a small gray-matter cortical reduction overall (7%) in schizophrenic patients compared to controls but no difference in white matter. Reductions varied according to the region studied, with prefrontal and frontotemporal showing the greatest deficits (8% and 9%, respectively) and parietal regions having smaller reductions (4%). Gray matter was weakly correlated with negative symptom scores as well. One of the more striking findings was that the controls showed a progressive loss of gray matter with age, accounting for 25% to 45% of the variance depending on the region. However, the loss of gray matter in patients was on top of this aging effect.

Gray-matter reductions are seen in first-episode patients but in some cases to a lesser degree (Gur et al., 1999; Zipursky et al., 1998). They are also seen in patients at risk for schizophrenia and in unaffected siblings of schizophrenic patients, although the pattern of loss sometimes varies (Cannon et al., 1998; Lawrie et al., 1999). Pearlson and Marsh (1999) point out that most of the regions showing gray-matter loss are part of the heteromodal association cortex: the planum temporale, the dorsolateral prefrontal cortex, Broca's area, and the inferior parietal lobule. However, differences are not limited to these regions.

Temporal lobes

Probably the most convincing demonstration of structural abnormalities in schizophrenia comes from Suddath et al. (1990), who studied 15 monozygotic twin pairs discordant for schizophrenia (8 males and 7 female pairs) recruited from the United States and Canada. Fourteen of the 15 affected twins had smaller left hippocampi whereas 13 of the affected twins had smaller right hippocampi when compared to their normal twin. Lateral ventricles were larger on the left in 14 of the affected twins and on the right in 13 of the affected twins. Third-ventricle enlargement was seen in 13 of the affected twins, a finding consistent with other ventricular studies of acute and chronic patients. None of these findings were evident in seven sets of monozygotic twins (three male and four female pairs) without schizophrenia. A study of pairs of twins concordant and discordant for schizophrenia found that hippocampal volumes did not differ among those affected by schizophrenia, suggesting similar etiologies in both types of twins (Weinberger et al., 1992b). Subsequent studies have shown that hippocampal volume is largely related to genetic factors, but environmental factors may be more important in schizophrenic patients and their relatives (van Erp et al., 2004).

There have been many other studies of temporal lobe structure in acute and chronic schizophrenic patients. Shenton et al. (2001) reported that 31 of 51 studies (about 61%) found smaller whole temporal-lobe volumes. About 74% of the 49 investigations found smaller medial temporal structures, including the amygdala–hippocampal complex and parahippocampal gyrus. Although it is difficult to completely separate the amygdala from the hippocampus, six of nine studies (about 67%) reviewed found smaller amygdala volumes on one or both sides in chronic patients. Ten of 15 studies (about 67%) found reductions in the superior temporal gyrus, which includes Heschl's gyrus, the primary auditory cortex, and Wernicke's area. The latter in turn includes the planum temporale, a region important in language processing. Five of 10 studies showed a reversal of greater-left-than-right asymmetry. The reductions in the medial temporal and hippocampal regions appear to be highly correlated and many of these differences can also be seen in the relatives of schizophrenic patients.

Several investigators have suggested that hippocampal and superior temporal gyrus volume reductions may be related to cognitive deficits, particularly memory-processing abnormalities in schizophrenic patients (Goldberg et al., 1994; Nestor et al., 1993). More recent work has correlated hippocampal volume reductions in first-episode schizophrenic patients with frontal neurological deficits

(Szeszko et al., 2002). There are some physiological and perinatal history correlates as well. Smaller left posterior superior temporal gyrus volumes have been associated with smaller left temporal P300 amplitudes in first-episode schizophrenic patients (McCarley et al., 2002). Stefanis et al. (1999) found reduced left hippocampal volume in patients who had severe pregnancy and birth complications but no family history of schizophrenia. McNeil et al. (2000) found a correlation between labor and delivery complications and smaller hippocampi on both sides in the affected twin of monozygotic twins discordant for schizophrenia.

Despite agreement among many investigators that temporal regions are involved in schizophrenia, several recent meta-analyses of MRI findings in this region have suggested that the effect sizes are likely smaller than those in neuropsychological and neurophysiological studies (Lawrie and Abukmeil, 1998; Nelson et al., 1998; Wright et al., 2000; Zakzanis et al., 2000). Effect sizes for medial temporal differences from controls were on the order of 0.40. Even though effect sizes were greater for the superior temporal lobes, there was an overlap of as much as 90% between schizophrenic and control groups on many volumetric measures.

Prefrontal and parietal regions

Andreasen et al. (1986) were the first to report smaller frontal lobes in schizophrenia. Among men in the sample, nearly 40% had markedly smaller frontal volumes than those of controls. Structural differences between schizophrenic patients and controls were not as strong in prefrontal and parietal regions in the studies that followed. Shenton et al. (2001) found 30 of 50 (60%) reported differences in the prefrontal region and 9 of 15 (60%) in the parietal region. Moreover, prefrontal deficits seem to correlate highly with hippocampal and temporal lobe volumes (Breier et al., 1992; Wible et al., 1995). As with other brain regions, the effect sizes for frontal differences were small, generally in the range of 0.4–0.5 (Davidson and Heinrichs, 2003).

Thalamus

The thalamus is technically more difficult to quantify on MRI, so there have not been as many studies in schizophrenic patients. However, Shenton et al. (2001) found 5 of 12 studies (about 42%) re-ported reductions in the thalamus in patients compared to controls. A meta-analysis including postmortem studies found that 91% of studies adjusted for brain size reported reductions in the thalamus, but the effect size was still small at 0.35 (Konick and Friedman, 2001). More recent investigations not included in these reviews have failed in one case to find a difference from controls in chronic patients (Deicken et al., 2002) but three other investigations of chronic and first-episode patients did find reductions (Byne et al., 2001; Ettinger et al., 2001; Kemether et al., 2003). Of particular interest was the finding that the reductions were primarily in nuclei connected with the association cortex (Byne et al., 2001; Kemether et al., 2003). Smaller thalamic volumes have also been found in first-degree rela-tives (Seidman et al., 1999; Staal et al., 1998).

Other brain regions

It is hard to think of a brain region that has not been looked at in schizophrenia. For brain regions other than those discussed above, the findings have usually been inconsistent. Noga et al. (1995) found a 3%–5% reduction in anterior cingulate cortex volumes, which was not clinically significant, whereas Takahashi et al. (2002) found a sig-nificant reduction in this region in only female schizophrenic pa-tients with a loss of normal asymmetry. Only four of nine MRI stud-ies (about 44%) of the occipital lobe have found differences from controls (Shenton et al., 2001). It is much the same story in the cere-bellum, with 4 of 13 studies (about 31%) reporting differences. More recent studies not included in the review have shown decreased cere-bellar volumes in schizophrenic patients (Ho et al., 2004; Ichimiya et al., 2001; Loeber et al., 2001). Patients with cerebellar tissue deficits also had cerebellar signs such as difficulties with coordina-tion of gait and stance (Ho et al., 2004) reminiscent of the soft neu-rological signs in Chapter 3.

Seventeen of 25 studies (about 68%) reviewed by Shenton et al. (2001) showed differences in the basal ganglia, but the increase in vol-ume was likely related to medication. More robust results have come from studies of the cavi septi pellucidi. The septum pellucidum is a membrane that separates the two frontal horns of the lateral ventricles. Abnormalities in the development of bordering structures such as the corpus callosum may result in a space or cavum in this membrane. Surprisingly, 11 of 12 studies (about 92%) reviewed by Shenton et al. (2001) found abnormalities in this membrane. The corpus callosum itself has also been found to be reduced in schizophrenic patients (David, 1994; Keshavan et al., 2002b). However, a meta-analysis of 11 studies found only a small difference in corpus callosum area rather than the length of the corpus callosum or corpus callosum/brain area ratio in schizophrenic patients (Woodruff et al., 1995).

Voxel-based studies

Abnormalities in brain structure in schizophrenia are at best subtle and difficult to quantify in three-dimensional space while allowing for variations in brain, size, shape, and composition among individuals. A number of techniques have been developed to transform images into a standard stereotactic space so that three-dimensional, voxel-based analysis can be done (Ashburner and Friston, 2000).

The results of these studies are fairly consistent with earlier efforts. Andreasen et al. (1994) were the first to report differences in the thalamus and nearby white matter of schizophrenic patients through use of a bounding-box technique. Wright et al. (1999) found significant reductions in the right and left temporal pole and insula, right amygdala, and left dorsolateral cortex. Other investigations have found temporal deficits along with differences in the anterior cingulate (Suzuki et al., 2002), thalamus (Ananth et al., 2002; Hulshoff Pol et al., 2001; Volz et al., 2000a), insula, and posterior cingulate (Holshoff Pol et al., 2001). A first-episode study found that only the superior temporal gyrus was significant after correction for multiple comparisons (Kubicki et al., 2002). Both increased and decreased cerebellar volumes have been reported (Marcelis et al., 2003; Volz et al., 2000a; Wilke et al., 2001). However, first-degree relatives of schizophrenic patients also have cerebellar deficits.

One advantage of the voxel-based approach is that it can be used to look at correlations across multiple locations. Using this methodology, Gaser et al. (2004) found significant negative correlations with the ventricle/brain ratio and voxels in the right and left thalamus, posterior putamen, left superior temporal gyrus, and insula. These findings indicate that enlarged ventricles in schizophrenia could be explained by tissue loss in these structures.

Relaxation times

No consistent results have emerged from studies of T_1 relaxation times (Andreasen, 1989). However, T_2 times were found to be decreased in frontal white matter, temporal cortex, and white matter as well as the hippocampus and basal ganglia in chronic patients (Williamson et al., 1992). These results confirm an earlier preliminary report of the temporal white matter in six patients (Andreasen, 1989). T_2 relaxation times can reflect a number of subtle tissue changes, including membrane abnormalities. We will address these changes in subsequent chapters through magnetic resonance spectroscopy studies.

Diffusion tensor imaging

Cell membranes, myelin sheaths, and white-matter tracts impede diffusion of water molecules. This effect can be detected in brain tissue with diffusion tensor imaging. Because water molecules tend to move further along paths that are parallel to fibers than along those that are perpendicular an ellipsoid distribution of water molecules is found, referred to as *anisotropy*. Generally, low anisotropy would imply tissue with low connectivity, but this is dependent upon whether the tissue contains tracts merging from different directions.

Buchsbaum et al. (1998) demonstrated lower levels of anisotropy in prefrontal white matter. Lower levels of anisotropy were subsequently shown to be widespread, extending from frontal to occipital regions, regardless of whether there was a deficit in white-matter volumes. In contrast, there does not seem to be any gray-matter anisotropy, even if there is gray-matter loss (Lim et al., 1999). All five subsequent studies have confirmed lower anisotropy in schizophrenic patients, although the difference was not statistically significant in one study (Davis et al., 2003; Lim and Helpern, 2002).

More recently, Burns et al. (2003) found reduced white-matter tract integrity in the left uncinate and arcuate fasciculi, which suggests frontotemporal and frontoparietal disconnectivity. In addition, Wang et al. (2004) found reduced fractional anisotropy in the anterior cingulum. Kubicki et al. (2003) have shown that decreased anisotropy in the cingulum bundle, the white-matter tract with input and output for the anterior cingulate, correlates with WCST abnormalities. Thus, there is considerable evidence that white-matter connections are deficient in schizophrenic patients, but the pattern varies considerably among different studies.

Laterality and gender

A number of studies have suggested that volumetric deficits may be more pronounced on the left side. Probably the most convincing evidence for this would appear to be volume losses in temporal regions associated with language, but even findings in this region are not consistent. Of 16 postmortem and imaging studies reviewed by Shapleske et al. (1999), only 5 (about 31%) showed reduced or reversed asymmetry of the planum temporale in schizophrenic patients. However, the portion of the corpus callosum that connects the temporal lobes may be smaller in schizophrenic patients (Woodruff et al., 1993). An MRI study that was specifically designed to examine the issue of laterality and gender effects in 102 schizophrenic patients found larger lateral and third ventricles, and smaller thalamic, hippocampal, and superior temporal volumes than those of comparison subjects but no significant effects of either laterality or gender (Flaum et al., 1995b). Thus, the evidence for a laterality or gender effect is not strong.

Clinical correlations

Ever since Crow (1980) suggested that there were two major syndromes in schizophrenia—type I, characterized by positive symptoms responding to medication and, type II, associated with large ventricles on CT, negative symptoms, and a poor outcome—there has been an intensive effort to try to find neuroanatomical correlates for symptom clusters in schizophrenia. Although early studies based on Crow's ideas were promising, the studies that followed did not find general support for the hypothesis (Pfefferbaum and Zipursky, 1991).

In recent years there have been many attempts to look at the correlates of negative symptoms through MRI. Wible et al. (2001) examined patients with a higher proportion of negative symptoms and found that these patients had smaller bilateral prefrontal white matter. Prefrontal volumes were also correlated with negative symptom severity and the volumes of medial temporal lobe regions. Sigmundsson et al. (2001) found prefrontal deficits in patients with predominantly negative symptoms but deficits were found in the medial temporal lobe (including hippocampus) and anterior cingulate as well, consistent with other investigations (Anderson et al., 2002; Pail-läre-Martinot et al., 2001). More recently, schizophrenic patients with high ratings of apathy have been found to have smaller bilateral frontal lobe volumes than those of contols (Roth et al., 2004).

When symptoms were divided into Liddle's three-factor model, psychomotor poverty negatively correlated with left prefrontal volumes (Chua et al., 1997). Findings with other techniques also correlated with negative symptoms. T_2 relaxation times in the left prefrontal cortex were increased in patients with high ratings of negative symptoms (Williamson et al., 1991b) and inferior frontal whitematter anisotropy was associated with the severity of negative symptoms (Wolkin et al., 2003). So while there are correlates with other regions, negative symptoms are most often correlated with prefrontal findings.

Volumetric correlates of positive symptoms seem more likely to be temporal, although thought disorder in children with schizophrenia has recently been correlated with nucleus accumbens volumes, a structure closely connected with the medial temporal lobe (Ballmaier et al., 2004). Barta et al. (1990) reported a correlation between the severity of auditory hallucinations and volume reductions of the left superior temporal gyrus, which has been replicated by others (Flaum et al., 1995a; Levitan et al., 1999). The volume and asymmetry of the left posterior superior temporal gyrus have correlated with measures of thought disorder in a number of studies (Holinger et al., 1999; Rossi et al. 1994; Shenton et al., 1992).

A recent voxel-based study of patients with and without prominent hallucinations has reported deficits in the left insula and adjacent temporal lobe (Shapleske et al., 2002). However, thalamic-volume deficits have also correlated with hallucinations and thought disorder (Portas et al., 1998). In a recent diffusion tensor imaging study (Hubl et al., 2004), patients prone to hallucinations had pronounced differences in the left hemisphere fiber tracts, including the cingulate bundle, when compared to patients without hallucinations. Findings suggested that during inner speech, abnormalities in white-matter tracts could lead to abnormal activation of regions involved in acoustical processing of external speech.

Correlations between MRI parameters and outcome have been somewhat mixed. In a study of patients with good and poor outcome,

Mitelman et al. (2003) found that the patients with poor outcome had significantly smaller gray-matter volumes in the temporal and occipital lobes but no differences in prefrontal regions. This finding is at odds with early studies that had found poor outcome to be associated with predominantly prefrontal deficits. Consequently, it is difficult to state a definitive relationship between either outcome or symptomatology and structural findings. The strongest linkages appear to be between negative symptoms and prefrontal deficits, and positive symptoms and temporal lobe deficits.

Specificity

There are many other psychiatric conditions associated with volumetric abnormalities. Probably the most problematic of these is alcoholism, as both lateral ventricular enlargement and gray-matter loss have been reported in these patients, and schizophrenic patients often abuse alcohol. However, in an elegant study of patients with schizophrenia or schizoaffective disorder with and without lifetime alcohol abuse or dependence, patients suffering from alcoholism, and healthy volunteers, both alcoholism and schizophrenia were associated with gray-matter deficits. But patients with both conditions had the most striking deficits, particularly in prefrontal and anterior superior temporal regions (Mathalon et al., 2003).

Ventricular enlargement is often reported in mood-disordered patients, with effect sizes in the range of 0.4. However, a comparison of these studies' results with those for schizophrenic patients suggests that the ventricular enlargement is greater in schizophrenic patients, although the effect size is small (Elkis et al., 1995). Studies using MRI have generally not found diffuse gray-matter loss in either major depression or bipolar disorder but there have been some differences from controls. These include bilateral temporal lobe reductions with loss of normal asymmetry and small but significant reductions in prefrontal volumes in bipolar patients. Bipolar patients also have cavum septi pellucidi abnormalities (Kwon et al., 1998). Results have been mixed for the hippocampus and thalamus in bipolar patients. Similarly, small frontal lobe and subgenual prefrontal cortical volume reductions have been found in patients with major depression. These patients do not seem to show volume reductions, with the possible exception of those with repeated episodes (Campbell et al., 2004; Sheline, 2003). Thus, medial and superior temporal lobe volumetric deficits do not seem to characterize mood-disordered patients, at least in the early stages of illness.

By contrast, patients with conditions related to schizophrenia show many of the same volumetric differences. In a review of 17 structural imaging studies on schizotypal personality disorder, abnormalities were found in the superior temporal gyrus, the parahippocampus, the temporal horn region of the lateral ventricles, the corpus callosum, and the thalamus in these patients. However, fewer differences from controls were seen in medial temporal structures (Dickey et al., 2002). While the failure to find medial temporal volume deficits in most mood-disordered patients and patients with schizotypal personality disorder could suggest that this is specific to schizophrenia, it is important to remember that hippocampal deficits can also be found in some patients with unrelated conditions such as posttraumatic stress disorder (Bremner et al., 1995).

Is There a Neuroanatomy of Schizophrenia?

There are a number of replicated findings in schizophrenia patients, most notably enlarged ventricles and gray-matter loss, particularly in temporal regions. Evidence for deficits in other regions such as the thalamus and cerebellum appears to be growing. Some findings such as posterior superior temporal deficits may be more specific to schizophrenia, but most findings are modest with considerable overlap with other psychiatric disorders and normal variation.

Although many of these deficits are associated with other findings, such as cognitive dysfunction and a history of perinatal trauma, it has been difficult to link specific regional deficits with symptomatology. Part of the reason for this may be that the symptoms of schizophrenia are subtle. Fortunately, many techniques have been developed over the last 20 years to study subtle aspects of brain function in living patients. The next chapter will address these findings.

8

Imaging Brain *Function* in Living Patients

Over the last 25 years remarkable advances have been made in quantifying brain chemistry and function in living patients. Beginning with primitive xenon techniques through to highly sophisticated positron emission tomography (PET) and functional MRI techniques, it has become possible to accurately determine cerebral blood flow changes in localized regions of the brain during performance of cognitive tasks. Other PET and single photon emission computed tomography (SPECT) techniques allow us to look at resting brain metabolism and receptor occupancy. The findings from these studies have changed the way we look at schizophrenia and have brought us much closer to understanding the neuronal circuits that could be involved.

Xenon Cerebral Blood Flow Studies

After either injecting or inhaling the radioactive tracer xenon-133, cerebral blood flow can be estimated by monitoring gamma-ray emissions with extracranial radiation detectors. In a landmark study using the injection technique, Ingvar and Franzen (1974) examined

20 chronic schizophrenic patients, one younger group (4 women and 7 men; mean age, 25 years) and an older group (9 women; mean age, 61 years). They found that the distribution of cerebral blood flow was largely normal in the younger schizophrenic patients with a predominance of higher flows to frontal regions. In older patients, a different pattern of *hypofrontality* was found with relatively low flows frontally and high flows occipitotemporally. In the older group and to some extent in the younger one, the intensity of psychotic symptoms correlated with mean hemispheric cerebral blood flow. Subsequent studies were somewhat mixed in the finding of resting hypofrontality, particularly in those patients early in their illness with acute symptoms (Berman and Weinberger, 1986).

Hypofrontality has usually been associated with negative symptoms but there also are some functional correlates of positive symptoms. Kurachi et al. (1985) examined patients with and without auditory hallucinations. Both groups had lower relative frontal flow bilaterally but patients with auditory hallucinations had higher left temporal flow, in keeping with some of the structural studies of this region. Gur et al. (1994) also found that some patients did not have the expected lateralized midtemporal increases with left-hemisphere (verbal) and right-hemisphere (facial memory) tasks. This was particularly evident on verbal tasks in patients with severe hallucinations, a finding supporting the link between the temporal lobe and positive symptoms. However, there are many other investigations using cognitive activation tasks which deserve discussion.

Activation studies

On the whole, xenon cerebral blood flow studies have been more consistent with activation paradigms. During mental tasks such as Raven's Matrices and digit-span-backward tests, Ingvar and Franzen (1975) found that severely ill patients tended to decrease rather than increase frontal flow. Weinberger et al. (1986), using inhalation xenon-133 in 20 medication-free, chronic patients, observed decreased dorsolateral prefrontal cerebral blood flow in patients while they were performing the Wisconsin Card Sorting Test (WCST), compared to that in 25 normal controls of similar age and handedness but higher levels of education. Performance on the task also correlated with cerebral blood flow in this region in patients. No differences in cerebral blood flow were seen between patients and con-

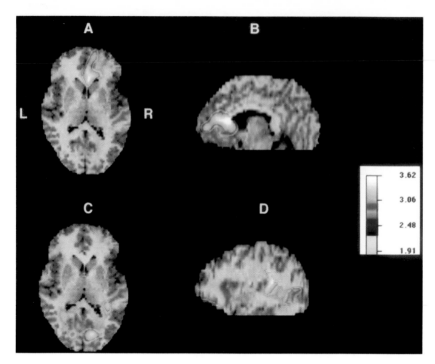

Color Plate 4–1. $^{15}O_2$-labeled PET cerebral blood flow increased in the anterior cingulate (*A, B*) and decreased in the hippocampus (*C, D*) in a schizophrenic patient given intravenous ketamine. Ketamine antagonizes *N*-methyl-D-aspartate receptors. Considering the wide distribution of these receptors in the brain, it is curious that other brain regions do not show differences. Used with permission, from Lahti et al. (1995a).

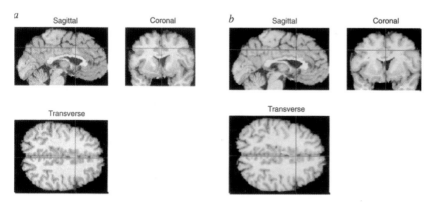

Color Plate 8–1. Brain regions showing a significantly greater $^{15}O_2$-labeled PET cerebral blood flow with cognitive activation (word fluency and repetition) in normal subjects compared to schizophrenic patients. In *a*, control subjects show significantly increased activation ($p < 0.05$ corrected) compared to that in schizophrenic patients on statistical parametric mapping. After injection of apomorphine, a dopamine agonist, in *b* a comparison of the groups shows that schizophrenic patients have an enhanced response to the same cognitive activation as in *a*. Used with permission, from Dolan et al. (1995).

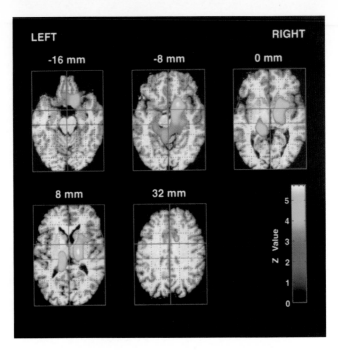

Color Plate 8–2. Brain areas with significantly increased $^{15}O_2$-labeled PET cerebral blood flow during auditory verbal hallucinations in five medicated, chronic schizophrenic patients. Note activations throughout the limbic system including the thalamus, hippocampus, parahippocampus, cingulate gyri, and orbitofrontal cortex. Used with permission, from Silbersweig et al. (1995).

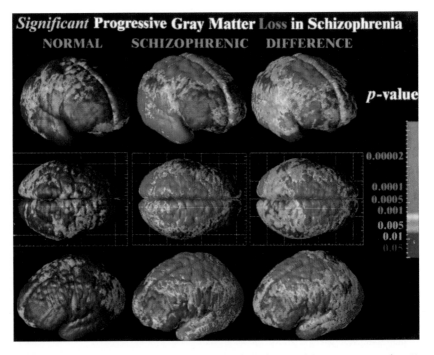

Color Plate 9–1. Dynamic gray matter loss in 12 schizophrenic adolescents compared to 12 normal adolescent volunteers, beginning in parietal regions and spreading over 5 years to include many frontal and temporal structures. Used with permission, from Thompson et al. (2001).

trols on a number-matching task, thus the findings could be specific to the prefrontal region and not related to effort. In a companion report, no differences in cerebral blood flow were seen between patients and controls on the Continuous Performance Test (CPT), indicating that findings were not likely due to differences in attention (Berman et al., 1986).

Twin studies

Berman et al. (1992) looked at 21 monozygotic twins—8 concordant for schizophrenia, 10 discordant for schizophrenia, and 3 normal twin pairs. Interestingly, hypofrontality during the WCST characterized *all* of the affected twins, compared to the unaffected twins. When MRI parameters were examined, the more an affected twin differed from the unaffected twin in left hippocampal volume, the more they differed in prefrontal cerebral blood flow during the WCST (Weinberger et al., 1992a). The results of these studies encouraged dozens of investigators around the world to make use of newer, more sensitive imaging techniques such as PET and SPECT.

Positron Emission Tomography and Single Photon Emission Computed Tomography Studies

In PET a radioactively labeled tracer is injected into the bloodstream of a patient. The tracer molecules are tagged with a positron emitter that is produced on-site in a cyclotron. When the positrons meet electrons in the subject's brain, two gamma-rays are released at 180° from each other that can be measured by scintillation detectors spaced diametrically in a ring around the subject's head. Images of radioactivity in sections of the brain as a function of time can then be constructed.

The earliest studies evaluated glucose metabolism in the brain with fluorodeoxyglucose (FDG), whereas later developments allowed the examination of cerebral blood flow with $H_2{}^{15}O$ and receptor occupancy with the various pharmaceutical labels for dopamine and serotonin described in Chapter 4. The first PET cameras had a spatial resolution much better than that of xenon-133 but still on the order of 15 mm. The present generation of PET scanners is closer to 3–5 mm or better in all three planes.

Single photon emission computed tomography is done in much the same way as PET in that a radioactively labeled tracer is injected into the patient. However, the tracer emits only a single photon, which means that a collimator (which allows radiation to enter from a specific direction) must be used in the detection ring around the patient to determine where the signal is coming from. Because SPECT does not require a cyclotron, it is much less expensive than PET, although many of the same parameters can be measured, such as cerebral blood flow, with tracers like 99m-hexamethyl-propylene-amine-oxime (HMPAO). Several pharmaceutical tracers have also been developed to measure dopamine and benzodiazepine receptors. Many of the initial problems with quantification have been overcome, and spatial resolution is approaching that of PET.

Resting findings

The finding of hypofrontality in schizophrenic patients by Ingvar and Franzen (1974) led to a large number of FDG studies of resting metabolism in schizophrenic patients. In a review of 25 of these studies, Buchsbaum and Hazlett (1998) found evidence of lower fronto-occipital ratios in 16 of 25 studies where this parameter was available, but it was significant in only 7 (about 32%). In studies in which a frontal/whole-slice ratio was available, levels were lower in 15 of 18 studies but again statistically significant in only 8 (about 44%). Including studies up to the end of 2001, Davidson and Heinrichs (2003) found an effect size of 0.65 for resting hypofrontality in schizophrenic patients. A more recent meta-analysis found a more modest effect size for resting hypofrontality when acute and chronic patients were pooled (Hill et al., 2004a). Nevertheless, prefrontal perfusion in schizophrenic patients and their asymptomatic high-risk relatives has been shown to correlate with other measures such as verbal memory and P300 (Blackwood et al., 1999).

The failure to convincingly demonstrate hypofrontality in the resting state with more sensitive techniques could be related to a number of factors, such as the effects of neuroleptic medication and chronicity. Yet careful analyses of available studies have demonstrated a modest effect of neuroleptic medication on global metabolism but not hypofrontality (Chua and McKenna, 1995; Hill et al., 2004a). While some investigators have found a correlation between chronicity and/or number of hospitalizations, most have not. Studies of drug-naïve patients have found both reduced and increased frontal metabolism (Andreasen et al., 1997; Buchsbaum et al., 1992; Cleghorn et al., 1989; Ebmeier et al., 1993; Vita et al., 1995). However, there may be an overall trend to find hypofrontality in chronic rather than acutely ill patients (Hill et al., 2004a).

Resting studies in other locations have been disappointing. Almost complete overlap between controls and schizophrenic patients was seen in resting temporal-lobe PET studies (Davidson and Heinrichs, 2003). Studies of subcortical structures have been equally disappointing, but thalamic metabolic activity has been linked with volumetric deficits on MRI (Buchsbaum et al., 1996).

Cognitive activation studies

Prefrontal tasks. Following up on the findings of Weinberger et al. (1986) with xenon cerebral blood flow during the WCST, Kawasaki et al. (1993) and Toone et al. (2000) developed similar paradigms for SPECT. However, they failed to find left dorsolateral deficits during the WCST as in the earlier studies. Many studies have used other paradigms to activate the prefrontal cortex. Differences from controls tend to fall in the same range as resting hypofrontality (Hill et al., 2004a). One of the problems with this type of study is that lack of activation could reflect poor performance or a lack of effort rather than dorsolateral prefrontal dysfunction. After all, schizophrenic patients generally perform poorly on these tests.

A way around the problem of poor performance on the task is to design a task that activates the left dorsolateral cortex and that patients do fairly well. Frith et al. (1995) did just this with a paced verbal-fluency task during PET in which patients and controls were asked to think of a word starting with a specific letter every 5 seconds. Using this approach, patients showed the same pattern of activation as the control subjects in the left dorsolateral prefrontal cortex. In the left superior prefrontal cortex, patients failed to show the normal decrease in activity during the fluency task. This was interpreted as reflecting abnormal connectivity between the frontal and temporal cortex.

Unfortunately, subsequent studies were unable to replicate abnormal temporal lobe activity with fluency tasks. However, they did suggest abnormal connectivity between the left dorsolateral prefrontal cortex and the anterior cingulate (Dye et al., 1999; Spence et al., 2000). A neural network analysis was able to correctly classify all 6 healthy subjects and 16 schizophrenic patients on the basis of abnormal connectivity between the left lateral frontal cortex and several brain regions (mostly temporal) during word generation (Josin and Liddle, 2001). It is not often that any measurement correctly classifies all schizophrenic patients; larger studies are necessary to confirm these findings.

Other investigators have looked at the pharmacological effects on brain activation during performance of fluency tasks. A dopamine agonist was found to enhance anterior cingulate activation during verbal-fluency tasks in schizophrenic patients (Dolan et al., 1995). In Color Plate 8–1, deficits are seen in patients in anterior cingulate activation during word fluency. After injection of apomorphine, a dopamine agonist, this deficit is reversed. Activation deficits in the anterior cingulate have also been found with attention-related tasks such as the Stroop task (Carter et al., 1997; Nordahl et al., 2001). On the other hand, it is possible that these observations may be related to a failure to engage this part of the brain in cognitively demanding tasks rather than to attentional deficits (Holcomb et al., 2000).

Memory tasks. Most PET and SPECT studies have found prefrontal and temporal activation deficits during declarative-memory tasks, including free recall of word lists and visual paired-associate learning (Ganguli et al., 1997; Nohara et al., 2000; Ragland et al., 1998). Prefrontal activation deficits during word-list learning can be related to task difficulty and performance in that deficits seem most apparent when the task is demanding (Fletcher et al., 1998). During word encoding, schizophrenic patients have shown left prefrontal and superior temporal activation deficits. However, left prefrontal activation deficits were also seen during word recognition, with additional differences in the left anterior cingulate, left medial temporal, and right thalamic regions (Ragland et al., 2001). Reduced hippocampal activation has been reported during conscious recollection of studied words along with robust activation of the dorsolateral prefrontal cortex during retrieval of poorly encoded material, thus findings are not entirely consistent (Heckers et al., 1998).

With the increasing research emphasis on working memory in recent years, a number of PET studies have assessed brain activation with cerebral blood changes during working-memory tasks such as the N-back task. All have demonstrated either activation deficits or abnormalities in the pattern of activation in schizophrenic patients (Carter et al., 1998; Kim et al., 2003; Meyer-Lindenberg et al., 2001). Prefrontal activation during these tasks was correlated with bilateral inferior parietal activation in controls but not patients, a finding suggesting abnormal prefrontal–parietal interaction in schizophrenia (Kim et al., 2003). Frontotemporal interaction deficits during working-memory tasks were found in another study. In fact, more than half the variance could be accounted for by a single pattern of inferotemoporal, parahippocampal, and cerebellar loadings for patients in contrast to dorsolateral prefrontal and anterior cingulate activity for comparison subjects (Meyer-Lindenberg et al., 2001).

Other investigators have implicated corticocerbellar–thalamic–cortical circuits. In a PET study with practiced- and novel-memory tasks, Crespo-Facorro et al. (1999) found decreased flow in the right anterior cingulate, right thalamus, and bilateral cerebellum during the novel-memory tasks and a similar patern involving the dorsolateral prefrontal cortex rather than the anterior cingulate for the practiced lists. Observations could not be accounted for by effort as similar performance on the tasks was seen in both groups. A follow-up study in chronic patients found a similar pattern (Kim et al., 2000).

A meta-analysis of 25 PET and SPECT studies of schizophrenia indicated that diminished physiological activity in the prefrontal cortex was the most significant finding. However, there was still a 53% overlap of patients and controls in the activation studies, compared to a 57% overlap in the resting studies. No comparable finding was found in the temporal-lobe activation studies, with a 73% overlap between patients and controls (Davidson and Heinrichs, 2003).

Laterality

The findings on language lateralization have been mixed. Reduced lateralization during verbal fluency has been found by some investigators (Artiges et al., 2000; Lewis et al., 1992) whereas others have found essentially no difference in language lateralization between schizophrenic patients and controls (Dye et al., 1999; Spence et al., 2000). There are technical problems in these studies in that some are paced and others are not. With unpaced studies, the patients may not be producing the same number of responses, leading to spurious activation patterns. However, the evidence for language laterality anomalies in schizophrenic patients is not overwhelming.

Clinical correlations

Probably the most cited investigation of symptom correlates is that by Liddle et al. (1992). In this study, 30 stable, medicated schizophrenic patients were examined with PET. Factor scores for psychomotor poverty, reality distortion, and disorganization were correlated with cerebral blood flow in various brain structures. Psychomotor poverty correlated negatively with dorsolateral prefrontal and anterior cingulate blood flow, which is in keeping with the role of the prefrontal cortex in planning and executive function. Positive correlations were seen with psychomotor poverty and dorsal striatal blood flow, which is closely connected with these regions. Disorganization was negatively correlated with right ventral prefrontal blood flow, perhaps reflecting the role of this part of the brain in attention and suppression of interference. Consistent with the MRI studies linking positive symptoms with temporal lobe structures, reality distortion correlated positively with the left parahippocampal region. These findings are illustrated in Figure 8–1. Similar correlations have been found using these symptom factors (Kaplan et al., 1993), but there have been many other imaging investigations of symptomatology using different approaches.

Negative symptoms. Most PET and SPECT studies have found a relationship between chronic negative or deficit symptoms and lower prefrontal metabolism at rest or during activation, which is consistent with Liddle's study (Andreasen et al., 1992; Heckers et al. 1999; Kawasaki et al., 1993; Lahti et al., 2001; Molina Rodriguez et al., 1997; Sabri et al., 1997; Schöder et al., 1996; Wolkin et al., 1992;). Other studies have found variable patterns with negative symptoms associated with relatively higher left midtemporal metabolism in one case (Gur et al., 1995) and lower temporal and ventral prefrontal metabolism in others (Potkin et al., 2002; Sabri et al., 1997). The deficit syndrome has also been found to correlate with hypometabolism in thalamic and parietal regions in addition to the prefrontal region (Tamminga et al., 1992).

Hallucinations. Studies of patients with frequent hallucinations have revealed a somewhat inconsistent pattern that has nevertheless been interpreted to reflect a failure of internal monitoring, as suggested by neuropsychological studies in Chapter 6. During a task in which pa-

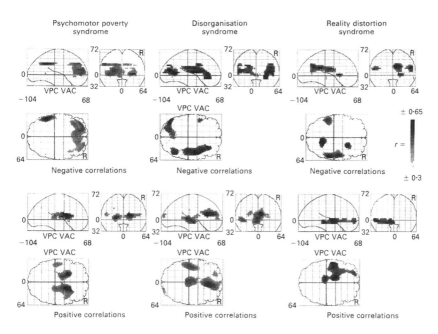

Figure 8–1. Statistical probability maps showing pixels with a significant correlation between cerebral blood flow and psychomotor, disorganization, and reality distortion syndrome scores. Used with permission, from Liddle et al. (1992).

tients were asked to imagine a sentence being spoken in another person's voice, frequent hallucinators had reduced activation in the left middle temporal gyrus and supplementary motor area, compared with that of infrequent hallucinators and controls (McGuire et al., 1995). In contrast to these findings, Busatto et al. (1995) found increased blood flow in the left basal ganglia during a memory task in frequent hallucinators. A limitation of using patients who report frequent hallucinations is that the patients may not be hallucinating at the time.

Several investigators have examined patients during actual auditory hallucinations. Using PET, Cleghorn et al. (1992) found that patients who reported hallucinations during the scan had significantly lower relative metabolism in the auditory cortex than that of patients who did not experience hallucinations. Hallucination scores also correlated positively with relative metabolism in the striatum and anterior cingulate regions. No activation was seen in Broca's area, which suggested that auditory hallucinations are not subvocalizations. However, a subsequent investigation did link activation in this area with the report of hallucinations (McGuire et al., 1993). Flow also tended to be higher in the left anterior cingulate and temporal lobe during hallucinations in this study.

More recent PET studies have implicated a much wider network of involvement during auditory hallucinations (Copolov et al., 2003; Sabri et al., 1997; Silbersweig et al., 1995). Silbersweig et al. (1995) examined five chronic schizophrenic patients with classic auditory verbal hallucinations despite antipsychotic medication. The investigators found the report of auditory hallucinations during scanning to be associated with activations throughout the limbic system including the thalamus, hippocampus, parahippocampus, cingulate gyri, and orbitofrontal cortex. These findings are shown in Color Plate 8–2. A patient who was experiencing visual as well as auditory hallucinations showed activation of visual- and auditory/linguistic-association cortices. Copolov et al. (2003) found that during auditory hallucinations, a network of cortical activations was demonstrated that included bilateral auditory cortex, left limbic regions, and right medial prefrontal regions.

Delusions. Curiously, a similar pattern of activation in mesotemporal and ventral striatal regions has been described in patients experiencing paranoid delusions (Epstein et al., 1999). Other symptoms seem to involve different regions. For example, schizophrenic patients with passivity phenomena (the delusion of being controlled by an outside force) showed hyperactivation of the parietal and cingulate cortices (Spence et al., 1997). Given that these brain regions are involved in attention to internal and external bodily space and the significance of sensory information, these observations make some sense.

Thought disorder. In a large study of 79 schizophrenic patients and 47 healthy controls, Schröder et al. (1996) found that disorganized cluster symptoms were associated with overactivity in the parietal cortex and motor strip, whereas activity in the corpus callosum was decreased. Kawasaki et al. (1996) found a somewhat different pattern with a negative correlation between thought disorder and left medial temporal activity.

Effects of treatment

As in the structural studies, there is always a concern that medication may account for the differences from controls. This does not seem to be the case. Torrey (2002) found very similar results in resting and activation PET/SPECT studies of never-treated schizophrenic patients, although there are obviously many fewer patients in these studies than in those with to more readily available medicated patients. If specific metabolic patterns seem to be associated with symptom clusters, one might expect that antipsychotic medication would have a predictable effect on metabolism as symptoms improve. This does, in fact, seem to be the case—convention neuroleptics tend to decrease prefrontal and cingulate cortex activity whereas striatal and thalamic activity is usually increased (Buchsbaum and Hazlett, 1998).

Somewhat different patterns were evident with atypical antipsychotic medications such as clozapine (Cohen et al., 1997; Potkin et al., 1994). Interestingly, clozapine but not haloperidol reversed abnormal task-activated cerebral blood flow patterns in the anterior cingulate cortex (Lahti et al., 2004). More recent studies have demonstrated that newer atypical neuroleptic medications such as risperidone decrease metabolism in many of the brain regions found to be activated with hallucinations, including the ventral striatum and thalamus (Liddle et al., 2000) and cerebellum (Miller et al., 2001b).

Specificity

Although PET studies measure more subtle brain features in schizophrenia, there is still an overlap with other conditions such as mood disorders. There are also some differences (Davidson et al., 1999b; Drevets, 2000; Videbech, 2000). Many studies have found decreased dorsolateral prefrontal activity in patients with major depression; however, the pattern of activity in the prefrontal cortex is different. In other ventral prefrontal regions such as the orbital prefrontal cortex and subgenual anterior cingulate there is actually an increase in PET metabolism, which to some extent normalizes with treatment with antidepressant medication (Mayberg et al., 1999). In contrast to schizophrenic patients, increases in metabolic activity have been found in the amygdala and thalamus in depressed patients (Drevets, 2000).

Increased activity in the amygdala has been seen in symptom provocation studies in some anxiety disorders and some posttraumatic stress disorders (Davidson et al., 1999b). Other regions such as the medial prefrontal region have also been reported to show decreased cerebral blood flow in posttraumatic stress disorders (Bremner et al., 1999). Obsessive-compulsive disorders show a somewhat different pattern involving both prefrontal and dorsal basal ganglia regions (Stein, 2000).

Patients with conditions closely related to schizophrenia symptomatically, such as schizotypal personality disorder, show activation deficits on PET during the WCST and word-list learning, much like schizophrenic patients. Interestingly, patients with schizotypal personality disorder tend to compensate by activativing alternative brain regions to do the task (Siever et al., 2002).

Functional Magnetic Resonance Imaging Studies

Functional MRI was developed in the early 1990s on the basis of blood oxygenation-level-dependent (BOLD) contrast effect (Ogawa et al., 1992). Simply stated, this effect is based on magnetic susceptibility caused by deoxyhemoglobin. The brain is like a muscle; when you use it the blood flow goes up. However, the vasculature in the brain is extremely well tuned, allowing very small regions to activate for any particular task. When they do, the vascular accommodates, the blood flow goes up, and the proportion of oxy-/deoxyhemoglobin changes. T_2 relaxation times also change because of the magnetic susceptibility caused by deoxyhemoglobin. If an image measured at rest is subtracted from an image collected during cognitive activation, it is possible to detect very subtle changes of blood flow, down to a spatial resolution of 1 mm^3 or less, associated with the task. Parametric mapping algorithms can then be applied to assess the significance of these changes. Functional MRI has a number of advantages over PET in that multiple images can be collected in less than a second, allowing the sequence of activation to be examined. Because the technique does not involve ionizing radiation, it can be done repeatedly in longitudinal studies even in children.

Activation studies

Although fMRI has great potential, not all of its potential has been used in studies of schizophrenic patients. In fact, almost all of the studies to date have covered very familiar territory from xenon cerebral blood flow and PET/SPECT investigations. Prefrontal activation deficits during verbal fluency tasks with variable effects in other brain regions have been reported (Curtis et al., 1998; Yurgelun-Todd et al., 1996b). Anterior cingulate abnormalities during the Stroop task have been described (Carter et al., 2001; Peterson et al., 1999). Several investigators have developed memory paradigms with findings similar to those of PET/SPECT in schizophrenic patients during working-memory and encoding tasks (Callicott et al., 2003; Hofer et al., 2003; Jessen et al., 2003; Manoach et al., 2000; Menon et al., 2001b; Perlstein et al., 2003).

During facial-emotion processing, deficits have been noted in the left amygdala and bilateral hippocampi in schizophrenic patients (Gur et al., 2002). Sensorimotor cortex abnormalities have also been reported with motor tasks (Kodama et al., 2001; Schöder et al., 1995; Wenz et al., 1994). Another study has examined patterns of coherence in fMRI data from the superior temporal cortex in medicated, chronic patients and healthy controls performing an auditory oddball task. Patients had greater synchrony in ventral and medial regions whereas controls had higher synchrony in dorsal and lateral regions. On the basis of these measurements, patients could be separated from controls with 97% accuracy (Calhoun et al., 2004).

Laterality

Schizophrenic patients have been found to have reduced cerebral blood flow in the left superior temporal gyrus and increased cerebral blood flow in the right middle temporal gyrus compared to controls while listening to speech (Woodruff et al., 1997). In a study of monozygotic twins discordant for schizophrenia, language lateralization was decreased in both the affected and unaffected twin compared to that in the healthy twin pairs (Sommer et al., 2004). This finding could suggest that failure to develop lateralization for language may be a genetic vulnerability marker. However, the findings were somewhat at odds with an earlier dichotic listening study in discordant twins, which found smaller right ear advantages only in the affected twin (Ragland et al., 1992).

In a study of first-episode schizophrenic patients, activation abnormalities during a working-memory task in the left dorsolateral prefrontal cortex, left thalamus, and right cerebellum while patients were acutely ill remained disturbed after stabilization 6–8 weeks later. Dysfunction of the right dorsolateral prefrontal cortex, right thalamus and left cerebellum, and cingulate gyrus normalized after stabilization on medication. The results suggested that dysfunction of the left frontothalamocerebellar circuit may be a stable characteristic of schizophrenia, whereas disturbance of right circuitry may be state-dependent (Mendrek et al., 2004). Several other fMRI investigations have examined clinical correlates.

Clinical correlates

Auditory hallucinations have been associated with activation in the inferior frontal/insular, anterior cingulate, bilateral temporal cortex, right thalamus, and left hippocampal/parahippocampal regions (Shergill et al., 2000a). A similar pattern was seen during auditory verbal imagery in schizophrenic patients (Shergill et al., 2000b). However, a different group found mostly bilateral superior temporal gyri, left inferior parietal cortex, and left middle frontal gyrus changes in association with auditory hallucinations (Lennox et al., 2000). Finally, activation of Heschl's gyrus and several other regions including the hippocampus and amygdala has been observed in association with auditory hallucinations (Dierks et al., 1999).

Reduced responsivity of the temporal cortex, especially the right middle temporal gyrus, to external speech has been seen during auditory hallucinations (Woodruff et al., 1997). Right dorsolateral prefrontal cortex dysfunction has also been associated with thought disorder and disorganization symptoms in chronic schizophrenic patients (Menon et al., 2001b; Perlstein et al., 2001). Reduced frontotemporal connectivity has been found in association with severity of hallucinations during a sentence completion task (Lawrie et al., 2002).

Formal thought disorder has been negatively correlated with fMRI signal changes in the left superior and middle temporal gyri and positively correlated with the cerebellar vermis, right caudate, and precentral gyrus (Kircher et al., 2001). Although the findings during auditory hallucinations are consistent with PET/SPECT studies, the disorganization and thought disorder correlates differ somewhat from earlier PET studies, which had implicated ventral prefrontal regions in disorganization.

Are There Patterns of Dysfunction?

There is considerable overlap between comparison subjects and schizophrenic patients on resting measures of metabolic activity across the functional techniques. The studies during activation and in association with particular symptoms are much more consistent. Prefrontal and temporal anomalies are seen with a variety of activation tasks, including those that tap executive function, word fluency, working memory, and encoding. Considering the poor performance of patients on these neuropsychological tests, activation deficits in brain imaging studies should not be too surprising.

Negative symptoms are most often linked with decreased prefrontal metabolic activity, but not in all cases. Most striking are the studies during actual auditory hallucinations, which are associated most often with widespread activation of limbic regions. Other symptom clusters such as disorganization show more lateralized changes involving the prefrontal cortex. Thus, both structural and functional imaging studies point to differences between schizophrenic patients and comparison subjects in prefrontal, temporal, subcortical, and possibly cerebellar regions. What happens to these parameters over time? We will examine the longitudinal changes in these measures and others in the next chapter.

9

Imaging Brain *Chemistry* and the Question of Neuronal Degeneration

In recent years, there has been a renewed interest in neuronal degeneration in schizophrenia (Deutsch et al., 2001; Keshavan, 1999; Knoll et al., 1998; Miller, 1989; Woods, 1998). This is not surprising, as marked deterioration in functioning led Kraepelin to separate dementia praecox from the manic-depressive psychoses. In fact, marked deterioration in social and occupational functioning remains a key criterion for schizophrenia in the DSM-IV. It is a difficult and all-too-common experience for a clinician to watch a patient deteriorate more and more with each breakdown until they are no longer the same person. In my own practice, I have watched high-functioning accountants, lawyers, and doctors become totally disabled and, in some cases, become chronic inpatients, incapable of relating to others in the community.

Another reason for the concept of neuronal degeneration in schizophrenia becoming popular is the suggestion that long-term morbidity in some patients with schizophrenia may be prevented if patients are treated early with neuroleptics (Wyatt, 1991, 1995). This has sparked considerable controversy, with some studies finding a relationship between duration of untreated psychosis and outcome and others, not (Black et al., 2001; Ho et al.; 2000; Loebel et al.;

1992; McEvoy et al., 1991; Norman and Malla, 2001; Rabiner et al., 1986; Szymanski et al., 1996; Waddington et al., 1995; Wyatt and Hunter, 2001; Wyatt et al., 1997).

This chapter will first review some of the longitudinal neuropsychological studies. Structural brain imaging findings in first-episode patients and longitudinal studies in chronic patients will then be discussed. To provide a perspective on the possible causes of longitudinal structural changes, findings from chemical imaging techniques will be reviewed. These techniques are phosphorus magnetic resonance spectroscopy (^{31}P MRS), which opens a window on membrane metabolites, and proton magnetic resonance spectroscopy (^{1}H MRS), which allows us to examine markers of neuronal integrity and glutamatergic metabolites in living patients.

Neuropsychological Investigations

Several investigations have suggested that there is a decline in functioning in schizophrenic patients from premorbid levels. The decline appears to occur in the very early years of illness, as chronic patients seem to have fairly stable scores in the later years of illness (Elliott and Sahakian, 1995; Frith, 1995, Hijman et al., 2003). There is also evidence that, at least in some patients, generalized intelligence after onset of the illness may not be that much different from levels before the illness (Russell et al., 1997). However, these may be the more severe cases; these patients had presented to a childhood psychiatric service and ended up with lower overall scores than those seen in most patients. Thus, there seems to be some difference of opinion as to whether schizophrenic patients show cognitive deterioration, as Kraepelin thought.

What there is some agreement on is that schizophrenic patients show a generalized neuropsychological deficit from the beginning of the illness (Bilder et al., 2000; Hill et al., 2004b). The deficit seems to include both generalized neuropsychological performance difficulties as well as problems with memory and executive function. Does this deficit correlate with the duration of untreated psychosis? Some investigators would argue that the question has not been properly answered because of a number of confounds (Norman and Malla, 2001), but several recent studies have failed to find a correlation with neuropsychological deficits on comprehensive test batteries (Barnes et al., 2000; Ho et al., 2003a; Hoff et al., 2000; Norman et al., 2001).

Despite the large number of neuropsychological investigations, there have been relatively few longitudinal studies. Rund (1998) reviewed 15 longitudinal studies of patients followed for at least 1 year. Almost all of these studies were of chronic patients and the main conclusion drawn was that after the onset of schizophrenia, cognitive deficits are relatively stable over long periods of time. Even patients early in the course of illness showed some stability across neuropsychological batteries with the possible exception of a decline in attentional performance (Bilder et al., 1991; Nopoulis et al., 1994). More recent studies of first-episode patients have generally confirmed these findings (Gold et al., 1999; Hoff et al., 1999). Thus, there seems to be a consensus that there is not much deterioration in cognitive functioning once the illness presents itself. However, this does not rule out the possibility that there are abnormalities in brain growth or neurodegeneration that predate illness onset leading to cognitive deficits at the beginning of the illness. It also does not rule out further changes in brain growth or neurodegeneration after onset of the illness that are not associated with appreciable changes in cognitive function in the traditional sense.

Structural Imaging

First-episode studies

One of the ways to evaluate the issue of progressive changes is to examine differences between schizophrenic patients and comparison subjects at the onset of illness or early on in the illness. The argument for this method is that differences at this stage may represent the effect of an early neurodevelopmental lesion. Torrey (2002) reviewed the CT and MRI findings from studies of never-treated patients and concluded that these patients do have significantly enlarged ventricles but differences in other structures are not as consistent. A similar conclusion was drawn by Shenton et al. (2001) in their review of MRI investigations, with 15 of 19 studies (about 79%) reporting ventricular differences from comparison subjects.

As noted in Chapter 7, the gray-matter deficits seen in first-episode patients are generally less striking than those seen in chronic patients (Gur et al., 1999; Zipursky et al. 1998). Only 5 of 11 studies (about 45%) of whole temporal volume in first-episode patients reviewed by Shenton et al. (2001) found reduced volumes. Eight of 10 (80%) studies found reduced hippocampal volumes but only 1 of 5 (20%) found reduced amygdala volumes. Seven of 10 studies (70%) showed differences in prefrontal volumes in contrast to somewhat weaker findings in chronic patients. Adding more recent reports to the review of Shenton et al. (2001), there is evidence of reduced thalamic volumes in 2 of 3 studies (about 67%), reduced hippocampal volume in 9 of 11 studies (about 82%), and reduced hippocampal and superior temporal gyrus volume in 3 studies (Gilbert et al., 2001; Szeszko et al., 2003). Whether these differences are due to an early neurodevelopmental lesion or to a progressive loss of neuronal tissue beginning just before the onset of symptoms is difficult to determine without longitudinal data.

Longitudinal studies

Early prospective studies of ventricle/brain ratio with computed tomography (CT) failed to show progressive increases after onset of the illness which would be expected with a neurodegenerative disorder (Illowsky et al., 1988; Nasrallah et al., 1986; Vita et al., 1988). Although there were some positive studies after these, there was not much enthusiasm for progressive volumetric changes in schizophrenia until magnetic resonance imaging (MRI) allowed more subtle changes to be examined (Woods, 1998). The first attempts to look at progressive MRI volumetric changes by DeLisi et al. (1992) were essentially negative but as cases were added to the group, progressive enlargement of the left lateral ventricle and reduction of the cerebral hemispheres, right cerebellum, and corpus callosum were detected (DeLisi et al., 1995, 1997b, 1998) with progressive ventricular enlargement in some patients for up to 10 years (DeLisi et al., 2004). Since these reports there have been 16 studies on longitudinal MRI data in schizophrenic patients. All but three (Garver et al., 2000; James et al., 2002; Keshavan et al., 1998) have found progressive changes in various brain structures.

As expected, ventricular enlargement over time was found in many of the longitudinal MRI studies (Cahn et al., 2002; Lieberman et al., 2001; Mathalon et al., 2001; Nair et al., 1997; Rapaport et al., 1997; Sporn et al., 2003). However, different patterns emerged in the various studies. Many found gray-matter changes involving the whole brain (Cahn et al., 2002; Sporn et al., 2003; Wood et al., 2001) whereas others found changes primarily in prefrontal (Ho et al., 2003b) or temporal structures (Jacobsen et al., 1998; Kasai et al., 2003a) or both (Mathalon et al., 2001; Pantelis et al., 2003; Thompson et al., 2001). One study found primarily white-matter loss (Gur et al., 1998). Progressive gray-matter loss has also been found in the parietal (Sporn et al., 2003), cingulate (Pantelis et al., 2003), cerebellar (Pantelis et al., 2003), and thalamic regions (Rapaport et al., 1997). In fact, one of the more dramatic studies found a *dynamic wave* of gray-matter loss beginning in parietal regions and spreading over 5 years to include many frontal and temporal structures (Thompson et al., 2001). Twelve adolescent schizophrenic subjects (mean age, 13.9 years at the first scan) were compared with the same number of healthy controls and patients with psychosis, not otherwise specified. These findings are illustrated in Color Plate 9–1.

The reason for different patterns of progressive changes is not entirely clear. All the studies except three (Garver et al., 2000; Mathalon et al., 2001; Nair et al., 1997) were done in first-episode patients or patients early in their illness. Ventricular enlargement was linked with poor outcome in one study (Lieberman et al., 2001) and frontal white-matter changes with negative symptoms in another (Ho et al., 2003b). Changes over time in the left Heschl guys and planum temporale in superior temporal gyrus have been linked to disorganization symptoms (Kasai et al., 2003b). Whether these changes are specific to schizophrenia is not known. The Kasai et al. (2003a) study did not find progressive changes in the superior temporal gyrus in a group of first-episode mood-disordered patients. However, the Pantelis et al. (2003) study found similar losses in the left parahippocampal, fusiform, orbitofrontal, and cerebellar cortices and cingulate gyri in patients who developed either schizophrenia or mood disorder with psychosis. These results are in keeping with reports of a correlation between illness duration and both gray-matter and hippocampal losses in mood-disordered patients (Lampe et al., 2003; MacQueen et al., 2003).

In such studies, there is an issue of whether progressive volumetric changes in schizophrenia could reflect the effects of medication. Unfortunately, this factor is very difficult to control for, because it is unethical to withhold treatment. Duration of medication treatment is generally not very helpful as this is usually directly related to the length of illness. However, many studies have commented on correlations between dose and volumetric changes. Only one study reported a clear relationship whereas six reported a negative correlation between dose and progressive changes (DeLisi et al., 1995; Gur et al., 1998; Ho et al., 2003b; Jacobsen et al., 1998; Sporn et al., 2003; Wood et al., 2001). Probably the best test of the effects of medication was in the Thompson et al. (2001) study, which included a psychosis, not-otherwise-specified, group. Patients in this group were exposed to neuroleptic medication but did not meet the criteria for schizophrenia. They showed less marked frontal gray-matter loss but no significant temporal gray-matter loss. These results suggest that temporal gray-matter loss might be specific to the development of schizophrenia and unrelated to the effects of medication. A subsequent report from the same research group demonstrated that patients with childhood-onset schizophrenia had significantly greater total frontal, temporal, and parietal gray-matter loss on follow-up after 2.5 years than pediatric patients with transient psychosis and behavior problems who had similar neuroleptic exposure (Gogtay et al., 2004b). Consequently, it does not appear likely that medication accounts for the volume changes.

Functional imaging studies have not provided much insight as to what might explain these progressive volumetric changes in schizophrenic patients. Hypofrontality is more frequently reported in chronic patients than patients ill for less than 2 years (Hill et al., 2004a). Concerns about exposure to ionizing radiation have limited longitudinal PET and SPECT studies, but there are some follow-up data from xenon cerebral blood flow studies. Cantor-Graae et al. (1991) found remarkable stability in hypofrontality in many of the patients from the original xenon cerebral blood flow studies after 18 years. However, this does not provide much information about the early years of illness or the basis of the volume changes. One technique that could provide some information about these observations is MRS.

Phosphorous Magnetic Resonance Spectroscopy Studies

Phosphorous MRS is a noninvasive technique for measuring high-energy phosphates and membrane phospholipid metabolism in the brain (Stanley et al., 2000). Levels of phosphomonoesters (PME) and phosphodiesters (PDE) reflect phospholipid synthesis and breakdown, respectively, whereas levels of adenosine triphosphate (ATP), phosphocreatine (PCr), and inorganic phosphorous (Pi) reflect metabolic activity generally. In recent years, it has become possible to examine the constituents of the PDE peak—phosphoethanolamine (PE) and phosphocholine (PC)—as well as the constituents of the PDE peak—glycerol-phosphoethanolamine (GPE) and glycerol-phosphocholine (GPC)—with proton decoupling or high-field strengths.

Low-field studies

Investigations of first-episode, never-treated schizophrenic patients have been fairly consistent in their findings of decreased PME and increased PDE in prefrontal (Pettegrew et al., 1991; Stanley et al., 1995b) and temporal (Fukuzako et al., 1999a) regions. In the first investigation of never-treated patients, 11 first-episode patients were compared with 10 healthy controls of comparable age, education, and parental education. The schizophrenic patients had significantly reduced levels of PME and Pi and significantly increased levels of PDE and ATP compared to the healthy controls. This pattern does not appear to characterize patients with other neuropsychiatric disorders. However, findings in chronic patients are far less consistent.

Levels of PME have been found to be either normal (Deicken et al., 1994; Volz et al., 1997, 1998, 2000b) or decreased (Fujimoto et al., 1992; Kato et al., 1995; Shiori et al., 1994; Williamson et al., 1991a) in prefrontal regions in chronic patients. Levels of PDE have been found to be both increased (Deicken et al., 1994) and decreased (Yacubian et al., 2002; Volz et al., 1997, 1998, 2000b) in prefrontal regions. Increased levels of PDE have been found in the temporal lobe in one study (Fujimoto et al., 1992) but other studies have failed to confirm this finding (Calabrese et al., 1992; O'Callaghan et al., 1991b; Volz et al., 2000b). Decreased levels of both PME and PDE have also been reported in the cerebellum (Volz et al., 2000b). Although findings are far from consistent, there does seem to be a pattern of increased membrane breakdown metabolites in first-episode, never-treated patients and decreased levels in chronic patients. The Yacubian et al. (2002) study is particularly interesting in that chronic, untreated patients were found to have decreased PDE levels, suggesting that medications did not influence this finding.

Proton decoupled and high-field studies

There have been few ^{1}H-decoupled and high-field ^{31}P MRS studies to date. Potwarka et al. (1999) demonstrated an increase in the broad component under the PDE peak (MP), which may be related to phospholipid vesicles (particularly higher-field strength) as well as a decrease in organic phosphate and PC in the prefrontal region in chronic patients. Bluml et al. (1999) found increased concentrations of GPC, GPE, and PCr in the parietal region. In a high-field (4 Tesla) study of never-treated, first-episode schizophrenic patients, increased levels of GPC were found in the anterior cingulate and decreased levels of PC and GPE in the left thalamus (Jensen et al., 2004). An earlier study of chronic, medicated schizophrenic patients (Jensen et al., 2002) found that GPE was decreased in the anterior cingulate, right prefrontal cortex, and left thalamus but was increased in the left hippocampus and cerebellum in schizophrenic patients. Levels of PE and GPC were decreased in the right prefrontal region and PC was decreased in the anterior cingulate. Thus, more sensitive measures of membrane metabolism seem to confirm the same pattern of increased membrane breakdown products in the anterior cingulate in first-episode patients, with deficits in membrane precursors in the same region in chronic patients. The finding of increased breakdown products in the hippocampus and cerebellum in chronic patients is somewhat unexpected but could be consistent with the progressive loss of volume seen in temporal regions in longitudinal volumetric studies.

What explains the membrane metabolite changes in schizophrenic patients? Some investigators have suggested that they reflect an exaggeration of synaptic pruning, consistent with postmortem reports of a loss of neuropil (Keshavan et al., 2000). Others have suggested that findings could reflect a neurodegenerative process (Williamson and Drost, 2003). Both explanations could be associated with progressive volume losses seen in the MRI studies. However, very different pathological processes are involved with a number of implications for treatment. Unfortunately, ^{31}P MRS is not specific to cell type and does not indicate whether glutamate is involved. ^{1}H MRS can provide some of this information and will be considered next.

Proton Magnetic Resonance Spectroscopy Studies

Proton MRS makes it possible to quantify N-acetylaspartate (NAA), glutamate, glutamine, choline-containing compounds (Cho), phosphocreatine/creatine (PCr), and other metabolites (Bovée, 1991; Miller,

1991). Since NAA is found only in neurons and not in mature glial cells, NAA levels were originally thought to reflect neuronal number (Urenjak et al., 1993). However, recent observations that NAA levels can recover in certain circumstances have suggested that NAA is more likely a marker of neuronal integrity or even mitochondrial dysfunction (Cendes et al., 1997; Clark, 1998; Vion-Dury et al., 1995). Cho contains a number of choline-containing compounds, mostly membrane in origin. Levels of PCr reflect both phosphocreatine and in varying proportions, thus it is difficult to make inferences about high-energy phosphate metabolism from these levels. Levels of NAA, Cho, and PCr can be easily quantified on any clinical magnetic resonance imager.

To quantify glutamate and glutamine, it is necessary to use a short-echo sequence with quantification based on prior knowledge of metabolites (Provencher, 1993; Stanley et al., 1995a). Glutamate is produced from glucose and glutamine. Only 15%–20% of total glutamate is available for release at the synapse (Erecinska and Silver, 1990). About 80% of the stimulus-released glutamate is derived from glutamine (Bradford et al., 1978), so glutamine may be a better indicator of physiological glutamatergic activity. The glutamine measured with ^{1}H MRS includes that from both neurons and glial cells. Glutamate signaling accounts for about 70% to 80% of brain energy consumption (Shulman, 2001).

N-acetylaspartate investigations

Most studies have looked at NAA in chronic patients. Six of 10 studies (about 60%) of temporal regions in medicated and unmedicated chronic patients have shown decreased NAA levels (Bertolino et al., 1996; Buckley et al., 1994; Deicken et al., 1998; Delamillieure et al., 2002; Fukuzako et al., 1995; Heimberg et al., 1998; Kegeles et al., 2000b; Maier et al., 1995; Nasrallah et al., 1994; Yurgelun-Todd et al., 1996a). Levels of NAA in the prefrontal cortex and anterior cingulate have been found to be decreased in only 5 of 10 studies (50%) of medicated and unmedicated patients (Bertolino et al., 1998; Block et al., 2000; Buckley et al., 1994; Bustillo et al., 2002; Cecil et al., 1999; Choe et al., 1994; Deicken et al., 1997; Heimberg et al., 1998; Lim et al., 1998; Stanley et al., 1996). In the thalamus, NAA has been found to be decreased in four of six, or about 67% of studies (Auer et al., 2001; Bertolino et al., 1996; Deicken et al., 2000; Delamillieure et al., 2000a; Ende et al., 2001a; Omori et al., 2000). In the cerebellum one of three studies (about 33%) have shown reduced levels (Deicken et al., 2001b; Eluri et al., 1998; Tibbo et al., 2000).

Studies of first-episode patients have included those on medication and never-treated patients. Renshaw et al. (1995) showed decreased NAA levels in temporal regions in first-episode, medicated patients. First-episode, never-treated patients have been found to have normal levels of NAA in prefrontal and anterior cingulate regions in three of four studies (75%) (Bartha et al., 1997; Cecil et al., 1999; Stanley et al., 1996; Théberge et al., 2003) and decreased levels in medial temporal regions in two of three studies (Bartha et al., 1999; Cecil et al., 1999; Fannon et al., 2003). Because there are fewer reports of decreased NAA levels in prefrontal regions in first-episode patients compared to levels in chronic patients, the possibility arises that neuronal integrity might be compromised with time in schizophrenic patients. There are some technical issues, however. The first-episode studies showing decreases and almost all the chronic studies were based on a ratio of NAA/PCr, which may not be as reliable as values based on the water signal used in studies that did not find differences. Another factor could be the collection techniques used. Differences in NAA T_2 values, which could cause spuriously lower NAA levels, have been reported in schizophrenic patients (Ke et al., 2003). The studies that did not find differences used shorter echo times, which are less vulnerable to this effect.

N-acetylaspartate levels have correlated negatively with length of illness in the anterior cingulate and thalamus (Ende et al., 2001b; Théberge et al., 2003), but no correlation has been found in the hippocampus or prefrontal regions (Deicken et al., 1999; Stanley et al., 1996). In a longitudinal study, frontal NAA levels were reduced at 1 year compared to baseline levels in frontal regions; further longitudinal studies are clearly necessary (Bustillo et al., 2002). Levels of NAA have been correlated with negative and disorganized symptom subtypes (Callicott et al., 2000; Delamillieure et al., 2000b; Fukuzako et al., 1999b), activation of working-memory cortical networks on PET (Bertolino et al., 2000b), and evoked release of striatal dopamine on PET (Bertolino et al., 2000a). Decreased NAA levels are not specific to schizophrenia and are found in a number of other neurological disorders such as Alzheimer disease (Keshavan et al., 2000).

Findings in other psychiatric disorders have been inconsistent, but there is a report of increased NAA levels in the thalamus (Deicken et al., 2001a) and decreased NAA levels in hippocampal and prefrontal regions in bipolar patients (Deicken et al., 2003; Winsberg et al., 2000). Decreased NAA levels have also been found in the caudate and thalamus in obsessive-compulsive patients (Bartha et al., 1998; Fitzgerald et al., 2000). Thus, NAA studies could indicate a loss of neuronal integrity, particularly in chronic patients, which correlates with some symptom types, working-memory deficits, and evoked release of dopamine. However, there are a number of technical issues that need to be resolved, and it appears that the decreased NAA levels can be found in some of the same regions in other conditions.

Glutamate and glutamine investigations

Few studies have attempted to measure glutamate or glutamine. However, Bartha et al. (1997) demonstrated increased glutamine levels in 10 first-episode, never-treated schizophrenic patients compared to 10 healthy volunteers of comaparable age, gender, handedness, and parental education. Increased glutamine levels were not observed in the dorsolateral prefrontal cortex or temporal region (Bartha et al., 1999; Stanley et al., 1996). Other groups have attempted to quantify the general peak region of glutamine, which also includes glutamine and GABA. Increases in this peak have been found in the hippocampus in first-episode, never-treated patients (Cecil et al., 1999) and in the hippocampus and prefrontal regions in chronic medicated and unmedicated patients (Choe et al., 1994; Kegeles et al., 2000b). These findings contrast with the finding of decreased levels for this peak in the anterior cingulate in depressed patients (Auer et al., 2000). These observations suggest that there could be increased glutamatergic activity in several parts of the limbic system that could be associated with decreased NAA and volumetric and phospholipid changes over time.

It is much more feasible to study glutamate and glutamine at higher field strengths that have much higher spatial and spectral resolution. Thus far, only one group has reported data on these metabolites in schizophrenic patients, using this technology. Théberge et al. (2002) found an increase in glutamine in both the left anterior cingulate and thalamus in first-episode, never-treated patients. The increase in glutamine likely indicated increased physiologically active glutamate, as 80% of glutamate released at the receptor is made from glutamine. Most glutamate measured by ^{1}H MRS is not physiologically active and is found throughout the cell. Curiously, chronic patients had decreased levels of both glutamate and glutamine, which could indicate a loss of neurons and/or neuropil (Théberge et al., 2003). While the effects of medication cannot be ruled out, they would be compatible with a degenerative process involving glutamate. Further studies are required to replicate these findings. It is of note that adolescents at high genetic risk for schizophrenia have increased glutamatergic metabolites in the right medial frontal lobe (Tibbo et al., 2004).

Developmental, Neurotrophic, or Excitotoxic?

In Chapter 3, some of the evidence that schizophrenia is a neurodevelopmental disorder was evaluated. While other interpretations are possible for some of the data, there is consensus that something goes wrong early in brain development in many schizophrenic patients. However, this does not exclude the possibility that there may be some sort of degenerative process just before and/or after the onset of the typical symptoms of the disorder. Is there evidence for such a process? Yes and no. There does not seem to be a progression in neuropsychological deficits and many volumetric changes are present in patients at the first episode. But there is striking evidence of volume losses in the first years of illness in an overwhelming number of longitudinal MRI studies. The problem is how to interpret this loss.

Some investigators have taken the view that progressive volume losses could reflect glutamatergic excitotoxic damage analogous to the damage caused by PCP in rats (Coyle, 1996; Deutsch et al., 2001; Olney and Farber, 1995). This view has been sharply criticized, largely because of the absence of gliosis in postmortem studies in schizophrenia, which would be expected with most types of excitotoxicity (Weinberger and McClure, 2002). While this is true, it has been pointed out that there are examples of tissue loss associated with apoptosis that do not necessarily lead to gliosis (Bredesen, 1995; Coyle, 1996; Margolis et al., 1994). As indicated in Chapter 4, reversible tissue loss in the hippocampus with stress is likely mediated by glutamatergic receptors and not associated with gliosis (McEwen, 1999). There is also evidence of glutamate-induced apoptosis at a synaptic level, which could account for the loss of neuropil without cell death observed in imaging and postmortem studies (Mattson et al., 1998). Another criticism made is that the genes associated with apoptosis are not found in postmortem studies (Weinberger and McClure, 2002). Because postmortem tissue is obtained in most cases from chronic patients, it would not be surprising to see that these genes were not activated, as the apoptotic process likely occurred many years before. Consequently, the possibility of excitotoxic damage cannot be completely ruled out.

Pettegrew et al. (1991) argued that the changes in membrane metabolites found on ^{31}P MRS at the onset of illness could reflect exaggerated cortical pruning leading to a loss of neuropil. Abnormal pruning could be caused by many genes regulating neurotrophic factors involved in normal brain growth and development. However, there is now some direct evidence of increased glutamatergic activity in first-episode schizophrenic patients from ^{1}H MRS studies (Théberge et al., 2002, 2003) indicating an increase in glutamatergic metabolites in the anterior cingulate and thalamus followed by low levels of these metabolites in chronic patients. It is also possible that regions showing volume loss and glutamatergic deficits over time may be functionally disconnected by the disease process, leading to plastic atrophic changes in these regions.

A more plausible explanation would be that there is both a neurodevelopmental and neurodegenerative process. A programmed loss of neuropil in the heteromodal cortex may lead to disinhibition of limbic regions, resulting in excitotoxic damage. The fact that the volume losses are widespread throughout the cortex whereas the glutamatergic changes seem to be localized to limbic stuctures such as the anterior cingulate and thalamus seems to be compatible with a two-stage disease process.

While the cause of volume losses in the first few years of illness is not clear, there can be little doubt that there are changes in the brain after the onset of symptoms not unlike the cascade of changes that occur in the heart and other parts of the body after the heart starts to fail. In the latter case, these changes became understandable with the circulatory system. It is now time to assemble the pieces of the puzzle in schizophrenia. The next chapter will examine the regions most likely to be part of the final common pathway that leads to symptoms such as hallucinations, delusions, and flat affect.

Pieces of the Puzzle: Likely Components of the Final Common Pathway

Have the brain imagers joined the neuropathologists and molecular biologists in the graveyard? One could conclude that this is indeed the case from the meta-analyses of both structural and functional findings in schizophrenic patients. Why do we see so many different patterns of findings in patients who presumably suffer from the same disorder? If there is a final common pathway, why do all patients not have the same findings? These are not easy questions to answer. Part of the answer has to be that multiple regions are affected in schizophrenia and these regions are interconnected in functional circuits. Damage to any part of the circuit would cause the entire circuit to fail.

A useful analogy would be the frontal lobe syndrome in neurology. Patients with this syndrome demonstate apathy, working-memory deficits, and deficits in executive function much like those in schizophrenic patients. Obviously, damage to the frontal cortex caused by a stroke or other diseases can lead to this syndrome. However, damage to subcortical regions including the caudate and dorsomedial thalamus or the white matter connecting these regions can also lead to this syndrome (Mesulam, 2002). The frontal lobes, caudate, and dorsomedial thalamus are connected by white-matter tracts, so when one part of this circuit is damaged, the whole circuit fails to perform its function and a frontal lobe syndrome results, even though the damage may be elsewhere. Thus, examination of the brain regions most often affected in schizophrenia could help us sketch out the neuronal circuits involved in this disorder. This chapter will highlight some of these regions and the evidence for their involvement.

Prefrontal Cortex

The most elegant case for the involvement of the prefrontal cortex in schizophrenia has been made by Goldman-Rakic (1999). Schizophrenic patients have difficulty with a number of tasks involving the prefrontal cortex, most notably working-memory tasks. These tasks are clearly dependent upon activation of the middle frontal gyrus. Interestingly, this region is also involved in the guidance of eye movements with which schizophrenic patients have trouble. Thus, Goldman-Rakic (1999) speculated that schizophrenia could be associated with abnormalities in the circuits necessary to keep information online. While the evidence for working-memory deficits and eye-tracking abnormalities in schizophrenia is good, not all schizophrenic patients perform poorly on working-memory or eye-tracking tasks.

The prefrontal cortex undergoes substantial revision during adolescence, particularly in regard to excitatory input to pyramidal cells in the supragranular layers, which may coincide with the onset of schizophrenia (Lewis, 1997). However, there is also evidence of abnormalities from postmortem studies done by Goldman-Rakic's group and others (Glantz and Lewis, 1997; Lewis et al., 2001; Selemon and Goldman-Rakic, 1999). Increased neuronal density was observed in prefrontal areas 9 and 46, suggesting a loss of neuropil in these regions, which contrasted with findings from patients with Huntington disease and schizoaffective disorders. Other investigators have found a reduction in synaptophysin reactivity consistent with disturbed synaptic transmission and deficits in parvalbumin-immunoreactive vararicosities in the prefrontal regions of schizophrenic patients, indicative of fewer projections from the mediodorsal prefrontal cortex (Glantz and Lewis, 1997; Lewis et al., 2001). Curiously, there was not a loss of neurons or glial cell changes in these regions but the cortex was found to be about 12% thinner in these studies. This amount approximates the difference seen between schizophrenic patients and controls in magnetic resonance imaging (MRI) studies (Selemon et al., 2002). One of the problems with this argument is that the MRI studies produced good evidence for gray-matter differences in the temporal lobe and other regions but the data for prefrontal differences were by far the weakest and were questionable at best. This raises the possibility that the postmortem studies were done on a small number of patients who were different in some way, or the volume losses may be a secondary phenomenon related to plastic and/or neurodegenerative processes in the brain.

Goldman-Rakic (1999) pointed out further evidence from functional imaging studies for the involvement of the middle prefrontal gyrus in schizophrenia. Patients often have diminished cerebral blood flow at rest and during cognitive activation in this region. However, as indicated in Chapter 8, this data are not very striking, with a 53% overlap between controls and patients on activation tasks (Davidson and Heinrichs, 2003). There also appears to be an issue of performance load. When the task is made easy enough for the patients to perform as well as controls, no activation deficits are seen in prefrontal regions (Frith et al., 1995). Performance on some of these tasks is dependent upon dopamine, which is clearly involved in schizophrenia. For example, it has already been pointed out that working-memory deficits can be reversed by D_1 receptor stimulation. Antipsychotic medications also likely impair working-memory performance by down-regulation of D_1 receptors in the prefrontal cortex (Castner et al., 2000). Yet the evidence for the involvement of D_1 receptors in schizophrenia is very weak. Postmortem evidence has not been convincing and early positron emission tomography (PET) studies have not been replicated.

Weinberger et al. (2001) have suggested that genetic polymorphisms affecting prefrontal function may be susceptibility alleles for schizophrenia. The candidate put forward was a functional polymorphism in the COMT gene that alters dopamine levels in the prefrontal cortex. As previously noted, both schizophrenic patients and normal subjects with this polymorphism perform poorly on the WCST (Egan et al., 2001). Unfortunately, case-control association studies with schizophrenia have been mixed (de Chaldée et al., 1999; Palmatier et al., 1999), but it is possible that this gene may be one of the many that increases the risk of developing schizophrenia, much as the apolipoprotein (APO) E4 allele increases the risk for Alzheimer disease.

Many investigators have linked structural and functional imaging findings with negative symptoms in schizophrenia with varying success (reviewed in Chapters 7 and 8). It would be surprising if connections were not found, as neurological patients with frontal lobe syndrome demonstrate many symptoms suggestive of negative symptoms such as apathy and problems with executive function and planning. However, no one would suggest that an older person with a frontal lobe syndrome caused by a stroke suffers from schizophrenia. Other symptoms are required but the greatest obstacle for the prefrontal theorists to overcome has been explaining how prefrontal dysfunction can lead to positive symptoms such as hallucinations.

Although striatal D_2 receptor hyperactivity has been linked to positive symptoms in schizophrenia, there is also evidence of hyperactivity of D_2 receptors in cortical regions. In fact, under conditions of NMDA and GABA blockade, D_2 receptor agonists cause burst firing of pyramidal neurons that can be reversed by haloperidol (Wang and Goldman-Rakic, 2004). Thus, the prefrontal cortex could play a role in positive symptoms. As indicated earlier in Chapter 2, the prefrontal cortex has *delay* neurons that order the sequence of neuronal activity by inhibition. If these neurons were not functioning properly (which would be expected with a loss of neuropil), then perseveration of neural activity in language modules of the prefrontal cortex could lead to a run-on thought process perceived as a hallucination (Goldman-Rakic, 1999). In support of this, it has been shown that bilateral lesions of the prefrontal cortex in primates prevent the development of hallucinatory-like behavior induced by amphetamines (Castner and Goldman-Rakic, 2003).

On the whole, the case for the involvement of the prefrontal cortex in schizophrenia is almost as strong as that for the involvement of dopamine. However, it is difficult for a prefrontal anomaly to be the sole cause of such widespread findings in these patients. The prefrontal cortex is connected to almost every other region hypothesized in schizophrenia, but how could a loss of neuropil or a genetic polymorphism in this region lead to all the other findings? Clearly other regions must also be involved in a primary way.

Anterior Cingulate Cortex

One of the regions closely connected to the prefrontal cortex is the anterior cingulate, which is a phylogenetically older part of the brain and part of the limbic system. The best evidence for the involvement of the anterior cingulate in schizophrenia comes from the post-mortem work of Francine Benes and her group. Essentially, there were three findings. First, an increase in glutamatergic vertical axons in the anterior cingulate was found. Second, a decrease in GABAergic interneurons leading to a compensatory up-regulation of GABA$_A$ receptors on postsynaptic pyramidal neurons was seen. Finally, a miswiring of dopaminergic afferents away from pyramidal neurons to GABAergic interneurons was suggested (Benes et al., 1987, 1991a, 1992a, 1992b, 1997). Increased concentrations of presynaptic proteins in the anterior cingulate cortex have also been observed by another group (Gabriel et al., 1997), which might be consistent with these findings.

Although some GABAergic abnormalities have been found in other psychiatric conditions, these observations have some interesting implications. Increased dopaminergic activity associated with stress would tend to exacerbate underlying deficits in GABAergic interneurons. These neurons are inhibitory and regulate glutamatergic pyramidal cell firing. Dopamine tends to inhibit GABAergic activity so an increased dopaminergic input would lead to increased glutamatergic activity and perhaps apoptosis and neurodegeneration similar to that seen with the PCP animal models in Chapter 4. Hyperinnervation of GABA cells by the dopamine system could explain why blockade of dopamine receptors leads to improvement in psychotic symptoms (Benes, 2000). Another explanation for decreased GABAergic activity in the anterior cingulate could be decreased NMDA stimulation. A recent study from Benes' group found a decreased density of GABA interneurons that express the NMDA NR$_{2A}$ subunit, although this decrease was also seen in bipolar patients (Woo et al., 2004). Tamminga et al. (2000) have suggested that the source of the deficient NMDA input may be the hippocampus. The two structures are closely connected and there is ample evidence implicating the hippocampus in schizophrenia, so this may be a possibility.

The impairment of normal habituation in schizophrenia manifested by prepulse inhibition and P50 and P300 event-related potentials (ERP) abnormalities would be consistent with deficient GABAergic activity in the anterior cingulate and other regions. The attentional deficits shown by these patients on tests such as the Continuous Performance Test (CPT) would also be consistent with anterior cingulate involvement in schizophrenia. The case for structural brain imaging abnormalities in the anterior cingulate is weak but functional imaging studies have been much more consistent, with activation deficits on the Stroop task (Carter et al., 1997; Nordahl et al., 2001) and the reversal of anterior cingulate deficits during word fluency tasks with a dopamine agonists. Magnetic resonance spectroscopy (MRS) studies also point to the anterior cingulate; an increase in glutamatergic metabolites was found in never-treated, first-episode patients and decreased levels in chronic patients with proton MRS (Théberge et al., 2002, 2003). Phosphorus MRS studies have found increased membrane breakdown products in first-episode patients, followed by a deficit in membrane metabolites in the anterior cingulate as well (Jensen et al., 2002, 2004). The MRS findings are consistent with the postmortem increase in vertical axons and a subsequent neurodegenerative process, as suggested by Benes (2000).

The anterior cingulate not only plays a role in attention and response selection but is also important in determining the salience of stimuli and integrating affect into behavior (Devinsky and Luciano, 1993). Consequently, it should play some role in negative symptoms. Liddle et al. (1992) found that both anterior cingulate and prefrontal cerebral blood flow correlated with psychomotor poverty symptoms. The functional imaging studies of hallucinating patients discussed in Chapter 8 have invariably found the anterior cingulate to be activated. However, almost all the limbic system is activated in association with hallucinations, so it is difficult to elucidate a special role for the anterior cingulate. As with the prefrontal cortex, the case is good for involvement, but not exclusive involvement, in schizophrenia.

Temporal Structures

Several temporal lobe structures have been implicated in the pathophysiology of schizophrenia: the hippocampus, amygdala, and superior temporal gyrus. Each will be considered separately below.

Hippocampus

It has long been known that the hippocampus must be involved in schizophrenia. Bogerts (1997) related the case of Ernst Wagner, a respected and successful teacher from a village near Stuttgart, Germany who in 1913 stabbed his wife and 4 children, shot and killed 8 villagers, wounded 12 others, and burned down several buildings.

Subsequent psychiatric evaluation revealed that he had suffered from long-standing persecutory ideas that eventually led him to destroy his imagined enemies. Kraepelin diagnosed him as suffering from paranoia arising from psychological distress from having practiced sodomy for 12 years. Schneider, another prominent psychiatrist, diagnosed a subtype of schizophrenia caused by a brain disease. It turned out that Schneider was right. Wagner's brain was found many years later in the Vogt collection of brain specimens. In his left posterior parahippocampal cortex was a clear invagination likely related to a disruption of limbic cortical development. Schizophrenia-like psychoses have also been reported in some patients with temporal lobe seizures affecting medial temporal structures. Often delusions, hallucinations, and thoughts of being controlled or influenced are seen in these patients (Slater and Beard, 1963).

The hippocampus is implicated by almost any line of investigation that has been attempted. It is vulnerable to hypoxia early in brain development, and animal lesion studies early in brain development lead to the development of dopaminergic hyperresponsivity (Lipska et al., 1992, Lipska and Weinberger, 1993). Postmortem studies have demonstrated atrophy, pyramidal loss, and pyramidal disarray and postmortem neurochemical studies have found increased dopamine concentrations, decreased GABA uptake, and glutamatergic dysfunction (Benes 2000; Bogerts, 1997). Studies in living patients have highlighted the problems that schizophrenic patients have with memory and context analysis. Bogerts (1997) argued that dissociation between higher neocortical cognitive activities and the phylogenetically older brain areas including the hippocampus leads to misinterpretation of surroundings and the positive symptoms of the illness.

There is ample evidence from structural and functional imaging as well. Most MRI studies of chronic and first-episode patients show decreased hippocampal volumes. The most striking of these are the studies of identical twins linking hippocampal deficits to prefrontal activation deficits (Suddath et al., 1990; Weinberger et al., 1992a). Some temporal activation deficits have been found on positron emission tomography (PET) and functional MRI with memory paradigms, but more convincing evidence comes from the examination of patients experiencing hallucinations, which almost always involves the hippocampus (see Chapter 8). However, hallucinations are also associated with activation throughout the limbic system and volumetric deficits are not limited to the hippocampus.

Amygdala

Like the hippocampus, the amygdala has interconnections with the cortex, the ventral striatum, thalamus, and brain stem. It has a much different function in that it plays a role in attaching emotional significance to environmental stimuli. When the amygdala is damaged on both sides in adults, the Klüver-Bucy syndrome results. This is primarily characterized by a lack of fear and an inappropriate tendency to explore all stimuli. Curiously, damage to the amygdala early in development in animals does not lead to these behaviors. In fact, the animals demonstrate withdrawal and passivity (Bachevalier, 1994). Damage to the amygdala in humans may also lead to symptoms suggestive of schizophrenia. Fudge et al. (1998) described a case of a young woman with prominent hallucinations and delusions who later developed negative symptoms. It was later found that she had scarring and hamartias in the basolateral nucleus of her left amygdala.

Schizophrenic patients have impaired emotional processing in tasks that require recognition of facial emotion and in social cognition. This could indirectly implicate the amygdala (Archer et al., 1992; Kohler et al., 2000; Walker et al., 1984). However, these findings may reflect broader performance deficits (Kerr and Neale, 1993). Most structural imaging studies of chronic schizophrenic patients have found smaller amygdala volumes than those of controls, although this does not appear to be the case for first-episode patients (Shenton et al., 2001). Functional studies are few but impaired amygdala activation has been found during visual emotional-processing tasks (Gur et al., 2002; Paradiso et al., 2003; Taylor et al., 2002; Williams et al., 2004). The amygdala is also known to regulate dopamine release in the ventral striatum (Haber and Fudge, 1997). Thus there is considerable evidence to add the amygdala to the list of brain regions that could be involved in schizophrenia.

Superior temporal gyrus

The superior temporal gyrus and its subdivisions, the Heschl gyrus and the planum temporale, are involved in language processing. Because auditory hallucinations are characteristic features of schizophrenia, abnormalities in these regions might be expected. However, only in recent years has this region been examined in any detail. Probably the strongest evidence comes from MRI volumetric studies. About 67% of studies show volume reductions in the superior temporal gyrus (Shenton et al., 2001). Both prominent hallucinations and thought disorder seem to be linked with these volume reductions (Barta et al., 1990; Shenton et al., 1992). While many other volumetric deficits seem to be found in mood-disordered patients, superior temporal deficits do not seem to characterize first-episode bipolar patients (Hirayasu et al., 2000).

More recently, postmortem studies have found reduced pyramidal cell somal volumes in layer 3 of areas 41 and 42 of the auditory association cortex, suggesting a deficit in the feedforward circuits to other parts of the cortex (Sweet et al., 2004). Functional imaging studies are not as convincing as structural studies. Activation deficits have been reported during word-encoding tasks in the superior temporal gyrus but are not limited to this region (Ragland et al., 2001). The association between volumetric deficits and hallucinations and thought disorder might be expected to predict superior temporal activation anomalies with positive symptoms. Superior temporal activation has been observed in association with auditory hallucinations in some but not all functional imaging studies. The more common pattern is widespread activation throughout the limbic system (see Chapter 8). However, the volumetric studies would be reason enough to consider this region in schizophrenia.

Ventral Striatum

As discussed in Chapter 2, the nucleus accumbens occupies a unique position in the brain. It integrates glutamatergic inputs from functionally different parts of the brain: the medial prefrontal cortex, the anterior cingulate cortex, and limbic structures in the temporal lobe such as the hippocampus and amygdala. Projections go to the mediodorsal and reticular nuclei of the thalamus, which in turn project back to the prefrontal and anterior cingulate cortices. This completes the limbic basal ganglia–thalamocortical neuronal circuit described in Chapter 2.

Stevens (1973) was one of the first investigators to point out the importance of the ventral striatum and other parts of the limbic system in schizophrenia. More recently, Heimer (2000) has reviewed the evidence for the involvement of the basal forebrain in this disorder. Postmortem data have suggested that there may be neuronal loss in this region (Pakkenberg, 1990). In contrast, a more recent study has shown an increase in volume (Lauer et al., 2001). In vivo studies are limited by virtue of the size of the nucleus accumbens and its location, which is associated with susceptibility artifacts on MRI. It is also difficult to anatomically separate the nucleus accumbens from the rest of the striatum. Even so, nucleus accumbens volumes have been correlated with thought disorder in childhood schizophrenia (Ballmaier et al., 2004).

The nucleus accumbens is the main projection target of the A10 dopamine neurons projecting from the ventral tegmentum. It is now possible to separate the ventral from the dorsal striatum with high-resolution PET. While this does not completely isolate the nucleus accumbens, there is evidence of increased ^{18}F fluorodopa uptake in the ventral striatum (McGowan et al., 2004). In Chapter 4, it was noted that all known antipsychotic drugs affect dopamine in some way, and the most likely site of action is the hyperpolarization of A10 dopaminergic neurons projecting to the nucleus accumbens. Consequently, there is considerable evidence for the involvement of the nucleus accumbens in schizophrenia.

Thalamus

Andreasen (1997) pointed out that the word *thalamus* in Greek means marriage bed, an appropriate term for a brain structure that facilitates connections. As indicated in Chapter 2, the thalamus is part of the basal ganglia–thalamocortical circuits. The thalamus plays a major role in gating or filtering information. Because it is common for patients to complain of sensory overload and difficulties in concentrating on neuropsychological tasks, thalamic dysfunction has been suggested in schizophrenia (Andreasen, 1997; Jones, 1997).

The thalamus is a complicated structure consisting of several nuclei with unique connections. The mediodorsal nucleus has connections with the dorsolateral prefrontal cortex and is important in memory and attention (Burgess et al., 2003; Krasnow et al., 2003). The pulvinar nucleus is connected to the prefrontal and temporal cortices and plays a role in visual and possibly auditory attention (Grieve et al., 2000; Wester et al., 2001). The centromedian nucleus, which is one of the intralaminar nucei, has sensorimotor and prefrontal connections. Damage to intralaminar nuclei can cause attentional and executive impairment similar to frontal lobe damage (Van der Werf et al., 2000). Finally, the reticular nucleus, which receives limbic input from the temporal lobe, surrounds the other nuclei and influences their activity, indicating a role in arousal and consciousness.

Postmortem studies have found abnormalities in several nuclei. Volumetric anomalies have been found in the mediodorsal (Byne et al., 2002; Danos et al., 2003; Pakkenberg, 1990; Popken et al., 2000; Young et al., 2000), pulvinar (Byne et al., 2002; Danos et al., 2003), and ventral lateral posterior nuclei (Danos et al., 2002). Abnormal glutamate receptor expression, vesicular and cell-surface transporters, and intracellular proteins associated with membrane-bound transporters have also been found in postmortem studies of the thalamus in schizophrenic patients (Meador-Woodruff et al., 2003).

Magnetic resonance imaging studies have also provided convincing evidence of thalamic abnormalities in schizophrenic patients, with the overwhelming majority finding volumetric deficits (see Chapter 7). Functional imaging studies have been less consistent but decreased glucose metabolism has been reported (Buchsbaum et al., 1996; Clark et al., 2001). Activation abnormalities in the thalamus during memory, object recognition, and attention tasks have been reported as well (Heckers et al., 2000; Manoach et al., 2000; Volz et al., 1999). A more recent study has attempted to assess the contribution of individual nuclei. Although there were no overall thalamic differences from controls, schizophrenic patients had significantly lower glucose metabolism in the mediodorsal and centromedian nuclei while glucose metabolism was higher in the pulvinar nucleus. Lower pulvinar metabolism was associated with hallucinations and lower mediodorsal metabolism was associated with negative symptoms (Hazlett et al., 2004).

The thalamus is central to attention, sensory processing, and conscious experience, all functions that could be involved in schizophrenia. It is also implicated by considerable direct evidence of postmortem and in vivo abnormalities.

Cerebellum

The cerebellum has traditionally been considered to play an exclusive role in the control of movements. While soft neurological signs are often seen in schizophrenic patients that implicate the cerebellum in schizophrenia, there is increasing evidence that the cerebellum is also critical for many cognitive processes because of the connections with the thalamus and prefrontal cortex (Middleton and Strick, 2000). Andreasen (1996) proposed that schizophrenic symptoms may be related to one or more neurodevelopmental defects leading to impaired connections between these regions and poor coordination of mental activity.

Although cerebellar abnormalities have been found in schizophrenic patients (Heath et al., 1979; Weinberger et al., 1980), a recent study has failed to find any global structural differences in volumes, cell numbers, or Purkinje cell volumes from controls (Andersen and Pakkenberg, 2003). Further evidence can be seen in structural CT and MRI studies but the findings are not overwhelming, with fewer than 50% of studies finding statistically significant differences. Somewhat more convincing is the finding of midline developmental abnormalities, which are found much more frequently and may be linked to the cerebellar abnormalities (see Chapter 7). Finally, several PET studies have found cerebellar activation deficits during tasks that engage the cerebellum in normal subjects (Crespo-Facorro et al., 1999; Kim et al., 2000). Consequently, the evidence seems to be mounting for the involvement of the cerebellum in schizophrenia.

So How Do They Fit Together?

Although there is considerable variability in the findings from any individual patient or study, there is also surprising agreement about the brain structures that are likely to be involved in schizophrenia: the prefrontal cortex, anterior cingulate, hippocampus, amygdala, superior temporal gyrus, ventral striatum, thalamus, and cerebellum. Some investigators might include the inferior parietal cortex and dorsal striatum, but the case for these brain structures is not convincing.

So how do they all fit together? We know that dopamine has to be accounted for in any model of schizophrenia. Many of the regions are connected by glutamatergic neurons. An early neurodevelopmental anomaly seems likely, but a reasonable case can also be made for a secondary neurodegenerative process of some type. What about the structural and functional brain imaging correlates of actual symptoms such as hallucinations? The next two chapters will consider some of the possible configurations of the final common pathway of schizophrenia.

Early Models of the Final Common Pathway I. Disconnection and Coordination

It is clear from the previous chapter that many brain regions are involved in schizophrenia. This chapter and Chapter 12 will examine some of the early attempts to put the clues together into a coherent whole, just as Harvey did when he realized that with venous valves, blood flowed not away from but back to the liver, thus raising the possibility of a circulatory system. Models that involve disconnection and coordination of information processing will be considered in this chapter, and the next chapter will examine models that depend on basal ganglia–thalamocortical circuits.

The models chosen for discussion include those that are based on some concept of how dysfunction in different parts of the brain could lead to the symptoms of schizophrenia. The list is not exhaustive but does highlight models that have either received considerable attention or offer a unique perspective on how various observations from postmortem psychophysiological and brain-imaging studies can be made understandable. Many investigators have come up with similar ideas about possible configurations. Wherever possible, these models are considered together under the same general explanation.

Aberrant Lateralization

One of the earliest attempts to put the pieces together suggested that schizophrenia reflects a failure to develop normal asymmetry. Modern interest in asymmetry in schizophrenia dates to Flor-Henry's (1969) observation that schizophrenia-like psychosis is more common in temporal lobe epilepsy when there is a left-sided focus. Gruzelier (1984, 1999) proposed a hemispheric-imbalance model in which symptoms reflecting relatively transient excitation were associated with right-hemisphere dysfunction whereas symptoms reflecting more persistent withdrawal were associated with underactivity of the left hemisphere. These asymmetries were suggested to arise from the influences of genes, hormones, and early experience.

Crow (1990a, 1990b, 1995, 1997a, 1997b, 1998) took the idea a step further. He reasoned that there is a genetic diversity in the evolution of the specifically human characteristic of language that has developed as a result of progressive hemispheric specialization. Because patients with schizophrenia often show lesser structural and functional asymmetries, symptoms may reflect a failure to develop language dominance on one side of the brain. He argued that hemispheric specialization allowed acoustically coded information to be retained for a few seconds in the dominant hemisphere so that a visuospatial sketch pad could be activated in the nondominant hemisphere, allowing an executive function to determine the direction of thought. If there was a disruption in the coordination of these two language processes, possibly caused by impaired callosal connections between the hemispheres, the result would be a disrupted train of thought and a breakdown in the distinction between *you* and *I*. The most likely location for the cerebral dominance gene (and genes causing schizophrenia) was suggested to be the pseudoautosomal region of the sex chromosomes.

Mechanism of symptoms

There have been many theories on how psychotic symptoms arise as a result of laterality anomalies. One of the more controversial ideas was proposed by Jaynes (1977), who argued that at one time humans were not truly conscious. Their brains were split in two: the executive part in the nondominant hemisphere was called *god* and the other part in the dominant hemisphere was *man*, which followed god. Considerable evidence for this view was marshalled from what we know about early civilizations. Sometime around 1200 BC, the nondominant hemisphere was inhibited by the present dominant hemisphere, leading to true consciousness and the development of civilization as we know it. Schizophrenia was seen as a throwback to the bicameral mind in which the voice of the nondominant hemisphere would be experienced as *god*.

Another interesting suggestion was offered by Nasrallah (1985). He argued that split-brain patients who had commissurotomies to treat their epilepsy actually have two distinct and separate selves. If schizophrenic patients had defective interhemispheric integration, the right hemisphere could become an alien intruder, leading to thought insertion and delusions of passivity. Interestingly, Nasrallah (1985) pointed out that there is a report of a paranoid patient who went into complete remission following a callosotomy.

The evidence

A variety of hemispheric anomalies in postmortem studies and in skin conductance, evoked-potentials, and electroencephalographic investigations in schizophrenic patients have supported anomalous lateralization in schizophrenia (Gruzelier and Flor-Henry, 1979). While neuropsychological investigations have found bilateral hemispheric impairment, an argument has been made that deficits are more prominent on tests sensitive to left temporal and parietal function (Abrams and Taylor, 1979). Subsequent CT studies have suggested that ventricular enlargement is greater on the left than on the right side. In some cases, even a reversal of asymmetry was found (Nasrallah, 1986).

There are now considerable CT and MRI imaging data for lateralized structural abnormalities in schizophrenia. Crow (1990b) found seven CT and MRI studies in which there was significant diagnosis by hemisphere interaction in temporal regions. Subsequent MRI studies also found some support for reduced or reversed cerebral asymmetries (Bilder et al., 1999; Bullmore et al., 1995; DeLisi et al., 1997a; Sharma et al., 1999). There is also structural brain-imaging evidence against the lateralization hypothesis. Probably the strongest contrary evidence comes from the National Institute of Mental Health (NIMH) MRI study of discordant twin pairs, which found changes in lateral ventricular and hippocampal volumes on both sides of the brain (Suddath et al., 1990). Crow (1999) pointed out that there was a left-sided loss of posterior temporal gray matter in the affected twin but there was no difference between discordant twins, affected and unaffected twins, on measures of Sylvian fissure asymmetry (Bartley et al., 1993). However, detailed postmortem and brain-imaging studies of the planum temporale have failed to find convincing evidence of reduced or reversed asymmetry (Shapleske et al., 1999). A more recent MRI investigation of cerebral asymmetry in familial and nonfamilial schizophrenic patients and their unaffected relatives has failed to replicate earlier findings as well (Chapple et al., 2004).

The findings from functional imaging studies reviewed in Chapter 8 have been somewhat stronger but still mixed. Gur et al. (1994) found impaired lateralization of xenon cerebral blood flow during verbal tasks sensitive to left-hemisphere function and facial memory tasks sensitive to right-hemisphere function. There is some PET and SPECT evidence of a lack of left–right asymmetry of dopamine transporter in the striatum in schizophrenic patients (Hsiao et al., 2003; Laasko et al., 2000). PET and SPECT studies of verbal fluency have found both lateralization anomalies (Artiges et al., 2000; Lewis et al., 1992) and normal lateralization during verbal tasks (Dye et al., 1999; Spence et al., 2000), although Crow (2000) argued that there may be more bilateral representation of word generation in patients than in controls in the Spence et al. (2000) study.

Functional MRI investigations have shown a decrease in cerebral blood flow on the left side along with an increase on the right side in schizophrenic patients listening to speech (Woodruff et al., 1997). Another fMRI study of discordant monozygotic twins has found decreased language lateralization for both affected and unaffected twins, which might be expected if a gene predisposing to schizophrenia is also related to the development of language lateralization (Sommer et al., 2004). However, the most interesting approach was offered by Mendrek et al. (2004), who suggested that dysfunction of the left dorsolateral prefrontal cortex, left thalamus, and right cerebellum may be a stable characteristic of schizophrenia, whereas dysfunction of the right dorsolateral prefrontal cortex, right thalamus, and left cerebellum may be state-dependent, an idea consistent with the hemispheric-imbalance model (Gruzelier, 1984).

Thus a case can be made for anomalies of language lateralization and/or impaired interhemispheric transfer in schizophrenia, but the evidence is not conclusive. It is possible that schizophrenia is caused by an abnormality of the genes that control cerebral dominance and language. So far, no gene in the pseudoautosomal or any other region has emerged (see Chapter 3). Rather, disturbed lateralization seems to be present in some patients, perhaps as a manifestation of an early neurodevelopmental insult of various etiologies that disturbs the normal process of hemispheric specialization, among other effects (Bullmore et al., 1997). Although an anomaly in the developmental process of brain lateralization has yet to be proved in schizophrenia, it is possible that lateralized dysfunction of various types may characterize schizophrenia. We will return to this idea in later chapters.

The Disconnection Hypothesis

While lateralization failure models viewed the transfer of information between the hemispheres to be fundamentally flawed in schizophrenia, the disconnection hypothesis saw the problem in schizophrenia as a more widespread failure of corticocortical and corticosubcortical connections. Earlier disconnection models emphasized the failure of connections between the prefrontal cortex and temporal lobe (Friston and Frith, 1995; Weinberger, 1991). It had been pointed out earlier that metachromatic leukodystrophy provided a useful analogy for frontotemporal disconnection in that patients with this disorder suffered from demyelination of subfrontal white matter. Generally, they presented early in life with complex auditory hallucinations and delusions similar to those of schizophrenic patients (Hyde et al., 1992). With the frontotemporal disconnection, there would be a failure to modulate intrinsically generated semantic and syntactical representations in the superior temporal regions. This in turn could result in the perception that formed utterances are extrinsic, that is, auditory hallucinations (Friston and Frith, 1995).

Later versions of the model (Friston, 1998, 1999) have looked at disconnection as a problem of cortical plasticity. From this viewpoint it is possible to include the effects of neurotransmitters such as dopamine on the development of connections and long-term potentiation. It is also possible to develop an explanation for negative symptoms if disconnection is seen to include impaired integration of the prefrontal cortex with the striatum and thalamus.

The evidence

A number of lines of evidence seem to point to disconnection in schizophrenia. Not the least of these is the phencyclidine (PCP) models of psychosis. Because most of the corticocortical and corticosubcortical connections are glutamatergic, blockage of NMDA receptors creates a type of disconnection that exacerbates both positive and negative symptoms in schizophrenic patients (see Chapter 4). Computer simulations of this type of disconnection also lead to *parasitic foci* that could lead to delusions and hallucinations (Hoffman and McGlashan, 1993; McGlashan and Hoffman, 2000). However, the brain-imaging evidence for frontotemporal disconnection has been mixed.

Studies using PET found a failure to suppress the superior temporal region during word fluency tasks in schizophrenic patients (Frith et al., 1995), but a subsequent study failed to replicate this finding (Dye et al., 1999). With the failure to replicate earlier findings, the model was modified to include the anterior cingulate. Activity in this region was found to modulate prefrontal inhibition of temporal regions (Dolan et al., 1999; Fletcher et al., 1999). To some extent, this modulation depends on dopamine, as apomorphine was shown to improve prefrontal inhibition of temporal regions (Dolan et al., 1995).

Probably the most convincing evidence comes from diffusion tensor imaging studies, which consistently show deficits in white tracks (see Chapter 7). The problem with these studies is that the changes seem to be widespread and no two patients seem to have the same pattern. White-matter differences from controls on MRI have also been inconsistent. There is no doubt that schizophrenia involves multiple brain regions and the connections between those brain regions are important. However, there are more specific models that integrate findings from other parts of the brain.

Imbalanced Brain Model

Grossberg (2000a) argued that the emotional centers of the brain, the amygdala and orbital prefrontal cortex, generate affective states, attend to emotionally salient events, and lead to motivated behaviors. Figure 11–1 shows some of these circuits and highlights their

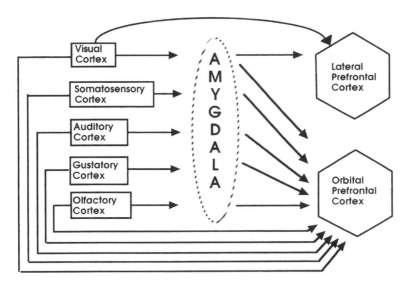

Figure II–I. The amygdala receives inputs from many sensory cortices and generates outputs to the prefrontal cortex. Used with permission, from Grossberg (2000a).

importance in mediating responses to sensory input. The amygdala receives input from all the sensory cortices and generates an output to the prefrontal cortex. Some of the processing could involve basal ganglia–thalamocortical neuronal circuits and the nucleus accumbens, but the model goes beyond this to consider direct connections between the amygdala and the prefrontal cortex.

The linkage between these emotional-processing centers and cognitive-processing centers supports conscious awareness. The emotional centers are calibrated by arousal level and depend on *gated dipoles* to process information. Arousal is viewed in a more general sense in this model, involving not just dopamine but multiple processes of habituation and motivational gating at subcortical and cortical levels. When emotional centers become depressed by either too much or too little arousal, symptoms like those of schizophrenia result. Negative symptoms of schizophrenia result from high levels of arousal (too much of a good thing) and positive symptoms result from underaroused gated dipoles. Essentially what happens is that diminished drive representations in the amygdala activated by sensory events leads to a failure to focus on relevant information, presumably resulting in misinterpretation.

ᵉ model is consistent with the effects of stress in schizophrenic
Either increased or decreased dopamine could depress
l-processing centers. However, the prediction is counterin-
...ive. Decreased arousal leads to hyperexcitability in the emotional-
processing centers. While this fits nicely with the beneficial effects
of stimulants in attention-deficit disorders, the response of schizophrenic patients is often quite different. If stimulants move the
processors to the normal range, why do so many patients experience
an exacerbation of their positive (not negative) symptoms? Part of
this dilemma could be explained by the state of habituation in the
dipole processors or regionally specific differences. However, what
makes schizophrenic patients different from others is not clear.

An interesting feature of the model is that it offers a unique perspective on hypofrontality in schizophrenia. Diminished drive representation in the amygdala may be one of the causes because of
close connections between these brain regions. Deficits in attention
and the PET studies showing aberrant emotional processing in schizophrenic patients (see Chapter 8) fit well with the model. However,
there is little evidence directly implicating either the orbital prefrontal cortex or the amygdala beyond this, and it would be difficult
for this model to account for changes in other parts of the brain
such as the cerebellum, which will be considered next.

Cognitive Dysmetria

Andreasen and her group have coined the term *cognitive dysmetria* to
call attention to the fact that the disturbances in schizophrenia include
not just executive functions but also memory, attention, emotion, and
motor activity (Andreasen, 1999; Andreasen et al., 1998). The anatomical substrate for cognitive dysmetria was proposed to be the corticocerebellar–thalamic–cortical circuit (Figure 11–2), which has been increasingly recognized for its role in cognitive coordination as well as
motor coordination (Middleton and Strick, 2000; Rapoport et al., 2000).

Andreasen (1999) suggested that schizophrenic patients have a
misconnection syndrome that leads them to make abnormal associations
between self and not-self or the important and the trivial. Consequently, internal representations may be attributed to the external
world, leading to hallucinations and delusions, a familiar theme that
almost all of the models refer to but have little direct evidence for.

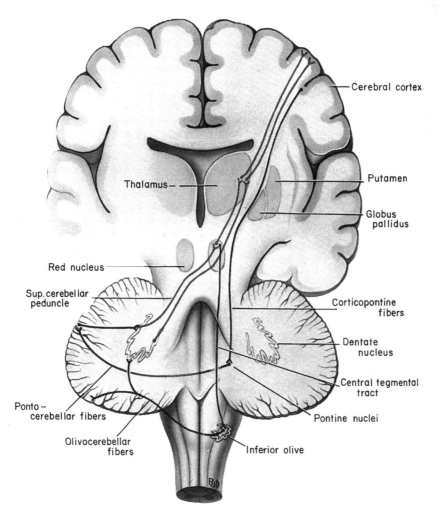

Figure II–2. Corticocerebellar–thalamic–cortical circuit: feedback loops between the cortex and the cerebellum. Used with permission, from Parent, A. (1996). *Carpenter's Human Neuroanatomy*, Williams and Wilkins, Baltimore, p. 613.

However, one recent piece of evidence that could offer an explanation is the finding that the cerebellum contains an auditory circuit for sound localization (Oertel and Young, 2004). Dysfunction in this circuit could link hallucinations more closely to the corticocerebellar–thalamic–cortical circuit. The explanation for negative symptoms from this model is that there is a failure to monitor, leading to negative symptoms in much the same way as when a computer locks and it cannot match signals sent at an incorrect rate.

There is considerable evidence pointing to structural abnormalities in the prefrontal cortex, thalamus, and cerebellum, but the studies are mixed and it is difficult to account for stronger structural findings in the temporal regions (see Chapter 7). The strongest evidence comes from a PET study showing activation deficits in the prefrontal–thalamic–cerebellar network during recall of complex narrative material (Andreasen et al., 1996). Other studies have also found evidence of cerebellar dysfunction during memory tasks (Crespo-Facorro et al., 1999; Kim et al., 2000; Mendrek et al., 2004; Meyer-Lindenberg et al., 2001). However, it is difficult to explain the diversity of imaging findings in prefrontal, temporal, and thalamic regions with abnormalities in the corticocerebellar–thalamic–cortical circuit alone.

What Is Missing?

The aberrant-lateralization, disconnection, imbalanced-brain, and cognitive-dysmetria models offer unique perspectives on schizophrenia. While there is evidence for impaired lateralization in schizophrenia, the question remains as to whether this is the fundamental defect in schizophrenia. It seems more likely that abnormalities in lateralization may be part of the final common pathway. In contrast, there seems to be little doubt that there is a failure of different parts of the brain to work together, as suggested by the disconnection model. However, the question is, which parts, and what is the nature of the disconnection? The imbalanced brain and cognitive dysmetria models implicate wide networks of neurons that interact together to control emotion and coordinate motor responses. What about other neuronal circuits? Basal ganglia–thalamocortical neuronal circuits are also involved in emotion and motor responses. The next chapter will consider some models focusing on these circuits and how they could be implicated in schizophrenia.

I2

Early Models of the Final Common Pathway 2. Basal Ganglia–Thalamocortical Circuits

The basal ganglia–thalamocortical neuronal circuits play an important role in learning new behaviors and integrating emotion into behavior (Alexander et al., 1990; Wise et al., 1996). Because these functions are often affected in schizophrenia, there may be a role for these circuits in the pathophysiology of the disorder. The behavior of patients with damage to regions associated with these circuits offers further evidence. Pantelis et al. (1992) highlighted the similarities between subcortical dementia and schizophrenia. Subcortical dementia as defined by Cummings (1986) is associated with slowness of thinking, impaired motivation, attention, and arousal, and sometimes depressed mood and psychotic symptoms. The syndrome occurs following lesions in the basal ganglia, thalamus, and brain-stem structures. With the exception of the brain stem, these structures are part of the basal ganglia–thalamocortical circuits.

Swerdlow and Koop (1987) drew attention to the fact that overactivity of the forebrain dopamine systems could result in the loss of lateral inhibitory interactions in the nucleus accumbens. This would cause disinhibition of palidothalamic efferents and a loss of focused corticothalamic activity. Underactivity could lead to difficulties in initiating activity as well as depression. Along a similar line of thinking, Robbins (1990) suggested that the excess subcortical and decreased prefrontal dopamine activity seen in schizophrenic patients may explain their deficiencies in willed action and monitoring of action. Other investigators have focused on the dorsolateral basal ganglia–thalamocortical neuronal circuit in schizophrenia (Bunney and Bunney, 2000).

The previous chapters have presented considerable evidence for the involvement of structures that are part of basal ganglia–thalamocortical neuronal circuits: the prefrontal and anterior cingulate cortices, the ventral striatum, and the thalamus. However, the functional aspects of these regions and the role of glutamate and dopamine have not been well integrated. The following four models attempt to integrate this information from different perspectives.

Corollary Discharge Systems

Corollary discharge and feed-forward are integrative mechanisms. They prepare for the consequences of self-initiated action allowing (at least with motor systems) the distinction to be made between self- and externally produced events in consciousness by the movement produced or not produced. Motor pattern generators may have comparable analogues in cognitive systems (Graybiel, 1997). A disruption in these cognitive pattern generators could explain hallucinations and delusions in schizophrenia (Feinberg and Guazzelli, 1999).

Although it is parsimonious to think that the brain may have similar systems for thought and action, Feinberg and Guazelli (1999) provided some interesting evidence from Penfield's neurosurgical studies. When the stimulation of the temporal lobes brought back memories into consciousness, the patients did not experience it as being self-produced but said, "You caused me to think that." Such a failure to establish self from externally produced events may be the basis for the delusions of passivity described so well by Kraepelin. Even hallucinations could be accounted for by a failure to recognize that internal speech is self-generated.

The circuitry of corollary discharge systems is not completely known, although Graybiel (1997) has suggested that the basal ganglia and their loop circuits with the frontal cortex and thalamus are essential for the retention and expression of cognitive pattern generators in the motor systems of thought. Dysfunction of innate cognitive pattern generators could explain the cross-cultural similarity of schizophrenic delusions and hallucinations and their fixed nature if cognitive pattern generators are able to override learned cognitive processes.

A failure of self-monitoring in schizophrenia has also been proposed by Frith (1995), albeit a somewhat different pathophysiology of symptomatolgy (Frith et al., 2000). In the case of delusion of control, the main problem is seen as a disconnection between the regions initiating actions in the prefrontal cortex and parietal regions involved in predicting the sensory consequences of action. Thus, movement in the absence of its predicted path is perceived as being produced by someone else. Some evidence for this idea is found in imaging studies in which the observation of movement is experimentally distorted. Normally the inferior parietal cortex is activated when subjects do not feel they are in control (i.e., the image of their self-initiated movement has been distorted). Schizophrenic subjects do not show parietal activation, which suggests that there could be a disconnection between prefrontal and parietal regions (Farrer et al., 2004). With regard to hallucinations, it has been proposed that there is a failure of self-monitoring of subvocal speech because of a disconnection between the prefrontal cortex and corollary discharge systems related to speech (Frith and Dolan, 1996). The PET data (see Chapter 8) do not entirely support these assertions. Findings in motor speech areas have been variable in association with hallucinations and there seems to be an increase, not a decrease, in parietal activity in association with delusions of control.

Functional MRI studies have shown more consistent abnormal activation patterns of the sensorimotor cortex (Schröder et al., 1995) and bilateral deficits in the posterior putamen, globus pallidus, and thalamus during a motor sequencing task, results supporting disrupted basal ganglia function (Menon et al., 2001a). There is also considerable evidence that the main efferent target of the basal ganglia, the thalamus, is involved in schizophrenia. However, it is difficult to elucidate whether the problem is due to abherrant cognitive pattern generators invoing the basal ganglia–thalamocortical neuronal circuits or to a corticocortical disconnection between the prefrontal and parietal regions. When we see a failure of modulated activation in the parietal cortex with distorted feedback from self-initiated movements, it does not necessarily mean that there is a frontal–parietal disconnection. A failure of integration at the sub-cortical level could also explain the findings.

Subcortical Neurotransmitter Imbalance

That schizophrenia is a subcortical neurotransmitter syndrome was first put forward by Carlsson and Carlsson (1990). Essentially the idea is that subcortical dopaminergic neurons are controlled by an *accelerator*, comprised of direct glutamatergic neurons from the cortex, and a *brake*, which is also glutamatergic but is inhibitory because the indirect pathway includes an intermediary GABA-ergic neuron (see Chapter 2 for direct and indirect pathways, and Fig. 12–1). Under normal conditions, the brake is stronger. If the release of dopamine is increased by amphetamine, feedback regulation will increase the activity of the brake. Treatment with an NMDA antagonist would be expected to enhance the amphetamine-induced release of dopamine. In schizophrenic patients, a glutamatergic deficiency would lead to a stronger accelerator and increased dopamine activity possibly resulting in psychotic symptoms (Carlsson et al., 1999).

Laruelle et al. (2003) have expanded this model. They argue that there there is good reason to believe that three phenomena take place in schizophrenia. First, there is an excessive stimulation of D_2

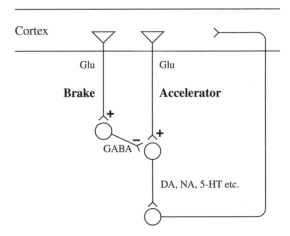

Figure 12–1. Cortical glutamate/GABA-mediated steering of subcortical systems by a brake and accelerator neuronal pathway. Used with permission, from Carlsson et al. (2000).

receptors in patients. The weight of the evidence discussed in Chapter 4 would appear to support this assertion. Secondly, there is deficient stimulation of prefrontal D_1 receptors. The evidence is not clear about D_1 abnormalities in schizophrenia, but there is some PET support for this. The many prefrontal neuropsychological deficits that depend on D_1 also support this concept. Finally, there is a deficiency of prefrontal connectivity involving NMDA receptors. While the postmortem evidence for this is not overwhelming, the effects of phencyclidine (PCP) and results from the animal models discussed in Chapter 4 are supportive. Thus, NMDA hypofunction in the prefrontal cortex may lead to a dysregulation of dopamine systems that would further weaken NMDA-mediated connectivity and plasticity.

The proof of this hypothesis lies in the effects of NMDA blockers such as ketamine on dopamine release measured by PET in humans. Ketamine has been found to have either no effect (Aalto et al., 2002; Kegeles et al., 2002) or a reduction in striatal D_2 receptor availability (Breier et al., 1998; Smith et al., 1998; Vollenweider et al., 2000). However, more important are its effects with amphetamine stimulation. Interestingly, ketamine caused an exaggerated response in healthy volunteers comparable to the response seen with amphetamine alone in schizophrenic patients (Kegeles et al., 2000a).

While the subcortical neurotransmitter imbalance model appears to have some support, it fails to integrate the many findings that are seen in temporal regions. Several investigators have attempted to integrate frontostriatal and dopaminergic regulation anomalies with temporal findings, and these ideas will be considered next.

Nucleus Accumbens Models

The neuropsychological literature recognized from an early stage that schizophrenic patients have an impaired ability to use stored information to interpret their current environment. Such impairment could lead to delusional thinking (Hemsley, 1987). The first investigators to translate this into a psychophysiological model were Gray and colleagues (1991). They reasoned that the limbic forebrain compares predictions with the actual world and sends *match* or *mismatch* messages from the subiculum to the nucleus accumbens. In schizophrenia, input from the subiculum to the nucleus accumbens is disrupted, leading to hyperactivity in the mesolimbic dopamine pathway and psychotic symptoms.

Although Gray (1998) revised his model to acknowledge the importance of the hippocampus in regulating the nucleus accumbens, it was really Grace and his group who developed the concept to its fullest potential on the basis of animal work carried out by this group (Grace, 2000; Moore et al., 1999; O'Donnell and Grace, 1998). As in Gray's model, the nucleus accumbens is seen as the key region where the prefrontal cortex, hippocampus, and amygdala come together to interact with one of the densest dopamine innervations in the brain. Neurons in the nucleus accumbens demonstrate a bistable membrane potential with a very negative resting state that is periodically disturbed by depolarizing events. The modulation of depolarizing events is largely under control of hippocampal (and likely amygdalar) neurons. Prefrontal input to the nucleus accumbens results in spike firing only when the neuron is in a depolarized state, so the hippocampus could control the flow to the prefrontal cortex, based on contextual information. The role of dopamine in the nucleus accumbens is complex; it is likely that it has an inhibiting and focusing effect by allowing passage of prefrontal information only through cells receiving strong hippocampal input. Another important feature of this model is that the accumbens output is directed to the reticular thalamic nucleus, which plays a critical role in regulating and filtering thalamocortical activity.

So how could this model explain the symptoms of schizophrenia? Figure 12–2 provides an explanation for the symptom clusters provided by Liddle (1987). Positive symptoms (reality distortion) are suggested to result from an increase in phasic dopamine activity. This would decrease accumbens shell excitability, and a decrease in tonic dopamine activity would reduce the spread of excitation in the accumbens via gap junctions. Thus, most of the prefrontal cortex would be unable to excite neurons in the nucleus accumbens. In spite of the hypofrontality or hippocampal deficit (shown by fewer arrows), it may still be possible for a particularly strong glutamatergic input to increase coupling. This would result in a small but inappropriate activation of accumbens neurons that would allow out-of-context information to traverse the system, resulting in delusions and hallucinations. Negative symptoms (psychomotor poverty) are seen to result from decreased (possibly dopamine) activity in the prefrontal cortex; a stronger inhibition of thalamic neurons then projects back

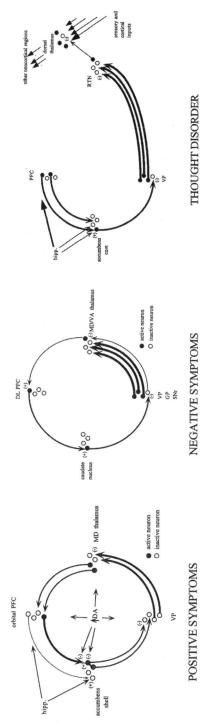

POSITIVE SYMPTOMS   NEGATIVE SYMPTOMS   THOUGHT DISORDER

Figure 12–2. Nucleus accumbens model explanations of Liddle's symptom clusters. DA, dopamine; DL, dorsolateral; GP, globus pallidus; hipp, hippocampus; MD, mediodorsal; PFC, prefrontal cortex; RTN, reticular thalamic nucleus; SNr, substantia nigra pars reticlata. Used with permission, from O'Donnell and Grace (1998).

to the prefrontal cortex. Essentially, this would lead to a perseveration state in the face of overall psychomotor retardation. Disorganization syndrome is seen to result from decreased activity in nucleus accumbens core neurons, leading to decreased activity in the reticular thalamic nucleus and a failure to suppress irrelevant incoming information passing through the thalamus (O'Donnell and Grace, 1998).

This is a very strong model—but do these predictions fit the data? The model of negative symptoms seems sound in that no one would dispute that decreased prefrontal activity seems to be associated with negative symptoms. However, whether there is decreased prefrontal dopamine in schizophrenia is not entirely clear. The explanation for disorganization syndrome is plausible but does not fit well with the findings of Liddle et al. (1992), who found a negative correlation between disorganization and right ventral prefrontal flow. The model does not account for a right-sided finding, nor is there any evidence that different parts of the nucleus accumbens are involved in particular syndromes in schizophrenia. The explanation for positive symptoms also seems to be at odds with almost all the imaging studies done during hallucinations, which have shown widespread increases (not decreases) in activity in limbic structures. Another problem with the model is that it does not account for the effects of stress and changes in symptoms over time.

Dopamine Sensitization

It has long been known that patients discharged home to emotionally overinvolved and critical families are more likely to relapse. Stress must therefore play a role in the illness. While several investigators have explored how this might be manifested in abnormalities in the response to stress in schizophrenic patients (Deutch, 1993; Laruelle, 2000; Moghaddam, 2002), the most comprehensive model has been proposed by Lieberman et al. (1997).

Lieberman et al. (1997) point out that psychostimulants can produce psychotic symptoms in healthy individuals and at low doses exacerbate psychotic symptoms in schizophrenic patients. Stimulant abusers after recovery from stimulant-induced psychosis exhibit a lower threshold for the induction of psychotic symptoms when reexposed to stimulants. This observation suggests that schizophrenic patients may develop sensitization to dopamine in much the same way that stimulant abusers or rats develop it when repeatedly exposed to amphetamine. In a sensitized limbic circuit, ventral tegmental stimulation to the nuceus accumbens is not opposed by prefrontal tonic inhibition of phasic dopamine release because of the uncoupling of these processes and decreased feedback inhibition by the nucleus accumbens on ventral tegmental neurons. The result is increased output from the accumbens through the pallidum, dorsal striatum, thalamus, and cortex, leading to increased cortical temporolimbic and temporolimbic striatal activity.

Figure 12–3 shows how normal or extreme stress in the presence of prefrontal and limbic neuropathology results in increased activity within the limbic circuit that exceeds compensatory capacity leading to psychosis. The process involves the following steps: (*1*) stimulation of the ventral tegmental area (VTA) produces an output to the nucleus accumbens (NA). (*2*) This stimulation is minimally opposed by cortical inhibition because of cortical deficits. (*3*) This results in decreased tonic inhibition of phasic dopamine release in the NA and increasing NA output to the pallidum and dorsal striatum through the thalamus to the cortex. (*4*) These effects produce

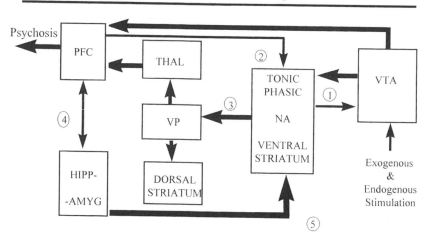

Figure 12–3. Neural circuits in normal, sensitized, and neuropathologic conditions. AMYG, amygdala; HIPP, hippocampus; PFC, prefrontal cortex; THAL, thalamus; VP, ventral pallidum; VTA, ventral tegmental area. Used with permission, from Lieberman et al. (1997).

increased temporolimbic activity and (5) temporolimbic striatal activity. The resulting pattern of activation leads to the expression of pathological behavior that eventually evolves to psychosis (Lieberman et al., 1997).

The model descried above makes sense from a number of perspectives. First, there are some neurodevelopmental events such as perinatal anoxia and prenatal stress that lead to increased vulnerability to the development of sensitization during adulthood (Brake et al., 1997; Henry et al., 1995). The PET data discussed in Chapter 4 also provide fairly convincing evidence that there is an exaggerated dopaminergic response to amphetamines in schizophrenic patients. Finally, the hypothesized increase in temporolimbic activity is consistent with the widespread increase in limbic activity during hallucinations on PET and possibly the degenerative changes seen on longitudinal MRI studies.

Thus all four basal ganglia–thalamocortical–based models appear to be strong candidates for the final common pathway of schizophrenia—but schizophrenia is not the only disorder to involve these neuronal circuits. While it is beyond the scope of this volume to consider all conditions, it is important to consider mood disorders, as Kraepelin's distinction between these two disorders forms the basis of modern psychiatry.

Are There Different Patterns in Mood Disorders?

Kraepelin separated manic-depressive psychoses from dementia praecox for a reason. Patients with mood disorders have different symptoms. They suffer from overwhelming depression lasting months or years, interspersed with periods of extreme mood elevation and euphoria. While these patients sometimes have psychotic symptoms, the symptoms are usually mood-congruent and patients recover to a large degree between episodes. Do we see a difference between the neuronal circuitry of mood disorders and that of schizophrenia?

Some differences have been noted between patients with mood disorders and patients with schizophrenia on neuropsychological test performance. Many patients with mood disorders perform poorly on frontal lobe and memory tasks but not as poorly as schizophrenic patients. Mood-disordered patients can have enlarged ventricles but do not usually demonstrate generalized loss of gray matter. They sometimes have prefrontal volumetric deficits but these tend to be sub-genual. Hippocampal volume loss is not often seen in first-episode patients (see Chapter 7). While decreased dorsolateral prefrontal activity has been observed in some functional imaging studies, a more typical finding is increased orbitofrontal, anterior cingulate, and amygdala activity in acutely depressed patients, which in some cases is reversed with treatment.

Several models have been proposed for the neuronal circuitry of depression (Drevets, 1998, Drevets and Raichle, 1992; Mayberg et al., 1999). In the model presented by Mayberg et al. (1999), vegetative-autonomic brain regions such as the subgenual prefrontal cortex and insula are believed to have a reciprocal relationship with dorsal cortical structures such as the right dorsal prefrontal cortex and anterior cingulate in mood disorders. With sadness, blood flow is increased in limbic-paralimbic regions (subgenual, anterior insula) and decreased in neocortical regions (right dorsolateral prefrontal, inferior parietal). With recovery from depression, the reverse pattern occurs (Mayberg et al., 1999). This relationship is illustrated in Figure 12–4.

The understanding of neuronal circuitry of mood disorders is no further along than that of schizophrenia, but even at this level of

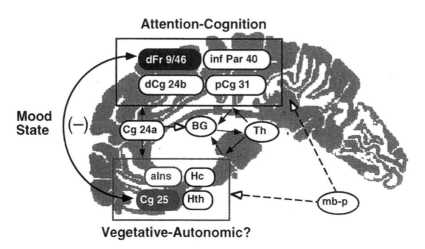

Figure 12–4. Regions mediating shifts in negative mood states. aIns, anterior insula; BG, basal ganglia; Cg24a, rostral anterior cingulate; Cg25, subgenual cingulate; dCg, dorsal anterior cingulate; dFr, dorsolateral prefrontal; Hc, hippocampus; Hth, hypothalamus; inf Par, inferior parietal; mb-p, midbrain-pons; pCg, posterior cingulate; Th, thalamus. Used with permission, from Mayberg et al. (1999).

knowledge there are important differences. The orbitofrontal and subgenual prefrontal cortices as well as the amygdala are more likely to be involved. Not surprisingly, these are the parts of the brain involved in emotional processing. There is some overlap with schizophrenia in the dorsolateral prefrontal cortex and hippocampus, but structures such as the nucleus accumbens and thalamus are less likely to be involved, perhaps suggesting that mood disorders are less likely to be associated with anomalies of perceptual and cognitive integration. This is consistent with the clinical picture of mood disorders, which is rarely associated with disturbances in the sense of self or perceptual disturbances. Thus there is certainly some involvement of structures that are are part of the basal ganglia–thalamocortical circuits in mood disorders, but the pattern is different.

Are We All Blind People?

Schizophrenia is a very complicated problem that can be viewed from many different perspectives. Maybe we are all blind people trying to understand what an elephant looks like from the part that we can feel. At this point in time, it would be impossible to accept or reject any of the proposed models. The dopamine sensitization and nucleus accumbens models do the best job of integrating diverse regional findings with dopamine and glutamate abnormalities. However, it is difficult to ignore findings that support aberrant-lateralization, cognitive-dysmetria, and the other models. The following chapter will compare these models from the viewpoint of what we know about the neuroanatomy, neurophysiology, neuropsychology, neurodevelopment, and longitudinal course of schizophrenia.

13

Do the Models Fit with What We Know about Schizophrenia?

Despite often conflicting data, we have learned a lot about schizophrenia since Kraepelin's description of the condition over a hundred years ago. There is considerable evidence that something goes wrong early in brain development. We are still arguing about whether dopamine receptors are increased or not, but there is agreement that there is dopaminergic hyperresponsivity. There seems to be some consensus that glutamate might be involved because patients given NMDA blockers experience an exacerbation of their symptoms.

Most investigators would accept that schizophrenic patients have difficulty with monitoring and willed action and are vulnerable to stress. Although the pattern may vary from patient to patient, we have a fairly good idea of what parts of the brain are affected. Not all would agree that there are progressive changes in schizophrenia, but the data for progressive volumetric loss in a substantial number of patients are convincing. This chapter will examine whether the proposed models fit with what we know about schizophrenia. It will also take a look at some of the things that we do not know about schizophrenia.

Neurodevelopmental Abnormalities

Most practitioners would accept that schizophrenia begins long before the onset of the characteristic symptoms. An early neurodevelopmental origin seems the most likely from evidence of abnormal cell migration in postmortem studies, the association with obstetric and perinatal complications or stress, and the many behavioral and soft neurological signs that patients show before the onset of the illness. However, there is no clear understanding of which structures might be affected. There is some evidence that the hippocampus could be affected and this would be consistent with the models proposing deficiencies in glutamatergic input to the nucleus accumbens. Damage to this structure early in animal brain development leads to findings seen in schizophrenic patients, such as the delayed onset of dopaminergic hyperresponsivity and abnormal prepulse inhibition (Lipska et al., 1992, 1995). Decreased hippocampal volume found in many schizophrenic patients with structural imaging adds further weight to the argument.

There is evidence of an early subplate abnormality from animal studies. These studies show delayed onset of dopaminergic hyperresponsivity and GABAergic abnormalities similar to postmortem findings in schizophrenic patients (Rajakumar and Rajakumar, 2003, Rajakumar et al., 2004). The subcortical neurotransmitter imbalance and dopamine sensitization models would be more consistent with this type of lesion. However, there are other lesions that lead to dopaminergic hyperresponsivity, the most notable of which are those caused by hypoxia and stress. Presumably, stress could also damage the hippocampus but it is likely that the damage would be more widespread. So it is difficult to rule out any of the models on the basis of their compatibility with an early neurodevelopmental lesion.

A case can be made for later neurodevelopmental events being involved in schizophrenia. During adolescence, about 50% of corticocortical connections are pruned. There is also extensive cortical sculpturing of the prefrontal cortex and myelination of corticocortical connections well into adolescence (Benes et al., 1994; Huttenlocher and Dabholkar, 1997; Keshavan et al., 2002a; Lewis, 1997; McGlashan and Hoffman, 2000; Penn, 2001). As previously noted, Feinberg (1982/1983) suggested that schizophrenia may be a result of anomalous cortical pruning at adolescence. Almost all of the models depend on cortical pruning as an explanation for the symptoms' onset later. The usual argument is that the defect is *uncovered* with loss of corticocortical connections at adolescence. Such an explanation is certainly viable for the disconnection, basal ganglia–thalamocortical, and cognitive-dysmetria models, but it is more difficult to understand how laterality differences might be uncovered, as lateralization occurs long before this. With this exception, the proposed models handle this hurdle fairly easily.

Dopaminergic Hyperresponsivity

There is one fact that no one would dispute about schizophrenia: dopamine is involved in some way. All of the drugs we use to treat schizophrenia affect D_2 receptors and dopaminergic agonists can produce hallucinations and delusions like those seen in schizophrenic patients. Although postmortem and PET/SPECT imaging studies often produce conflicting results about whether the number of D_2 receptors is increased in schizophrenia, almost all investigators have found increased presynaptic dopamine activity and hyperresponsivity with pharmacological stimulation subcortically. So far, dopaminergic findings in the cortex have been mixed (see Chapter 4). However, it seems clear that dopamine is involved in the stress response, and we do know that schizophrenic patients tend to relapse under stress.

Predictive value of models

How do the proposed models fare with regard to predictions about dopamine activity in schizophrenia? Although there is dopaminergic asymmetry in the brain (Reynolds, 1983), it is difficult to see how aberrant lateralization in the brain could lead to dopaminergic hyperresponsivity, which does not seem to be limited to one side of the brain. Interestingly, the opposite may be a possibility—hyperdopaminergia could lead to reduced lateralization. Mice lacking the dopamine transporter gene have persistent hyperdopaminergia and impaired lateralization of paw preference (Morice et al., 2005). It remains to be seen whether this finding is relevant to schizophrenia. The cognitive-dysmetria and corollary-discharge models do not provide a good account of how abnormalities in these circuits could lead to dopamine abnormalities. The disconnection model discusses the role of dopamine with cortical plasticity. However, it is necessary to address corticosubcortical circuits, which are better accounted for by other models in explaining dopaminergic hyperresponsivity through the disconnection hypothesis.

The other models address well the increased subcortical dopaminergic activity and hyperresponsivity with pharmacological stimulation. The subcortical neurotransmitter imbalance model attributes increased dopamine activity to the absence of a glutamatergic brake from the cortex whereas the nucleus accumbens model suggests that faulty control from the hippocampus or amygdala is to blame for the dopamine abnormalities. Dopamine abnormalities are obviously the core of the dopamine sensitization and imbalanced-brain models. In the dopamine sensitization model, deficits in multiple control dopamine mechanisms involving the prefrontal cortex and temporal lobe structures could lead to dopamine abnormalities, whereas the imbalanced-brain model is not very specific about the way in which dopamine hyperresponsivity or hyperarousal comes about. Both models offer an explanation for patients experiencing an exacerbation when they are under stress. Schizophrenia follows a variable course characterized by exacerbations of hallucinations, delusions, or thought disorder interspersed with periods of relative remission often associated with some degree of flattened affect and lack of motivation. Although none of the models fully account for these longitudinal changes, the dopamine sensitization and imbalanced-brain models at least integrate the effects of stress on dopamine that could explain some of the variability. They do not provide a good explanation for patients experiencing high levels of negative and positive symptoms at the same time.

How do dopamine abnormalities lead to positive symptoms?

It is always taken as self-evident that increased dopamine activity leads to hallucinations and delusions. Is this really the case? Not everyone given psychostimulant drugs becomes psychotic. In fact, a very small number become psychotic; these drugs are still used widely to treat obesity, narcolepsy, and even depression. Lieberman et al. (1987) reviewed 36 studies of the effects of psychostimulant drugs in schizophrenia and found only 40% evidence of a psychotogenic response. Factors affecting the response included degree and type of psychopathology, stage of illness, and pharmacological status at the time of testing.

PET/SPECT correlations. The PET/SPECT studies offer the best opportunity to look at dopamine and symptomatology. While the receptor studies may not be able to directly look at dopamine activity, presynaptic dopamine and stimulant response studies should be able to detect a relationship between dopamine activity and symptomatology. Surprisingly, the findings are not clearcut. Hietala et al. (1999) found a weak correlation between paranoid symptoms and activity in the right putamen but no correlation was found with symptoms in other studies (Dao-Castellano et al., 1997; Hietala et al., 1995; McGowan et al., 2004). Even a SPECT dopamine depletion study failed to find a correlation between positive symptoms and striatal D_2 receptor occupancy (Abi-Dargham et al., 2000). The exception appears to be the stimulant response studies, which detected an exacerbation of positive symptoms (Abi-Dargham et al., 1998; Breier et al., 1997b; Laruelle, 2000), but these studies were limited in their spatial resolution. The McGowan et al. (2004) study examined the ventral and dorsal striatum and failed to find a correlation with positive symptoms. Patients experiencing an exacerbation are more likely to experience positive symptoms with stimulation than patients in remission (Laruelle et al., 1999), so stage of illness may be a factor.

Mechanisms. How does increased dopamine activity lead to hallucinations and delusions? The explanations, some of which have been mentioned in previous chapters, are many and range from effects in the thalamus and striatum to the cortex. Dopamine is known to affect sensory gating at the levels of nucleus accumbens, reticular thalamic nucleus, and cortex (Grace, 2000; Grunwald et al., 2003; Krause et al., 2003), but this finding provides only a partial explanation. It has been suggested that increased dopamine activity could lead to neuroplastic adaptions downstream from the mesolimbic dopaminergic synapse. In this way, dopamine would be seen as a trigger unleashing hard-wired prefrontal–ventral, striatal–ventral, pallidal–mediodorsal, thalamic–prefrontal loops associated with positive symptoms (Laruelle, 2000; O'Donnell and Grace, 1998).

It is likely that dopamine mediates the salience of environmental events and internal representations. It has been proposed that delusions may result from the aberrant assignment of salience to experiencial events, whereas hallucinations may arise from the aberrant salience of internal representations (Kapur, 2003). While this explanation may have some merit with regard to delusions, it is difficult to see how this could really account for the clear experience of hearing more than one voice commenting on what is happening at the time. In many cases, these perceptions are not associated with much affect.

From the viewpoint of the cortex, Goldman-Rakic (1999) has suggested that dysfunction of delay neurons in the prefrontal cortex could lead to run-on in language circuits and the perception of hallucinations. Grossberg (2000b) also highlighted the importance of the cortex in hallucinations with his suggestion that hallucinations arise from hyperactivity of the top-down control of sensory processing, which allows more efficient processing by using learned prototypes. In other words, we have a set of learned expectations that form our experience by interacting with bottom-up sensory input. When this process becomes tonically hyperactive, these cortical modules can fire on their own without willful control. It is possible that dopamine may play a role in the regulation of some the circuits related to this type of sensory processing.

If we view hallucinations as being run-on in the prefrontal circuits or some hard-wired prefrontal–striatal–thalamic–prefrontal loop, how do we explain the widespread activity of almost every part of the limbic system and auditory cortex in association with hallucinations and other positive symptoms in the imaging studies (see Chapter 8)? An interesting observation about hallucinations comes from studies that have looked at the location of brain lesions associated with hallucinations in different sensory modalities (Braun et al., 2003). The lesion is always located in the brain pathway of the sensory modality—i.e., visual hallucinations have lesions in the vision pathways and auditory hallucination in the auditory pathways. After the lesion has occurred, a compensatory overactivation of tissue may take place in the nearby brain sensory pathway. This could explain why the correlations between actual tissue loss in the auditory cortex and auditory hallucinations are stronger than in functional studies, which do not always show activations in these regions in association with hallucinations. It would also be consistent with anecdotal reports of visual pathway activation with visual hallucinations in schizophrenic patients (see Chapter 8).

It is noteworthy that pretreatment with neuroleptics has not been found to significantly reduce positive symptoms produced with NMDA antagonists in healthy volunteers (Krystal et al., 1999; Lipschitz et al., 1997). Chronic treatment with neuroleptics is also ineffective in blocking the effects of NMDA antagonists in schizo-phrenic patients, although atypical agents may blunt the response (Lahti et al., 1995b; Malhotra et al., 1997). Thus it appears that we have a lot to learn about positive symptoms. Dopamine may be only one of the factors to be considered.

The Role of Glutamate

The case for glutamate in the pathophysiology of schizophrenia is also strong. Drugs that block NMDA receptors cause both positive and neg-ative symptoms in healthy volunteers and patients, unlike dopamine agonists, which cause only positive symptoms. Postmortem studies have shown increased glutamatergic receptors and uptake sites in some pre-frontal regions, whereas other investigators have found evidence of glutamatergic hypofunction in the prefrontal cortex and temporal re-gions (see Chapter 4). Proton MRS studies have shown increased glu-tamatergic metabolites in the anterior cingulate and medial prefrontal regions in first-episode patients and decreased levels in chronic pa-tients. This suggests that stage of illness may be a factor (see Chapter 9). When large doses of NMDA antagonists such as PCP are given to animals, there is a widespread loss of neurons throughout the limbic system. The loss is more severe but not incompatible with some of the changes seen in schizophrenic patients in postmortem studies. Chronic, lower doses of NMDA antagonists lead to dopaminergic hy-perresponsivity like that seen in schizophrenic patients.

All of the models discussed can account for the glutamate ob-servations to some extent. The aberrant lateralization and discon-nection models rely on connections between the prefrontal cortex and temporal lobe as well as connections with other brain regions on either side of the brain. Naturally, a disruption in glutamatergic neurotransmission would lead to dysfunction, as most of these con-nections are glutamatergic. Similarily, a disruption in glutamatergic neurotransmission would lead to abnormalities if it specifically in-volved the hippocampal/amygdalar or prefrontal cortical connec-tions to the nucleus accumbens, as in the nucleus accumbens and imbalanced-brain models, or the various connections of the corti-cocerebellar–thalamic–cortical circuit associated with cognitive dys-metria. It therefore comes down to whether the glutamatergic ab-normalities are widespread or localized to a specific region.

Self-monitoring and Willed Action

Many investigators from Kraepelin on have noticed that patients seem to have a poverty of will and a failure to self-monitor. However, Frith (1995) expanded these concepts and suggested that a poverty of will could explain negative symptoms and the difficulties that schizo-phrenic patients have with neuropsychological tasks such as word fluency. Moreover, a failure of self-monitoring could lead to positive symptoms such as thought insertion (failure to recognize one's own thoughts) and auditory hallucinations (attribution of internal speech to someone else). As discussed in Chapter 6, a failure of self-monitoring may reflect a more widespread failure of linking current stimuli with higher-order cognitive functions or action plans, i.e., encoding.

Almost all of the models attempt to provide some sort of explanation for poverty of will or negative symptoms—usually in some way related to the prefrontal cortex. Most models also attempt to explain positive symptoms as a failure to self-monitor in some way, although the brain structures and explanations vary widely. Recently, much has been learned about the structures in the brain that are important in distinguishing self from nonself. It may be helpful in reviewing these structures before comparing the models with regard to this aspect.

Brain structures involved in distinguishing self from non-self

As we saw in Chapter 2, there are many brain structures involved in self-perception. Self-representation allows additional behavioral flexibility by separating representation of internal states from perceptions of the external world (Churchland, 2002). In humans, self-recognition begins in infancy, in concert with the myelination of fibers in the frontal lobe (Kinney et al., 1988). At the other end of the life span, patients with frontotemporal dementia seem to show deficits in self-concepts when the nondominant frontal lobe is involved in the disease process (Miller et al., 2001a). Is there other evidence to implicate the right prefrontal cortex in self-representation? When subjects rate adjectives according to whether they apply to themselves or others, the right prefrontal cortex seems to activate more with self-ratings (Craik et al., 1999). Activation of the right dorsomedial prefrontal cortex has been found with self-ratings of traits regardless of the emotional valence of the trait (Fossati et al., 2003). Similar self-statement studies found activations on both sides in the medial prefrontal cortex but more often on the right side (Johnson et al., 2002; Kelley et al., 2002). When activation was found in the posterior cingulate, it was bilateral (Johnson et al., 2002). More general tasks, such as rating how pictures make one feel, led to both increases and decreases in medial prefrontal activity on both sides of the brain (Gusnard et al., 2001).

The association with right-sided prefrontal activation with self-ratings is interesting. However, it appears that self-representation is widely distributed in the brain. When subjects view themselves, there is activation throughout the right limbic system (hippocampus, insula, anterior cingulate) and the left prefrontal and superior temporal cortices (Kircher et al., 2000). Other structures are also involved. For example, when subjects view a virtual hand that is manipulated to correspond or not correspond to the subject's actual movements, the more the movements are out of control, the more the right parietal cortex is activated. The reverse was observed in the insula (Farrer et al., 2003). In another study, hypnotized subjects' active movements attributed to an external source resulted in higher parietal and cerebellar activation than did identical movements correctly attributed to the self. The hypnotic suggestion was seen as impairing the functioning of the cerebellar–parietal network (Blakemore et al., 2003). Self-initiated movement has been associated with cerebellar activation as well (Blouin et al., 2004). Thus, the cerebellum may play a role in self-initiated tasks, in keeping with the cognitive dysmetria model.

One of the first attempts to look at self-representation in schizophrenia was *theory of mind,* or the ability to infer what other people are thinking and feeling. This appears to involve the medial prefrontal, superior temporal, and inferior frontal (Frith and Frith, 1999) regions and possibly the cerebellum (Calarge et al., 2003). While deficits with this ability are more characteristic of autism, there are also reports of difficulties in schizophrenic patients (Frith and Frith, 1999). However, there is more direct evidence of abnormalities with internal monitoring in schizophrenia. Frith (1987) argued that hallucinations may be understood as a deficit in an internal monitoring mechanism that regulates internal speech, whereas others have proposed that hallucinating patients have a response bias to attribute internal events to an external source (Bentall, 1990).

There is support for an internal monitoring deficit from the imaging literature in that hallucinating patients have reduced activation on PET in the left middle temporal gyrus and rostral supplementary areas (both regions involved in monitoring speech) when asked to imagine sentences spoken in another person's voice (McGuire et al., 1995). A more recent study demonstrated that schizophrenic patients with active persecutory delusions showed a marked absence of rostral–ventral anterior cingulate activation together with increased posterior cingulate activation during evaluation of neutral and threatening self-referential statements (Blackwood et al., 2004). The psychological literature provides further support for the proposal that schizophrenic patients have a response bias to external attribution of internal events (Brébion et al., 2000; Morrison and Haddock, 1997) but there is little support for the idea that hallucinators are unable to distinguish inner imagined speech from real external speech (Evans et al., 2000).

Monitoring deficits may be seen in motor tasks as well. When schizophrenic patients were asked to perform simple wrist and finger movements while watching an image of either their own hand or an alien hand executing the same or different movements, they were more impaired in discriminating their own hand from the alien one and tended to misattribute the alien hand to themselves (Daprati et al., 1997). Patients with delusions of influence were particularly impaired on this task (Franck et al., 2001). This would suggest that the problem was not so much one of monitoring internal events; rather, it was a problem with the *who* system in schizophrenia (Georgieff and Jeannerod, 1998), which involves the structures activated during self-representation and self-initiated tasks.

Relevance to models of schizophrenia

How does all of this information relate to our models? It is curious that many of the structures involved in self-representation are lateralized. In a way, the aberrant-lateralization model could explain schizophrenic symptoms better if the focus were self-representation rather than language. It is also interesting that the cerebellum is activated in self-initiated and theory-of-mind tasks. This is not a structure that would immediately come to mind in self-representation: its involvement adds some validity to the cognitive-dysmetria theory. Whereas the other theories touch on the regulation of structures such as the right prefrontal cortex associated with self-representation in various ways, none provide good explanations for the obvious difficulties that these patients have in distinguishing self from nonself.

Heterogeneity of Neuropsychological and Brain Imaging Findings

There is general agreement about the parts of the brain that show structural changes in schizophrenic patients: most likely the hippocampus, superior temporal gyrus, and thalamus and possibly the prefrontal cortex, anterior cingulate, cerebellum, and midline structures such as the corpus callosum. There is also some consensus from neuropsychological studies about the structures that might be involved: probably the prefrontal cortex and temporal lobe structures and possibly the anterior cingulate, thalamus, and cerebellum. The problem is that no two patients or studies seem to find exactly the same thing! The effect sizes for neuropsychological and brain-imaging studies are usually in the range of 0.4–1.0. Even at the higher end, only about 25% of patients would score outside the normal range on any given variable if the scores were normally distributed. Somehow, this remarkable degree of heterogeneity has to be accounted for in our models of schizophrenia.

The concept of malfunctioning circuits helps to some degree in dealing with heterogeneity. Damage to any part of the circuit would lead the whole circuit to fail and one might expect the damage to differ between individuals. However, one might also expect some consistency in the correlates with actual symptoms that presumably reflect the failure of particular circuits. To some extent, there is consistency. Both neuropsychological studies and imaging studies point to the prefrontal cortex as being important in negative symptoms and the activation of the entire limbic system with hallucinations and other positive symptoms. Studies of patients with a predominance of these symptoms over time (rather than direct time-related correlations) are not as consistent. However this would be expected, considering other factors that could come into play with this type of study.

Can the proposed models account for heterogeneity? Some seem to do better than others. For example, the aberrant-lateralization model might have difficulty accounting for the majority of patients who do not show clear signs of aberrant lateralization. It would be difficult for the corollary discharge and corticocerebellar–thalamic–cortical models to explain changes in the temporal lobes and other parts of the brain not directly linked to these circuits. Likewise, the hippocampal/amygdalar input to the nucleus accumbens accounts for temporal and subcortical findings but has difficulty with changes in some patients in the prefrontal cortex and superior temporal gyrus. The two models that seem to do better with heterogeneity are the subcortical neurotransmitter imbalance model and the sensitization model, which allow for the multiple regulators of dopamine; damage to any of these could lead to the same result.

Longitudinal Findings

There has been increased interest in the idea that there are changes in the brain after the onset of the illness. The MRI data showing progressive structural deficits are now as overwhelming as the dopamine findings. The increase in glutamate metabolites and membrane breakdown products in first-episode patients, followed by deficits in chronic patients in MRS studies, raises the possibility of neurodegeneration, as first proposed by Kraepelin. However, most investigators would lean toward other explanations, such as a programmed loss of neuropil due to some sort of genetic abnormality. Regardless, the proposed models have to account for longitudinal changes in patients.

The aberrant-lateralization and corollary discharge brain models do not fit well with longitudinal changes. These circuits are functional long before the onset of symptoms and it is difficult to see how dysfunction could lead to longitudinal volumetric changes. The subcortical neurotransmitter imbalance, nucleus accumbens, imbalanced-brain, and cognitive-dysmetria models also do not address this problem. The disconnection hypothesis addresses plastic changes in synaptic connections in the postnatal period but does not address changes after the onset of the illness. There has been increasing interest in genetically programmed changes in brain development throughout adolescence. The finding of reduced neuropil in the prefrontal cortex could be explained by a number of abnormalities in the genes that support synaptic connections during development and throughout life (Bullmore et al., 1997; Frankle et al., 2003; Sawa and Snyder, 2002). Unfortunately, any one of hundreds (if not thousands) of genes could be involved.

The dopamine sensatization model is the only model that attempts to integrate a three-stage model—early cortical pathology, neurochemical sensation, followed by neurotoxicity. In this model, repeated stress leads to an exaggerated dopamine response as well as increased glutamatergic activity that eventually becomes neurotoxic via an apoptotic mechanism and may not necessarily be associated with gliosis (Lieberman, 1999). This model could explain some of the progressive volumetric changes as well as the glutamatergic and membrane metabolite findings with MRS (see Chapter 9).

Are We There Yet?

We have some good models of schizophrenia. While the aberrant-lateralization, cognitive-dysmetria, imbalanced-brain, disconnection, and corollary-discharge models have more limited explanatory power, we do have three models that are able to bridge most of what we know about neurodevelopment, dopamine, and glutamate in schizophrenia: the subcortical neurotransmitter imbalance, nucleus accumbens, and dopamine sensitization models. Of these, the subcortical neurotransmitter imbalance and dopamine sensitization models seem to address heterogeneity best, but the dopamine sensitization model may be unique in its explanation of longitudinal changes.

There seems to be general agreement that there is a problem with the cortical regulation of dopamine, which is likely related to some early neurodevelopmental or genetic factor. This could be glutamatergic, as most of the corticosubcortical projections are glutamatergic, but it could also be GABAergic because of the effects of interneurons on these projection neurons. Depending on the model, origin of the projection neurons is from the prefrontal cortex, hippocampus/amygdala, or cerebellum. Irrespective of the origin, involvement of the nucleus accumbens and thalamus appears to be important. The imaging findings on the whole find abnormalities in all of these structures. While the pattern varies from patient to patient, this is not necessarily a problem, as dysfunction in any part of a circuit generally leads the whole circuit to fail.

So what do we not know? One problem to reconcile is that the core of most models—dopamine hyperresponsivity—is found in only a minority of patients. However, the greatest problem with all of the models is integrating the actual symptoms of schizophrenia with the physiology. We all accept that increased dopamine activity causes hallucinations, but it is very difficult to provide unequivocal evidence of this. The link between negative symptoms and impaired prefrontal function is strong but not consistently found in all studies (see Chapter 8). Although the patterns of activation with positive symptoms also vary, there is generally widespread activation of all parts of the limbic system with hallucinations. It is difficult to see how existing models could explain this. There are not many studies of passivity phenomena, but linkage to centers involved in self-representation is also weak.

Despite these limitations, the models raise important questions and force us to look at schizophrenia in different ways. Some of the models also suggest new ways of approaching treatment. Our treatments to date have focused on dopamine, but most of the models emphasize the importance of glutamatergic and GABAergic connections. The following chapter will examine some novel approaches to treatment that would be compatible with some of the proposed models.

14

Implications for Treatment

It could be argued that the treatment of patients with schizophrenia began with the discovery of chlorpromazine in the early 1950s. Before that time, anyone with this illness had a greater than even chance of spending the rest of their life in an institution. With antipsychotic medication, most patients are able to live in the community, even though they may be unable to work or have a family because of persistent negative and, in some cases, positive symptoms.

The short-term benefits of neuroleptic medications are widely accepted, but fewer than half of patients reach full remission and only 70%–80% would be characterized as responding well to neuroleptics (Kane, 1989). Long-term follow-up studies have yet to demonstrate unequivocally any effect of treatment on the natural history of schizophrenia (McGlashan, 1988). Others have pointed out that there is some evidence that schizophrenia is becoming more benign (Hare, 1974; Zubin et al., 1983). We do not see catatonia or hebephrenia as frequently, and one of the likely reasons for this is treatment with neuroleptics (Mahendra, 1981; Morrison, 1974). Consequently, there is no doubt that our current treatments are beneficial, but there is clearly a long way to go.

The realization that the effectiveness of antipsychotic medications was correlated with D_2 receptor blockade led to an intensive search for other medications that might also block dopamine with fewer side effects than those from chlorpromazine. These so-called atypical antipsychotic medications had a number of other actions besides their effect on dopamine. This chapter will review some of what we know about the actions of currently used antipsychotic medications. It will explore some of the possibilities for new antipsychotic medications and treatments based on pharmacological, electromagnetic, and neurosurgical manipulations of some of the neuronal circuits suggested to be involved in schizophrenia.

Newer Dopaminergic Medications

The finding of consistently low levels of D_2 receptor blockade in patients who showed an excellent clinical response to clozapine did not fit with other antipsychotic medications and led to a search for other mechanisms of action (Pilowsky et al., 1992). Meltzer et al. (1989) proposed that the ratio of $5\text{-}HT_{2A}$ to D_2 receptor affinities characterized atypical antipsychotic medications such as clozapine, risperidone, quetiapine, and olanzapine. However, the failure of $5\text{-}HT_{2A}$ antagonists to improve schizophrenic symptoms seemed to go against this idea.

Neuroimaging data suggest that optimal D_2 receptor occupancy between 65% and 80% is necessary for the clinical effectiveness of atypical neuroleptics without motor side effects. At occupancy levels higher than this, extrapyramidal motor symptoms emerge. However, animal data indicate that a rapid dissociation from the D_2 receptor may be more characteristic of atypical neuroleptics than receptor occupancy (Kapur and Seeman, 2001). If this is the case, the problem of low D_2 occupancy by clozapine could be understandable if the dissociation levels were comparable to other atypical neuroleptics.

Other investigators have suggested that somatodendritic autoreceptors may also play a role in actions of some atypical antipsychotic medications by regulating the firing rate of dopamine neurons. Aripiprazole occupies up to 95% of striatal D_2 receptors at clinical doses, yet patients have almost no side effects. The reason for this is likely the drug's weak partial agonist effect on the autoreceptors (Gründer et al., 2003a).

Theoretically, aripiprazole should be the ideal antipsychotic agent. It is believed to decrease dopamine activity in the nucleus accumbens where dopamine neurons are likely hyperresponsive while protecting or enhancing dopaminergic activity in mesocortical dopaminergic neurons in prefrontal regions, which could improve negative symptoms. It also has partial agonist effects on serotonin 5-HT$_{1A}$ receptors, and is an antagonist at 5-HT$_{2A}$ receptors, so it should be both a serotonin and dopamine stabilizer (Carlsson et al., 2000). This sounds good on paper, but is there any evidence of improved efficacy over other antipsychotic agents? Although aripiprazole is clearly a good antipsychotic agent with few side effects, the evidence from short-term trials comparing aripiprazole with other agents suggests that its efficacy is similar to that of risperidone and haloperidol (Argo et al., 2004; Crismon et al., 2003; Kane et al., 2002).

It is quite possible that longer trials of aripiprazole may establish superior efficacy to that of current antipsychotic agents. It is also possible that other similar agents may be developed. However, the pathophysiological models discussed in Chapters 11 and 12 would predict other approaches beyond dopamine. Most investigators suggest that NMDA neurotransmission may be deficient in some way in schizophrenia. If this is the case, there are many agents that may enhance NMDA neurotransmission that could be used in schizophrenic patients.

Glutamatergic Agonists

There is still general agreement in the field that clozapine in the most effective treatment for schizophrenia. While only about 30% of patients resistant to conventional antipsychotic medications show improvement on clozapine, the effects on negative symptoms are sometimes striking (Kane et al., 1988). How does it work beyond its effects on dopamine, which appear to be minimal? Unfortunately, this question has never been satisfactorily answered. It is of interest that clozapine interacts with NMDA receptors (Arvanov et al., 1997; Lidsky et al., 1993; Ninan and Wang, 2003; Ossowska et al., 1999). Recently, it has been shown that clozapine modulates midbrain dopamine neuron firing by interacting with the NMDA receptor complex. Clozapine could possibly be acting as an agonist at the glycine site of the NMDA receptor or as an inhibitor of the glycine transporter (Schwieler et al., 2004). Another possibility is that one of the metabolites of clozapine could potentiate NMDA receptors via its effect on muscarinic M_1 receptors (Sur et al., 2003).

Glycine

There are several other agents that affect NMDA receptors. Of these, the most widely studied have been glycine, D-serine, and D-cycloserine (D'Souza et al., 1995; Goff and Wine, 1997; Javitt, 2004; Krystal et al., 1999; Tsai and Coyle, 2002). Glycine potentiates NMDA receptor–mediated neurotransmission by acting on a site on the NMDA receptor. Glycine has been found to reverse prepulse inhibition deficits and methamphetamine-induced locomotor activity in neonatal ventral hippocamapal–lesioned rats (Kato et al., 2001; Le Pen et al., 2003). A number of studies have attempted to improve negative symptoms in schizophrenic patients by adding glycine to conventional treatment. The first three failed to show statistically significant differences (Costa et al., 1990; Rosse et al., 1989; Waziri, 1988) but a few patients seemed to show improvement and other studies were carried out with more positive results. The first high-dose double-blind, placebo-controlled trial showed only a 15% improvement in negative symptoms with high-dose glycine versus placebo (Javitt et al., 1994), but a later study by the same group showed a 36% reduction in negative symptoms (Heresco-Levy et al., 1996). Subsequent studies have shown similar effects of glycine on negative symptoms (Heresco-Levy et al., 1999; Javitt et al., 2001; Leiderman et al., 1996).

D-cycloserine

One of the problems with glycine is that it does not cross the blood-brain barrier easily. D-cycloserine crosses the blood-brain barrier readily. Originally used an an antimicrobial agent to treat tuberculosis, it was observed to improve depression and apathy but side effects sometimes included psychosis (Goff and Wine, 1997). Over a narrow range of concentrations, D-cycloserine is a relatively selective partial agonist at the glycine modulatory site. Goff et al. (1995) found that negative symptoms were reduced by about 21% when D-cycloserine was added to conventional neuroleptics in chronic schizophrenic patients. Later studies found similar effects when

D-cycloserine was given alone or in combination with conventional or atypical neuroleptics (Evins et al., 2002; Goff et al., 1999; van Berckel et al., 1996). The exceptions to this included one study in which the dose was likely too low (Rosse et al., 1996) and another in which D-cycloserine was used with clozapine (Goff et al., 1996). Patients in the later study actually became worse, which suggests that D-cycloserine may act as an antagonist at the glycine site in the presence of clozapine. Worsening of psychotic symptoms was also observed with high doses of D-cycloserine (Cascella et al., 1994).

D-serine

In contrast to D-cycloserine, D-serine is a full agonist at the glycine site. Patients who were treated with D-serine in addition to a variety of conventional and atypical antipsychotic medications showed significant improvements in both positive and negative symptoms. Their cognitive symptoms and performance on the Wisconsin Card Sorting Test (WCST) improved as well (Tsai et al., 1998). This finding would be in keeping with the suggestion that full glycine agonists such as glycine and D-serine are more effective than partial agonists such as D-cycloserine (Heresco-Levy and Javitt, 2004).

Glycine transport inhibitors

The doses necessary to demonstrate a therapeutic response in schizophrenia for both glycine and D-serine are in grams rather than milligrams because of absorption limitations. One of the ways to increase brain levels is to use glycine transport inhibitors that raise synaptic glycine levels by preventing its removal from the synaptic cleft. Drugs which have this effect have been shown to reverse PCP-induced and dopaminergic hyperactivity in rodents (Harsing et al., 2003; Javitt et al., 2003).

Only one trial of a glycine transporter inhibitor has been reported in the treatment of schizophrenia. Tsai et al. (2004) used N-methylglycine as an addition to stable antipsychotic regimes in a placebo-controlled trial in 38 schizophrenic patients. Significant improvements were seen in both positive and negative symptoms as well as cognitive symptoms, but further trials will be necessary to evaluate this approach.

Glutamatergic Antagonists

It is quite possible that some existing neuroleptics are neuroprotective. Many argue that outcome is better with fewer episodes and treatment with neuroleptics (Wyatt, 1991). It is also interesting to look at some of the studies of patients before and after the introduction of neuroleptics. In one study, the primary clinical correlate of the duration of initially untreated psychosis was muteness (Waddington et al., 1995). Patients who have anterior cingulate damage present as being mute and there is evidence of increased glutamergic activity in the anterior cingulate in first-episode patients that could lead to excitotoxic damage (Théberge et al., 2002). Could other agents provide more effective neuroprotection?

Lamotrigine

Lamotrigine was introduced as an anticonvulsant, but like many anticonvulsants was found to have other effects. It stabilizes neuronal membranes and attenuates cortical glutamate release via its effects on sodium, potassium, and calcium channels (Grunze et al., 1998; Leach et al., 1991; McNaughton et al., 1997). While the effect is probably small, some benefit has been reported in amyotrophic lateral sclerosis, Alzheimer disease, and stroke, possibly because of decreased excitatory amino acid–mediated neuronal degeneration (Eisen et al., 1993; Leach et al., 1993; Tekin et al., 1998).

When healthy subjects were given lamotrigine 2 hours before ketamine, perceptual abnormalities, including both positive and negative symptoms, were significantly reduced. Subjects also performed better on a learning and memory task with lamotrigine pretreatment (Anand et al., 2000). Studies in schizophrenic patients are limited thus far to treatment-resistant patients, but the findings are promising.

The first open trial of adding lamotrigine to clozapine in six partially responsive schizophrenic patients demonstrated improvement on the Brief Psychiatric Rating Scale (Dursun et al., 1999). A subsequent nonrandomized trial of lamotrigine or topiramate added to clozapine, risperidone, olanzapine, or flupenthixol in 26 treatment-resistant patients found a significant improvement on the Brief Psychiatric Rating Scale in those patients who were treated with clozapine and lamotrigine. When lamotrigine was added to the other neuroleptics, no significant effects were observed. The addition of topiramate was not beneficial with any of the neuroleptics, although only nine patients were studied (Dursun and Deakin, 2001).

The first randomized, placebo-controlled trial of the addition of lamotrigine to clozapine produced more convincing results. Thirty-four hospitalized treatment-resistant, chronic schizophrenic patients received 200 mg/day of lamotrigine in a 14-week crossover design with placebo. On the Positive and Negative Syndrome Scale, lamotrigine was more effective in reducing positive and general psychopathology scores than placebo, but surprisingly no differences were found with negative symptoms (Tiihonen et al., 2003). While preliminary, these results suggest that there may be a role for lamotrigine in treatment-resistant patients.

Topiramate

High levels of glutamate acting via kainate or AMPA receptors can result in oxidative stress and possibly apoptosis. Topiramate blocks kainate and AMPA receptors and potentiates GABA (Shank et al., 2000). In an animal model, topiramate was able to inhibit behaviors induced by MK-801, an analogue of PCP (Deutsch et al., 2002) so it would seem to be a good candidate for use in schizophrenia. Case reports of adding topiramate to antipsychotic medications have been mixed. The first found a dramatic improvement in negative symptoms (Drapalski et al., 2001), but others have found significant worsening of symptoms with the addition of topiramate (Millson et al., 2002).

In an open-label study of the addition of topiramate to schizophrenic patients with prominent negative symptoms on stable antipsychotic medication levels, significant improvement was noted in scores on the Positive and Negative Syndrome Scale, mostly on the basis of an improvement in negative symptoms. However, a selective but reversible worsening of verbal fluency performance was also seen with the addition of topiramate (Deutsch et al., 2003). It is difficult to draw any conclusions from these results until double-blind studies are attempted.

GABAergic Drugs

In most of the basal ganglia–thalamocortical neuronal circuit models and the dopamine sensitization model, a deficiency of GABA activity in the anterior cingulate or prefrontal cortex would have the same effect as a deficiency in NMDA activity. Both would lead to increased glutamatergic activity and problems with dopamine regulation. Thus would increasing GABAergic activity pharmacologically improve positive and negative symptoms? In addition to topiramate, a number of drugs that affect GABA have been used in schizophrenia, including benzodiazepines and valproic acid (Wassef et al., 1999).

Benzodiazepines

Early studies of benzodiazepines in schizophrenia found mixed results. However, 9 of 14 double-blind studies of benzodiazepines alone showed an improvement in many symptoms, including negative symptoms. When benzodiazepines are used as adjunctive agents with antipsychotic drugs, nearly two-thirds of studies reported since 1975 have shown beneficial effects (Wolkowitz and Pickar, 1991). However, the effects tended to be short-lived and the majority of trials did not demonstrate improvements in positive symptoms.

Valproic acid

The most widely studied and used GABAergic agent is valproic acid. In fact, a survey indicated that 28% of schizophrenic patients in New York State facilities were being treated with this medication in addition to their neuroleptics (Citrome et al., 2000). Valproic acid enhances GABAergic transmission, possibly via inhibition of dopaminergic activity in the mesolimbic system and stimulation of dopaminergic activity in the mesofrontocortical tract (Wassef et al., 1999).

Early, mostly open-label trials of valproic acid in schizophrenic patients provided some support of clinical benefit (Chong et al., 1998; Mori§igo et al., 1989, Wassef et al., 1989). Double-blind trials have had mixed results with both positive (Wassef et al., 2000, 2001) and negative (Dose et al., 1998; Hesslinger et al., 1999; Ko et al., 1985) effects with the addition of valproic acid to neuroleptics. A very large double-blind, multicenter trial involving 249 schizophrenic patients experiencing an acute exacerbation of their illness randomly assigned patients to receive olanzapine or risperidine alone or in combination with valproic acid for 28 days. Improvements were noted as early as day 3 on the total Positive and Negative Syndrome Scale score (Casey et al., 2003). However, Boylan and Labovitz (2004) pointed out that there was no statistically significant difference between the combination and monotherapies at 28 days, suggesting that it was actually a negative trial.

Basan et al. (2004) did a meta-analysis of the five randomized trials completed to date and were unable to confirm any overall superiority of adjunctive therapy with valproate when compared to neuroleptics alone. Thus, the clinical benefits of available GABAergic drugs have yet to be demonstrated.

Metabotropic Receptor Drugs

One of the problems with ionotropic glutamate receptors like NMDA, kainate, and AMPA is that they are found throughout the cortex. Any drug that acts on them would be expected to have a large number of unwanted effects. Metabotropic glutamate receptors offer a potential way around this in that the three types, groups I–III, show some degree of regional distribution with group II receptors more commonly found in forebrain regions (Conn and Pin, 1997; Petralia et al., 1996). Recent reports have suggested a role for metabotropic glutamate receptors in long-term potentiation, long-term depression, and neural sensitization (Anwyl, 1999; Feenstra et al., 1998). In fact, metabotropic glutamate receptors may be necessary for the development of sensitization with amphetamine (Kim and Vezina, 1998).

In animals treated with PCP, a group II metabotropic receptor agonist was able to attenuate the disruptive effects of PCP on working memory, stereotypy, locomotion, and cortical glutamate efflux while increasing the release of dopamine in the cortex (Moghaddam and Adams, 1998). Other investigators have found metabotropic glutamate receptor agonists to protect the rat retrosplenial cortex from the effects of NMDA antagonists (Okamura et al., 2003). Postmortem metabotropic glutamate receptor mRNA expression has not been found to be abnormal in the thalamus in schizophrenic patients (Richardson-Burns et al., 1999). In healthy subjects, a group II metabotropic glutamate receptor agonist has been shown to attenuate ketamine-induced working-memory deficits (Krystal et al., 2003). This kind of profile would suggest beneficial effects in schizophrenia. So far, no reports have been published about their use in schizophrenic patients; part of the reason for this may be the bioavailability of some of the agents currently in use. Other agents are currently in development (Bruno et al., 2001).

Transcranial Magnetic Stimulation

About 25%–30% of schizophrenic patients experience auditory hallucinations that are resistant to traditional antipsychotic drugs (Shergill et al., 1998). An option for these patients is transcranial magnetic stimulation (Hoffman and Cavus, 2002). Low-frequency (~1 Hz) transcranial magnetic stimulation for extended periods (>15 minutes) has been shown to reduce cortical activation (Chen et al., 1997). Because widespread activation has been seen throughout the limbic system and auditory cortex in patients experiencing hallucinations (see Chapter 8), the application of a low-frequency magnetic field could be therapeutic.

The first report of the use of transcranial magnetic stimulation in schizophrenic patients with persistent auditory hallucinations was positive (Hoffman et al., 1999). Three patients improved and two of the three had near-total cessation of their hallucinations for 2 weeks or more with left temporoparietal stimulation. Subsequent trials in mostly treatment-resistant patients were also encouraging, although not all patients responded to treatment (d'Alfonso et al., 2002; Hoffman et al., 2000; Schoenfeldt-Lecuona et al., 2001). When improvement was seen, the lasting effects were variable but often went on for several weeks after treatment.

The most extensive trial to date has included 24 schizophrenic or schizoaffective patients with treatment-resistant auditory hallucinations. Transcranial magnetic stimulation was delivered to the left temporoparietal cortex for up to 16 minutes for 9 days. Compared to the sham condition, patients who had received stimulation showed significant improvement in the frequency and severity of their hallucinations. Nine of 12 in the active treatment group had a 50% or greater improvement on the Hallucination Change Scale and just over half maintained improvement for at least 15 weeks (Hoffman et al., 2003). Balancing these encouraging findings is a more recent double-blind investigation of 16 patients with treatment-resistant hallucinations, which found no difference between real and sham treatments (McIntosh et al., 2004).

The rationale for a response makes sense from the brain-imaging studies that have found increased activity in the auditory cortex with hallucinations. However, the response is a little surprising from the perspective of the nucleus accumbens models. Although the magnetic field is delivered over the auditory cortex, the region is difficult to localize and usually extends for 2 or 3 centimeters. It is hard to believe that some of the deeper structures such as the hippocampus would not be affected. If they are, why does this not make the hallucinations worse by impairing the regulation of basal ganglia–thalamocortical circuits? Considering that mostly treatment-resistant patients have participated in these studies, the results are encouraging and will likely improve with refinements in the technique.

Psychosurgery

Psychosurgery has a very checkered past in psychiatry. Frontal lobotomies introduced in the United States by Walter Freeman in 1936 were proposed as a way of isolating the *diseased* frontal lobe from the rest of the brain. Unfortunately, they lead to emotional flatness, euphoria, and a lack of judgment. With the introduction of better treatments such as chlorpromazine, psychosurgery has been all but abandoned. However, some investigators argue that there may be a role for cingulatomy in very refractory cases (da Costa, 1997).

Variations on surgical approaches to neurological diseases such as Parkinson disease raise some interesting alternatives to the classic approaches in schizophrenia. Central lateral thalamotomy and anterior medial pallidotomy have been suggested as alternatives for intractable schizoaffective, obsessive-compulsive, and mood disorders on the basis of their possible effects on dysrhythmias caused by hyperpolarization of thalamic relay and/or reticular cells (Jeanmonod et al., 2003). Psychotic symptoms improved in four patients, but seven other patients with intractable depression, anxiety, and obsessive symptoms also improved, so the treatment may not be specific to schizophrenia.

Of particular interest is the use of chronic electrical stimulation of the subthalamic nucleus in medically refractory Parkinson disease, a treatment that has been associated with lasting benefits in many patients (Krause et al., 2004; Romito et al., 2003). The precise mechanism of effectiveness is not known, but it is likely that the stimulation leads to diminished inhibitory outflow of the internal segment of the globus pallidus onto the motor thalamus, resulting in some improvement in the motor symptoms of the disease.

Is it possible that deep brain stimulation could be offered to refractory schizophrenic patients? Many of these patients face a lifetime in seclusion. I would not doubt that many would choose to take the risks of surgery if one were available. Unfortunately, no procedures are available, but it is likely only a matter of time before one is developed.

Is There Any Reason to Be Hopeful?

Over the last 50 years, the only option in the treatment of schizophrenia has been drugs that block D_2 receptors. As models of schizophrenia have developed, some other possibilities have started to emerge. The early attempts to find drugs that decrease dopamine subcortically and without decreasing dopamine cortically have been disappointing, but there are now some other approaches targeting glutamate, GABA, and other neurotransmitters. Of these, drugs that affect the glycine receptor and lamotrigine look promising, but many more are in development (Miyamoto et al., 2005). One of the limitations of the glutamatergic drugs is that ionotropic receptors are ubiquitous in the brain. Metabotropic receptors may be more regionally specific but we do not as yet know if they have any antipsychotic properties.

Probably the most hopeful sign in treatment is that we are now starting to think about ways of preventing deterioration in patients, not just providing acute treatment of their symptoms. Many of the drugs already available such as lamotrigine have the potential to prevent deterioration by virtue of their neuroprotective properties. However, long-term studies are required to demonstrate these benefits. This research is not something that the drug companies are eager to do, but it is essential if we hope to change the course of this disorder.

There is a long way to go in developing better practical treatments for schizophrenia. There is also a long way to go in our understanding of the final common pathway of the disorder. The last chapter will offer some directions that could be taken in our quest.

15

The Way Forward

None of the models for the final common pathway of schizophrenia described thus far can approach the explanatory power that the circulatory system offers for heart failure. Yet we have some emerging principles. It seems highly likely that there is some deficit in either GABAergic or NMDA receptor circuitry related to an early neurodevelopmental genetic, viral, or hypoxic anomaly. The deficit is then manifested with cortical pruning at around adolescence, leading to dysregulation of dopamine release, particularly in response to stress. Whether there are further degenerative changes after the onset of illness remains debatable, but there is certainly ample evidence that the loss of gray matter proceeds for several years in many patients.

A perplexing problem, raised by many in the field, is the heterogeneity of findings. Some patients have large lateral ventricles and some do not. Some show frontal lobe activation deficits and others have temporal lobe activation deficits. Some have postmortem glutamatergic deficits and others show excesses. Even dopaminergic abnormalities are difficult to demonstrate in most patients. Why is this so? It may be that we are not thinking about the problem from the proper perspective. To return to the analogy of heart failure, we know that the heart is there to pump blood to the body so that oxygen and nutrients can enter body tissue. What is the equivalent relationship in schizophrenia? Obviously the brain is not pumping blood but it is processing information via signal transduction in complex networks of neurons. More importantly, the function of the brain is to connect disparate pieces of information about the environment into a coherent whole so that an appropriate response can be selected. Clearly, something is going wrong with this process in schizophrenia.

Where does this leave us? Some have argued that we have already discovered the genes responsible for schizophrenia; it is just a matter of time until we figure out how these genes translate into symptoms. Others take the approach that we can never understand schizophrenia because of its heterogeneity, so we should try to understand the physiological basis of dimensions such as psychomotor poverty, disorganization, and reality distortion. This chapter will argue that schizophrenia is *more* than the sum of its syndromes. It will also suggest that what is missing is the ways in which the brain streams and binds information. A better understanding of this process would have implications not just for schizophrenia but for the nature of consciousness as well.

Waiting for a Miracle?

The last two decades of schizophrenia research have been dominated by molecular genetic research. Almost every year, the gene for schizophrenia is discovered, only to be followed by the inevitable negative report. This is not to say that there have been no findings, but it is increasingly clear that no single genetic abnormality is likely to account for the large degree of the variance (Harrison and Owen, 2003; Harrison and Weinberger, 2005; Owen et al., 2004; Waterworth et al., 2002). It is possible that more careful evaluation of the genes involved in brain development could lead to more reliable findings. For example, abnormalities in genes that regulate the subplate early in brain development could lead to many of the findings characteristic of schizophrenia. As indicated in Chapter 3, animal models have demonstrated delayed development of dopaminergic hyperresponsivity, abnormal prepulse inhibition, and postmortem decreases in prefrontal GABA neurons and thalamic neurons in rats subjected to neonatal subplate lesions (Rajakumar and Rajakumar, 2003;

Rajakumar et al., 2004). However, the marked heterogeneity of findings in schizophrenia indicates that no single gene is likely to be the
smoking gun.

Even if we could determine the dozen or more genes that are
likely to be involved in schizophrenia, would this information help
us very much? For example, could we predict who is likely to get
schizophrenia? Not likely—as with many other disorders, having a
particular gene would probably carry variable risks. Would such genetic information help us to treat schizophrenia better? Possibly. Perhaps the best example to date is that of COMT gene polymorphisms,
which have been shown to be associated with performance on the
Wisconsin Card Sorting Test (WCST) as well as that on other tests
of processing speed and attention, factors found to be abnormal in
schizophrenia (Bilder et al., 2002; Egan et al., 2001). Individuals with
the *Met/Met* COMT genotype appear to be at increased risk for development of impaired neuropsychological performance if they take
an amphetamine (Mattay et al., 2003). However, it should be pointed
out that these studies were done in individuals who happened to
have this genotype but did not have schizophrenia. In fact, linkage
with the COMT gene is weak and very dependent upon the ethnic
background of the subjects (Glatt et al., 2003; Harrison and Owen,
2003). Much the same can be said for the metabotropic receptor
modulating gene *GRM3*. The linkage to schizophrenia is tenuous
and neuropsychological deficits associated with the polymorphism
can be seen in both normal and affected populations (Harrison and
Weinberger, 2005).

As time goes on, it is likely that a number of genes will be weakly
linked to schizophrenia. Some of these may convey vulnerability to
stress. Others may result in brain neurodevelopmental anomalies.
The brain develops epigenetically, much like an unfolding flower:
damage at one stage cannot be reversed at another stage. Even if we
find a gene with a strong association with schizophrenia, it would
not likely be reasonable to treat perfectly well individuals or withhold a certain type of treatment on the basis of genotype. The fact
that identical twins have only about 50% concordance would suggest
that prediction of the development of schizophrenia is very difficult
even in high-risk populations. While characterization of the genes
involved in schizophrenia will no doubt be helpful, it is likely that
schizophrenia is best understood at a different level: the level of neuronal circuits.

Schizophrenia Is *More* Than the Sum of Its Syndromes

A popular approach to schizophrenia over the last 10 to 15 years has been to accept heterogeneity and simply try to understand the physiological basis of individual syndromes. This attempt began with the positive-negative, type I-type II, and deficit-nondeficit (Andreasen, 1982; Crow, 1989; Tamminga et al., 1992) approaches. These did not fare well in factor analytic studies of symptoms that tend to go together. While many investigators favor four or more factors (Kay, 1991), the system that has taken hold is that of Liddle (1987), which characterized psychomotor poverty, disorganization, and reality distortion syndromes. Efforts to link these syndromes have had mixed results. Patients with chronic symptoms related to these syndromes show only weak correlations to either neuropsychological tests or volumetic findings (see Chapters 6 and 7). The link to patterns of cerebral blood flow is much stronger, but studies of specific symptoms are not consistent. On the whole, there does seem to be a link between negative symptoms and prefrontal activity. Similarly, widespread limbic activity seems to be associated with auditory hallucinations and other positive symptoms, but the pattern varies considerably from subject to subject.

These studies have contributed much to the understanding of schizophrenia. However, in a way, they miss the essence of schizophrenia. Hallucinations, delusions, and negative symptoms occur in a variety of different disorders, such as strokes, dementia, drug intoxication, and mood disorders. In many cases, the symptoms are indistinguishable from those of schizophrenia, but these patients do not have schizophrenia. The disorder described by Kraepelin was a combination of these symptoms, with an onset usually early in life, characterized by a variable chronic course that often includes considerable deterioration in social and cognitive functioning. Examination of the correlates of individual syndromes may be helpful in determining the brain circuits that may be more or less affected in an individual patient but they do not capture the whole picture. It should also be recognized that all patients show unique combinations of these syndromes. We do not see patients with only reality distortion or with only psychomotor poverty.

An examination of the link between characteristic symptom clusters offers an opportunity to look at the whole picture. Probably the best example of this would be the revised dopamine theory (see

Chapter 4). Stated simply, too much subcortical dopamine activity leads to positive symptoms whereas too little cortical activity leads to negative symptoms. Many of the models discussed in Chapters 11 and 12 are variations on this theme, with the addition of NMDA hypofunction in various parts of the brain. These models account for much of what we know about schizophrenia but fall short in few areas. Most noteworthy is the rather weak link between dopamine and positive symptoms. The majority of subjects given amphetamine do not get psychotic and even schizophrenic patients show an exaggerated response to dopamine agonists in only 30% of cases. Nor are dopamine agonists the only way to induce positive symptoms. NMDA antagonists seem to be able to do this even when dopamine is blocked by antipsychotic drugs (see Chapter 13). Is it possible that both dopamine and glutamate are simply factors that control another process in the brain that is leading the symptoms?

A Problem of Connection Rather Than Disconnection?

Much has been said about disconnection in schizophrenia—not just disconnection between the prefrontal and temporal cortices, but also the loss of connections involved in cortical control of subcortical structures such as the nucleus accumbens or even a more widespread loss of corticocortical connections that may be genetically based and account for the loss of gray matter observed in brain imaging studies. There is good reason to believe that disconnection is present in schizophrenia, but as with almost everything in schizophrenia, the patterns of disconnection may differ considerably between cases. All of these regions converge on the ventral striatum and thalamus, regions known to integrate current and past emotional and perceptual information about the organism and its environment into conscious awareness. Dysfunctional input from any of these regions could lead to errors in this integration, which may explain why the findings and the symptoms of schizophrenia vary so much among individual cases. Maybe the problem in schizophrenia may not be so much disconnection as connection—a problem of streaming and binding information.

No one knows how information is bound into the coherent whole that we experience as consciousness. It is quite an accomplishment when one thinks of the complexity of the task. Information from all five senses must be blended across time with past experience, emotional valence, and internal thought processes. No single cortical area has been shown to support consciousness. Rather, corticocortical connectivity seems to be essential for the conscious integration of information. Some investigators have argued that thalamocortical loops, the hippocampus, and even basal ganglia are critical for understanding consciousness (Tononi and Edelman, 1998b). It is of interest that NMDA receptors are likely involved in the maintenance of intracortical and thalamocortical reentrant loops related to conscious perception. In fact, ketamine's use as an anesthetic may arise from its ability to impair consciousness without depressing cortical activity (Tononi and Edelman, 1998b). Thus, there are several brain regions that could be associated with binding, but the problem is even more complicated.

Gray (2004) suggests that there are at least two versions of the binding problem. The first is the multimodal problem—we are always experiencing more than than one sense. Yet the senses come together in a unified whole, leading to distinctive qualitative features of conscious experience referred to as *qualia*. For example, we do not perceive a tree as a jumble of colors heard to rustle in the wind. We see it as a tree. The second version is the intramodal problem. It is curious that vision can be clearly divided into a conscious perceptual system that can suffer visual illusions and an unconscious or action system that does not. The two systems are perceived as one in consciousness. The movement of the kite cannot be separated from its color. There is reason to believe that other senses are also structured in a similar way. In the auditory pathway, the streams for *what* and *where* seem to be quite different (Rauschecker and Tian, 2000). Yet it is not likely that schizophrenia is related to an intramodal binding problem. The patients with impaired conscious perceptual deficits and unconscious action deficits do not hallucinate or believe that someone else is controlling their actions (Goodale and Milner, 2004), but there may be a case for a multimodel problem in schizophrenia.

The possibility that schizophrenia and other neuropsychiatric conditions may arise from a failure of thalamocortical reentrant loops to integrate perception and cognition has been raised by others (Green and Nuechterlein, 1999; Gruzelier, 1999; Llinás et al., 1999; Tononi and Edelman, 2000)—but how does this occur? The nucleus accumbens and reticular thalamic nucleus have been highlighted by some models of schizophrenia (Lieberman et al., 1997;

O'Donnell and Grace, 1998). Both the nucleus accumbens and reticular thalamic nucleus have been suggested to play a unique role in streaming and binding information (Newman and Grace, 1999). Gruzelier (1999) suggested that lateralized imbalances in thalamocortical and callosal arousal system may be central to schizophrenia. Others (Llinás et al., 1999) have suggested that thalamocortical dysrhythmia associated with low-frequency resonances in thalamocortical circuits results from either bottom-up or top-down changes in voltage-gated conductances in thalamic relay and/or reticular cells. These low-frequency loops interact with higher-frequency loops, leading to clinical symptoms. Anormalities of bottom-up input result in neurological conditions like Parkinson disease, whereas top-down anomalies result in neuropsychiatric conditions like depression and possibly schizophrenia. The recent observation of abnormalities in the synchrony of fast activity in schizophrenic patients (Spencer et al., 2003; 2004) is consistent with this idea but we are at a very early stage of understanding how the thalamus works. It is likely that intralaminar and a newly identified matrix of calbindin-immunoreactive neurons extending throughout the thalamus and projecting to the superficial layers of the cortex may also be important (Jones, 2001).

We could think of consciousness as a spinning wheel where streams of affective, sensory, and intentional information are spun together into a single thread and stored for future use on the bobbin. Thalamocortical reentry loops could be seen as the wool spinning around, and the hippocampus would be the bobbin while the nucleus accumbens and reticular thalamic nucleus are the spinners allowing the different colors of cognition, perception, and affect to be spun into a single thread. Although there are other candidates for the spinner, nowhere else does affective information from the limbic system and cognitive information from the prefrontal cortex come together as merging streams with current perceptual information and past experience. It is not difficult to think of many of the symptoms of schizophrenia as a failure to effectively integrate cognition, perception, and affect; an irelevant piece of information linked with fear can become paranoia; an internal thought gets disconnected from self-monitoring in the brain and becomes a hallucination. But is it just the nucleus accumbens and thalamus that participate in binding? Let us take another look at the neuropsychological and imaging literature and some of the preliminary models.

Schizophrenia Reconsidered

The neuropsychological literature is compatible with schizophrenia as a failure of binding. To some extent, all core explanations of deficits in schizophrenic patients depend on encoding. In order to do any task, information has to be held on-line and compared to previous information to execute a self-initiated plan—all elements in which binding information about current and past sensory and affective information as well as intention is essential. Considering the central nature of these processes, it is little wonder that the cognitive deficits are so diffuse in schizophrenia.

The imaging literature would suggest that there are many possible abnormalities in schizophrenic patients that could lead to deficit glutamatergic input from the temporal lobe or prefrontal cortex to the ventral striatum and thalamus, all of which could result in affective and perceptual abnormalities. The nature of the faulty input may lead to the unique character of an individual's illness. At the same time, all patterns of illness would share the same basic failure to bind these elements of consciousness.

Perhaps it is no accident that almost all of the models proposed for schizophrenia include regions most often implicated in binding. A particularly appealing model is the nucleus accumbens model (Grace, 2000; Moore et al., 1999; O'Donnell and Grace, 1998): the nucleus accumbens streams information into the reticular nucleus of the thalamus, which in turn influences the activity of all the thalamic nuclei and reentrant thalamocortical loops necessary for consciousness. The dopamine sensitization model (Lieberman et al., 1997) also proposes a central role for the nucleus accumbens. However, the focus on dopamine is different. Instead of suggesting disturbed gating caused by deficient input to the nucleus accumbens from the hippocampus and/or amygdala, it suggests that the problem with dopamine is due to dopamine sensitization that is unregulated by cortical inhibition. In either case, output to the thalamus and presumably streaming and binding of information could be disturbed. Where both models fall short is the explanation of why certain inputs are periodically excluded, such as self- and intentional information.

If self-monitoring information is routed through the nucleus accumbens, then the nucleus accumbens and dopamine sensitization models may provide an explanation for how this information is affected in schizophrenia. Some of the brain-imaging evidence implicates brain regions that project to the nucleus accumbens. The right medial prefrontal cortex is activated during self-monitoring (see Chapter 13) and the anterior cingulate clearly is involved with intention. Patients with damage to the anterior cingulate are often mute and amotivated. However, it is worth remembering that not all the inputs to the thalamus are gated through the nucleus accumbens. In fact, the nucleus accumbens handles the input from the medial prefrontal regions and anterior cingulate, but most of the traffic from the other parts of the prefrontal cortex go to the dorsal striatum and then the thalamus through the direct and indirect pathways (see Chapter 2).

Some of the regions that project to the dorsal striatum have been implicated in other models of schizophrenia and also in self-monitoring tasks. The corollary-discharge model (Feinberg and Guazzelli, 1999) has implicated the various basal ganglia–thalamocortical pathways involved in prediction of action. The cognitive-dysmetria model (Andreasen, 1999; Andreasen et al., 1998) has suggested that structures such as the cerebellum play a role in self-monitoring. Finally, the laterality (Crow, 1990a, 1990b, 1995, 1997a, 1997b, 1998; Gruzelier, 1984, 1999), disconnection (Weinberger, 1991; Friston and Frith, 1995), and imbalanced-brain (Grossberg, 2000a) models have implicated problems with corticocortical and subcortical integration involving the transfer of information between the hemispheres, prefrontal and temporal cortices, and sensory regions.

So the question as to where the binding anomalies occur in schizophrenia remains unanswered. The nucleus accumbens and the thalamus are probable sites, but much larger networks of brain activity such as the cortical pathways that coordinate perception, affect, and movement cannot be ruled out. Another question that remains unanswered is why schizophrenia occurs naturally only in humans.

Why Is Schizophrenia a Uniquely Human Disorder?

While it is clear that lesioned or stressed animals can have some findings associated with schizophrenia, they do not demonstrate the clinical features of the disorder. Part of the reason may be that schizophrenia is a disorder of human consciousness. No doubt, animals are conscious, but they do not seem to have a sense of self nor do they seem to experience time in the same sense. They also do not use language in the way that we do. Indeed, the emergence of higher-order consciousness seems to be tied to the emergence of language (Tononi and Edelman, 1998b). It is curious that these qualities are represented in schizophrenic symptoms.

The possibility that language (and laterality) may be central to schizophrenia has often been commented on. However, no one has provided a good explanation as to why patients are more likely to experience auditory rather than visual or olfactory hallucinations. Delirium does not seem to follow this pattern in most species and visual hallucinations usually predominate. Is there something unique about the way auditory signals enter consciousness in humans? Or is this related to the linkage between intentionality (self) and perception? A large prefrontal cortex allows anticipation and planning but has to be integrated with older structures in the brain designed to respond to affective cues. Many investigators have pointed to the imbalance between these two parts of brain in schizophrenia over the years. When activity in the limbic inputs through the nucleus accumbens overwhelms the input through the dorsal striatum, critical information about self-monitoring could be lost to conscious appraisal, leading to positive symptoms. The observation that the entire limbic system becomes hyperactive on the PET during hallucinations is compatible with this suggestion. Negative symptoms could reflect the opposite state, where self-monitoring is intact but affective integration is missing.

What we need to do now is develop a better understanding of how the limbic brain coordinates its activity with the cognitive brain. At what level or levels does this occur? The reticular nucleus of the thalamus would seem to be a good bet. It receives input from the nucleus accumbens and influences all the nuclei of the thalamus, including those which process information from the dorsolateral and lateral orbital prefrontal cortex. However, a good case can also be made for a failure of the integration of larger corticocortical networks involving many prefrontal and temporal structures. Part of the reason that we have not been able to answer this question may be that it is actually very difficult to study consciousness with current imaging techniques. The time frame is much too long. Electroencephalographic techniques are better from this perspective but have limited spatial resolution for subcortical structures. Magnetoencephalography has more spatial resolution and the potential to examine some of these questions, but it is at a very early stage of application. Nevertheless, it is interesting that functional imaging studies that have looked at correlations between brain regions have shown a disconnection between limbic structures such as the anterior cingulate and the dorsolateral prefrontal cortex during fluency tasks, which activates both regions normally (Dye et al., 1999; Spence et al., 2000). This could suggest a disconnection between limbic and cortical basal ganglia–thalamocortical neuronal circuits.

Another question worth thinking about is the course of the disorder. Does the disconnection between the limbic and cognitive brains occur gradually as the extended prodromal phase in many patients suggests? The longitudinal volumetric and MRS data suggest that the disinhibition of limbic and subcortical structures could be associated with degeneration. Some of these structures such as the medial prefrontal region are involved in both self-perception and affect. If there is gradual damage to these structures, could neuroprotective agents be helpful? There is already some evidence that this might be the case. All too often patients are left with severe disabilities with conventional treatment. We now have the tools to begin to answer these questions.

Some Final Thoughts

If we look at schizophrenia as a problem of streaming and binding perceptual, cognitive, and affective information, much of what we know about schizophrenia makes sense. The prefrontal cortex, anterior cingulate, temporal lobes, and associated structures comprise the main inputs to the ventral and dorsal striatum which in turn projects to the thalamus and back to the cortex. Damage to any part of these circuits could affect reentrant circuits critical for consciousness. Dopamine and glutamate would also be expected to be involved. Dopamine regulates the neuronal circuits involving these regions and glutamate is the main neurotransmitter involved in both corticocortical and cortical–subcortical connections. Little wonder that two anesthetics that affect dopamine and NMDA receptors have had such an impact on the history of schizophrenia research: chlorpromazine and ketamine.

Another study correlating some postmortem, structural, or functional finding to schizophrenia is not going to help much. We already know which regions are more likely to have abnormalities, and chances are that some patients will have the finding and others will not. Schizophrenia is a heterogenous disorder not unlike heart failure. Like heart failure, it may well have a common final pathway, and all indicators point to the brain structures that stream and bind perceptual, cognitive, and affective information. While understanding how this occurs in the brain is going to be a challenge, it is likely more feasible in our generation than understanding the extremely complex interactions between environmental factors, the dozens of genes that predispose to schizophrenia, and brain development. It is also likely that in the course of these investigations, we may learn as much about what makes us human as we learn about schizophrenia.

References

....

Aalto, S., Hirvonen, J., Kajander, J., Scheinin, H., Någren, K., Vilkman, H., Gustafsson, L., Syvälahti, E., and Hietala, J. (2002). Ketamine does not decrease striatal dopamine D_2 receptor binding in man. *Psychopharmacology*, **164**, 401–406.

Abel, K.M., Allin, M.P.G., Hemsley, D.R., and Geyer, M.A. (2003). Low dose ketamine increases prepulse inhibition in healthy men. *Neuropharmacology*, **44**, 729–737.

Abi-Dargham, A., Gil, R., Krystal, J., Baldwin, R.M., Seibyl, J.P., Bowers, M., van Dyck, C.H., Charney, D.S., Innis, R.B., and Laruelle, M. (1998). Increased striatal dopamine transmission in schizophrenia: Confirmation in a second cohort. *American Journal of Psychiatry*, **155**, 761–767.

Abi-Dargham, A., Krystal, J., Laruelle, M., D'Souza, D., Zohbi, S., Brenner, L., Gil, R., Sernyak, M., Baldwin, R.M., Zubal, G., Hoffer, P.B., Charney, D.S., and Innis, R.B. (1995). SPECT imaging of the benzodiazepine receptor in schizophrenics and healthy subjects. *Schizophrenia Research*, **15**, 75.

Abi-Dargham, A., Mawlawi, O., Lombardo, I., Gil, R., Martinez, D., Huang, Y., Hwang, D-R., Keilp, J., Kochan, L., Van Heertum, R., Gorman, J.M., and Laruelle, M. (2002). Prefrontal dopamine D_1 receptors and working memory in schizophrenia. *Journal of Neuroscience*, **22**, 3708–3719.

Abi-Dargham, A., Rodenhiser, J., Printz, D., Zea-Ponce, Y., Gil, R., Kegeles, L.S., Weiss Cooper, T.B., Mann, J.J., Van Heertum, R.L., Gorman, J.M., and Laruelle, M. (2000). Increased baseline occupancy of D2 receptors by dopamine in schizophrenia. *Proceedings of the National Academy of Science of the United States of America*, **97**, 8104–8109.

Abrams, R. and Taylor, M.A. (1979). Laboratory studies in the validation of psychiatric diagnoses. In J.H. Gruzelier and P. Flor-Henry (Eds.), *Hemispheric asymmetries of function in psychopathology* (pp. 363–372). Amsterdam, Elsevier.

Ackerknecht, E.H. (1968). *A short history of medicine.* New York, Ronald Press.

Addington, J., Addington, D., and Maticka-Tyndale, E. (1991). Cognitive functioning and positive and negative symptoms in schizophrenia. *Schizophrenia Research*, **5**, 123–134.

Aggleton, J.P. (Ed.) (1992). *The amygdala: Neurobiological aspects of emotion, memory, and mental dysfunction.* New York, Wiley-Liss Inc.

Akbarian, S., Bunney, W.E., Potkin, S.G., Wigal, S.B., Hagman, J.O., Sandman, C.A., and Jones, E.G. (1993a). Altered distribution of nicotinamide-adenine dinucleotide phosphate-diaphorase cells in frontal lobe of schizophrenics implies disturbances of cortical development. *Archives of General Psychiatry*, **50**, 169–177.

Akbarian, S., Kim, J.J., Potkin, S.G., Hagman, J.O., Tafazzoli, A., Bunney, W.E., and Jones, E.G. (1995). Gene expression for glutamic acid decarboxylase is reduced without loss of neurons in prefrontal cortex of schizophrenics. *Archives of General Psychiatry*, **52**, 258–266.

Akbarian, S., Vinuela, A., Kim. J.J., Potkin, S.G., Bunney, W.E., and Jones, E.G. (1993b). Distorted distribution of nicotinamide-adenine dinucleotide phosphate-diaphorase neurons in temporal lobe of schizophrenics implies anomalous cortical development. *Archives of General Psychiatry*, **50**, 178–187.

Akil, M., Pierri, J.N., Whitehead, R.E., Edgar, C.L., Mohila, C., Sampson, A.R., and Lewis, D.A. (1999). Lamina-specific alterations in the dopamine innervation of the prefrontal cortex in schizophrenic subjects. *American Journal of Psychiatry*, **156**, 1580–1589.

Aleman, A., Hijman, R., de Haan, E.H.F., and Kahn, R.S. (1999). Memory impairment in schizophrenia: A meta-analysis. *American Journal of Psychiatry*, **156**, 1358–1366.

Alexander, G.E., Crutchner, M.D., and De Long, M.R. (1990) Basal ganglia-thalamocortical circuits: Parallel substrates for motor, oculometer, "prefrontal" and "limbic" functions. In H.B.M. Uylings, C.G. Van Eden, J.P.C. De Bruin, M.A. Corner, and M.G.P. Feenstra (Eds.), *The prefrontal cortex: its structure, function and pathology.* New York, Elsevier (Published as *Progress in Brain Research*, **85**, 119–146).

American Psychiatric Association. (2000). *Diagnostic and statistical manual of mental disorders,* fourth edition, text revision. American Psychiatric Association, Washington, DC.

Anand, A., Charney, D.S., Oren, D.A., Berman, R.M., Hu, Z.S., Cappiello, A., and Krystal, J.H. (2000). Attenuation of the neuropsychiatric effects of ketamine with lamotrigine: support for the hyperglutamatergic effects of *N*-methyl-D-aspartate receptor antagonists. *Archives of General Psychiatry,* **57**, 270–276.

Ananth, H., Popescu, I., Critchley, H.D., Good, C.D., Frackowiak, R.S.J., and Dolan, R.J. (2002). Cortical and subcortical gray matter abnormalities in schizophrenia determined through structural magnetic resonance imaging with optimized volumetric voxel-based morphometry. *American Journal of Psychiatry,* **159**, 1497–1505.

Andersen, B.B. and Pakkenberg, B. (2003). Stereological quantification in cerebella from people with schizophrenia. *British Journal of Psychiatry,* **182**, 354–361.

Anderson, J.E., Wible, C.G., McCarley, R.W., Jakab, M., Kasai, K., and Shenton, M.E. (2002). An MRI study of temporal lobe abnormalities and negative symptoms in chronic schizophrenia. *Schizophrenia Research,* **58**, 123–134.

Andreasen, N.C. (1976). The artist as scientist: Psychiatric diagnosis in Shakespeare's tragedies. *Journal of the American Medical Association,* **235**, 1868–1872.

Andreasen, N.C. (1982) Negative symptoms in schizophrenia: Definition and validation. *Archives of General Psychiatry,* **39**, 784–788.

Andreasen, N.C. (1989). Nuclear magnetic resonance imaging. In N.C. Andreasen (Ed.), *Brain imaging: applications in psychiatry* (pp. 67–121). Washington, DC, American Psychiatric Press.

Andreasen, N.C. (1996). Pieces of the schizophrenia puzzle fall into place. *Neuron,* **16**, 697–700.

Andreasen, N.C. (1997). The role of the thalamus in schizophrenia. *Canadian Journal of Psychiatry,* **42**, 27–33.

Andreasen, N.C. (1999). A unitary model of schizophrenia: Bleuler's "fragmented phrene" as schizencephaly. *Archives of General Psychiatry,* **56**, 781–787.

Andreasen, N.C., Arndt, S., Swayze, V., Cizadlo, T., Flaum, M., O'Leary, D., Ehrhardt, J.C., and Yuh, W.T.C. (1994). Thalamic abnormalities in schizophrenia visualized through magnetic resonance imaging averaging. *Science,* **266**, 294–298.

Andreasen, N., Nasrallah, H.A., Dunn, V., Olsen, S.C., Grove, W.M., Ehrhardt, J.C., Coffman, J.A., and Crossett, J.H.W. (1986). Structural abnormalities in the frontal system in schizophrenia: A magnetic resonance imaging study. *Archives of General Psychiatry,* **43**, 136–144.

Andreasen, N.C., O'Leary, D.S., Cizadlo, T., Arndt, S., Rezai, K., Boles Ponto, L.L., Watkins, G.L., and Hichwa, R.D. (1996). Schizophrenia and cognitive dysmetria: A positron-emission tomography study of dysfunctional prefrontal-thalamic-cerebellar circuitry. *Proceedings of the National Academy of Sciences of the United States of America,* **93**, 9985–9990.

Andreasen, N.C., O'Leary, D.S., Flaum, M., Nopoulos, P., Watkins, G.L., Ponto, L.L.B., and Hichwa, R.D. (1997). Hypofrontality in schizophrenia: Distributed dysfunctional circuits in neuroleptic-naïve patients. *Lancet,* **349**, 1730–1734.

Andreasen, N.C., Paradiso, S., and O'Leary, D.S. (1998). "Cognitive dysmetria" as an integrative theory of schizophrenia: A dysfunction in cortical-subcortical-cerebellar circuitry? *Schizophrenia Bulletin,* **24**, 203–218.

Andreasen, N.C., Rezai, K., Alliger, R., Swayze, V.W., Faum, M., Kircher, P., Cohen, G., and O'Leary, D.S. (1992). Hypofrontality in neuroleptic-naïve patients and in patients with chronic schizophrenia: Assessment with xenon 133 single-photon emission computed tomography and the Tower of London. *Archives of General Psychiatry,* **49**, 943–958.

Anwyl, R. (1999). Metabotropic glutamate receptors: Electrophysiological properties and role in plasticity. *Brain Research Reviews,* **29**, 83–120.

Archer, J., Hay, D.C., and Young, A.W. (1992). Face processing in psychiatric conditions. *British Journal of Clinical Psychology,* **41**, 45–61.

Argo, T.R., Carnahan, R.M., and Perry, P.J. (2004). Aripiprazole, a novel atypical antipsychotic drug. *Pharmacotherapy* **24**, 212–228.

Arnold, S.E. and Rioux, L. (2001). Challenges, status, and opportunities for studying developmental neuropathology in adult schizophrenia. *Schizophrenia Bulletin,* **27**, 395–416.

Artiges, E., Martinot, J.L., Verdys, M., Attar-Levy, D., Mazoyer, B., Tzourio, N., Giraud, M.-J., and Paillère, M.-L. (2000). Altered hemispheric functional dominance during word generation in negative schizophrenia. *Schizophrenia Bulletin,* **26**, 709–721.

Arvanov, V.L., Liang, X., Schwartz, J., Grossman, S., and Wang, R.Y. (1997). Clozapine and haloperidol modulate N-methyl-D-aspartate- and non-N-methyl-D-aspartate receptor-mediated neurotransmission in rat prefrontal cortical neurons in vitro. *Journal Pharmacology and Experimental Therapeutics,* **283**, 226–234.

Ashburner, J. and Friston, K.J. (2000). Voxel-based morphometry: The methods. *Neuroimage,* **11**, 805–821.

Auer, D.P., Putz, B., Kraft, E., Lipinski, B., Schnill, J., and Holsboer, F. (2000). Reduced glutamate in the anterior cingulate cortex in depression: An in vivo proton magnetic resonance spectroscopy study. *Biological Psychiatry,* **47**, 305–313.

Auer, D.P., Wilke, M., Grabner, A., Heidenreich, J.O., Brouisch, T., and Wetter, T.C. (2001). Reduced NAA in the thalamus and altered membrane and glial metabolism in schizophrenic patients detected by ^{1}H-MRS and tissue segmentation. *Schizophrenia Research,* **52**, 87–99.

Avila, M.T., Weiler, M.A., Lahti, A.C., Tamminga, C.A., and Thaker, G.K. (2002). Effects of ketamine on leading saccades during smooth-pursuit eye movements may implicate cerebellar dysfunction in schizophrenia. *American Journal of Psychiatry,* **159**, 1490–1496.

Bachevalier, J. (1994). Medial temporal lobe structures and autism: A review of clinical and experimental findings. *Neuropsychologia,* **32**, 627–648.

Baddeley, A. (1992). Working memory. *Science,* **255**, 556–559.

Ballmaier, M., Toga, A.W., Siddarth, P., Blanton, R.E., Levitt, J.G., Lee, M., and Caplan, R. (2004). Thought disorder and nucleus accumbens in childhood: A structural MRI study. *Psychiatry Research: Neuroimaging,* **130,** 43–55.

Barnes, T.R., Hutton, S.B., Chapman, M.J., Mutsata, S., Puri, B.K., and Joyce, E.M. (2000). West London first-episode study of schizophrenia: Clinical correlates of duration of untreated psychosis. *British Journal of Psychiatry,* **177,** 207–211.

Barr, C.E., Mednick, S.A., and Munk-Jorgensen, P. (1990). Exposure to influenza epidemics during gestation and adult schizophrenia. *Archives of General Psychiatry,* **47,** 869–874.

Barta, P.E., Pearlson, G.D., Powers, R.E., Richards, S.S., and Tune, L.E. (1990). Auditory hallucinations and smaller superior temporal gyral volume in schizophrenia. *American Journal of Psychiatry,* **147,** 1457–1462.

Bartha, R., Al-Semaan, Y.M., Williamson, P.C., Drost, D.J., Malla, A.K., Carr, T.J., Canaran, G., Densmore, M., and Neufeld, R.W.J. (1999). A short echo proton magnetic resonance spectroscopy study of the left temporal lobe in first-onset schizophrenic patients. *Biological Psychiatry,* **45,** 1403–1411.

Bartha, R., Stein, M., Williamson, P.C., Drost, D.J., Carr, T.J., Canaran, G., Densmore, M., Anderson, G., Neufeld, R.W.J., and Siddiqui, A-R. (1998). A short ^{1}H echo magnetic resonance spectroscopy and volumetric MR imaging study of the basal ganglia in patients with obsessive-compulsive disorder and healthy controls. *American Journal of Psychiatry,* **155,** 1584–1591.

Bartha, R., Williamson, P.C., Drost, D.J., Malla, A., Carr, T.J., Cortese, L., Canaran MacFabe, G., Rylett, R.J., and Neufeld, R.W.J. (1997). Measurement of glutamate and glutamine in the medial prefrontal cortex of never-treated schizophrenic patients and healthy controls using proton magnetic resonance spectroscopy. *Archives of General Psychiatry,* **54,** 959–965.

Bartley, A.J., Jones, D.W., Torrey, E.F., Zigun, J.R., and Weinberger, D.R. (1993). Sylvian fissure asymmetries in monozygotic twins: A test of laterality in schizophrenia. *Biological Psychiatry,* **34,** 853–863.

Basan, A., Kissling W., and Leucht, S. (2004). Valproate as an adjunct to antipsychotics for schizophrenia: A systematic review of randomized trials. *Schizophrenia Research,* **70,** 33–37.

Baxter, R.D. and Liddle, P.F. (1998). Neuropsychological deficits associated with schizophrenic syndromes. *Schizophrenia Research,* **30,** 239–250.

Bazin, N., Perruchet, P., Hardy-Bayle, M., and Feline, A. (2000). Context-dependent information processing in patients with schizophrenia. *Schizophrenia Research,* **45,** 93–101.

Bearden, C.E., Hoffman, K.M., and Cannon, T.D. (2001). The neuropsychology and neuroanatomy of bipolar affective disorder: a critical review. *Bipolar Disorders,* **3,** 106–150.

Benes, F.M. (2000). Emerging principles of altered neural circuitry in schizophrenia. *Brain Research Reviews,* **31,** 251–269.

Benes, F.M., Majocha, R., Bird, E.D., and Marrotta, C.A. (1987). Increased vertical axon numbers in cingulate cortex of schizophrenics. *Archives of General Psychiatry*, **44**, 1017–1021.

Benes, F.M., McSparren, J., Bird, E.D., Vincent, S.L., and SanGiovanni, J.P. (1991a). Deficits in small interneurons in prefrontal and cingulate cortices of schizophrenic and schizoaffective patients. *Archives of General Psychiatry*, **48**, 996–1001.

Benes, F.M., Sorenson, I., and Bird, E.D. (1991b). Reduced neuronal size in posterior hippocampus of schizophrenic patients. *Schizophrenia Research*, **17**, 597–608.

Benes, F.M., Sorensen, I., Vincent, S.L., Bird, E.D., and Sathi, M. (1992a). Increased density of glutamate-immunoreactive vertical processes in superficial laminae in cingulate cortex of schizophrenic brain. *Cerebral Cortex*, **2**, 503–512.

Benes, F.M., Todtenkopf, M.S., and Taylor, J.B. (1997). Differential distribution of tyrosine hydroxylase fibers on neuronal subtypes in layer II of anterior cingulate cortex of schizophrenic brain. *Synapse*, **25**, 80–92.

Benes, F.M., Turtle, M., Khan, Y., and Farol, P. (1994). Myelination of a key relay zone in the hippocampal formation occurs in the human brain during childhood, adolescence, and adulthood. *Archives of General Psychiatry*, **51**, 477–484.

Benes, F.M., Vincent, S.L., Alsterberg, G., Bird, E.D., and SanGiovanni, J.P. (1992b). Increased GABA receptor binding in supragranular layers of schizophrenic cingulate cortex. *Journal of Neuroscience*, **12**, 924–929.

Bentall, R.P. (1990). The illusion of reality: A review and integration of psychological research on hallucinations. *Psychological Bulletin*, **107**, 82–95.

Berger, H. (1929). Über das Elektrenkephalogramm des Menschen. *Archiv für Psychiatrie*, **87**, 527–570.

Berman, K.F., Torrey, E.F., Daniel, D.G., and Weinberger, D.R. (1992). Regional cerebral blood flow in monozygotic twins discordant and concordant for schizophrenia. *Archives of General Psychiatry*, **49**, 927–934.

Berman, K.F. and Weinberger, D.R. (1986). Cerebral blood flow studies in schizophrenia. In H.A. Nasrallah and D.R. Weinberger (Eds.), *Handbook of schizophrenia, volume 1: The neurology of schizophrenia* (pp. 277–307). Amsterdam, Elsevier.

Berman, K.F., Zec, R.F., and Weinberger, D.R. (1986). Physiological dysfunction of dorsolateral cortex in schizophrenia: II. Role of neuroleptic treatment, attention, and mental effort. *Archives of General Psychiatry*, **43**, 126–135.

Bertolino, A., Breier, A., Callicott, J.H., Adler, C., Mattay, V.S., Shapiro, M., Frank, J.A., Pickar, D., and Weinberger, D.R. (2000a). The relationship between dorsolateral prefrontal neuronal N-acetylaspartate and evoked release of striatal dopamine in schizophrenia. *Neuropsychopharmacology*, **22**, 125–133.

Bertolino, A., Callicott, J.H., Elman, I., Mattay, V.S., Tedeschi, G., Frank, J.A.,

Breier, A., and Weinberger, D.R. (1998). Regionally specific neuronal pathology in untreated patients with schizophrenia: a proton magnetic resonance spectroscopic imaging study. *Biological Psychiatry*, **43**, 641–648.

Bertolino, A., Esposito, G., Callicott, J.H., Mattay, V.S., Van Horn, J.D., Frank, J.A., Berman, K.F., and Weinberger, D.R. (2000b). Specific relationship between prefrontal neuronal *N*-acetylaspartate and activation of the working memory cortical network in schizophrenia. *American Journal of Psychiatry*, **157**, 26–33.

Bertolino, A., Sawroz, S., Mattay, V.S., Barnett, A.S., Duyn, J.H., Moonen, C.T.W., Frank, J.H., Tedeschi, G., and Weinberger, D.R. (1996). Regionally specific pattern of neurochemical pathology in schizophrenia as assessed by multislice proton magnetic resonance spectroscopic imaging. *American Journal of Psychiatry*, **153**, 1554–1563.

Bilder, R.M., Goldman, R.S., Robinson, D., Reiter, G., Bell, L., Bates, J.A., Pappadopulos, E., Wilson, D.F., Alvir, J.M.J., Woerner, M.G., Geisler, S., Kane, J.M., and Lieberman, J.A. (2000). Neuropsychology of first-episode schizophrenia: Initial characterization and clinical correlates. *American Journal of Psychiatry*, **157**, 549–559.

Bilder, R.M., Kipschultz-Broch, L., Reiter, G., Mayerhoff, D., Loebel, A., Degreef, G., Ashtari, M., and Lieberman, J.A. (1991). Neuropsychological studies of first-episode schizophrenia. *Schizophrenia Research*, **4**, 381–397.

Bilder, R.M., Mukherjee, S., Reider, R.O., and Pandurangi, A.K. (1985). Symptomatic and neuropsychological components of defect states. *Schizophrenia Bulletin*, **11**, 409–419.

Bilder, R.M., Volavka, J., Czobor, P., Malhotra, A.K., Kennedy, J.L., Ni, X., Goldman, R.S., Hoptman, M.J., Sheitman, B., Lindenmayer, J.-P., Citrome, T.B., McEvoy, J.P., Kunz, M., Chakos, M., Cooper, T.B., and Lieberman, J.A. (2002). Neurocognitive correlates of COMT Val[158]Met polymorphism in chronic schizophrenia. *Biological Psychiatry*, **52**, 701–707.

Bilder, R.M., Volavka, J., Lachman, H.M., and Grace, A.A. (2004). The catechol-*O*-methyltransferase polymorphism: Relations to the tonic-phasic dopamine hypothesis and neuropsychiatric phenotypes. *Neuropsychopharmacology*, **29**, 1943–1961.

Bilder, R.M., Wu, H., Bogerts, B., Ashtari, M., Robinson, D., Woerner, M., Lieberman, J.A., and Degreef, G. (1999). Cerebral volume asymmetries in schizophrenia and mood disorders: A quantitative magnetic resonance imaging study. *International Journal of Psychophysiology*, **34**, 197–205.

Black, K., Peters, L., Rui, Q., Milliken, H., Whitehow, D., and Kopala, L.C. (2001). Duration of untreated psychosis predicts treatment outcome in an early psychosis program. *Schizophrenia Research*, **47**, 215–222.

Blackwood, D.H.R., Glabus, M.F., Dunan, J., O'Carroll, R.E., Muir, W.J., and Ebmeier, K.P. (1999). Altered cerebral perfusion measured by SPECT in relatives of patients with schizophrenia. *British Journal of Psychiatry*, **175**, 357–366.

Blackwood, N.J., Bentall, R.P., Ffytche, D.H., Simmons, A., Murray, R.M., and Howard, R.J. (2004). Persecutory delusions and the determination of self-relevance: An fMRI investigation. *Psychological Medicine*, **34**, 591–596.

Blakemore, S-J., Oakley, D.A., and Frith, C.D. (2003). Delusions of alien control in the normal brain. *Neuropsychologia*, **41**, 1058–1067.

Block, W., Bayer, T.A., Tepest, R., Träber, F., Rietschel, M., Muller, D.J., Schulze, T.G., Honer, W.G., Maier, W., Schild, H.H., and Falkai, P. (2000). Decreased frontal lobe ratio of N-acetyl aspartate to choline in familial schizophrenia: A proton magnetic resonance spectroscopy study. *Neuroscience Letters*, **289**, 147–151.

Blouin, J-S., Bard, C., and Paillard, J. (2004). Contributions of the cerebellum to self-initiated synchronized movements: A PET study. *Experimental Brain Research*, **155**, 63–68.

Bluml, S., Tan, J., Harris, K., Adatia, N., Karine, A., Sproull, T., and Robb, B. (1999). Quantitative proton-decoupled ^{31}P MRS of the schizophrenic brain in vivo. *Journal of Computer Assisted Tomography*, **23**, 272–275.

Bogerts, B, (1997). The temporolimbic system theory of positive schizophrenic symptoms. *Schizophrenia Bulletin*, **23**, 423–435.

Bogerts, B., Meertz, E., and Schonfeldt-Bausch, R. (1985). Basal ganglia and limbic system pathology in schizophrenia: A morphometric study of brain volume and shrinkage. *Archives of General Psychiatry*, **42**, 782–791.

Boks, M.P.M., Liddle, P.F., Burgerhof, J.G.M., Knegtering, R., and van den Bosch, R-J. (2004). Neurological soft signs discriminating mood disorders from first episode schizophrenia. *Acta Psychiatrica Scandinavica*, **110**, 29–35.

Boksa, P. and El-Khodor, B.F. (2003). Birth insult interacts with stress at adulthood to alter dopaminergic function in animal models: Possible implications for schizophrenia and other disorders. *Neuroscience and Biobehavioural Reviews*, **27**, 91–101.

Boronow, J., Pickar, D., Ninan, P.T., Roy, A., Hommer, D., Linnoila, M., and Paul, S.M. (1985). Atrophy limited to third ventricle only in chronic schizophrenic patients: Report of a controlled series. *Archives of General Psychiatry*, **42**, 266–271.

Bovée, W.M.M.J. (1991). Quantification of glutamate, glutamine and other metabolites in in vivo proton NMR spectroscopy. *NMR in Biomedicine*, **4**, 81–84.

Boylan, L.S. and Labovitz, D.L. (2004). Unbalanced statistical analysis of combined divalproex and antipsychotic therapy for schizophrenia. *Neuropsychopharmacology*, **29**, 636.

Bradford, H.F., Ward, H.K., and Thomas, A.J. (1978). Glutamine—a major substrate for nerve endings? *Journal of Neurochemistry*, **30**, 1453–1459.

Braff, D.L. and Geyer, M.A. (1990). Sensorimotor gating and schizophrenia: Human and animal model studies. *Archives of General Psychiatry*, **47**, 181–188.

Brake, W.G., Boksa, P., and Gratton, A. (1997). Effects of perinatal anoxia on the acute locomotor response to repeated amphetamine administration in adult rats. *Psychopharmacology*, **133**, 389–395.

Bramon, E., Rabe-Hesketh, S., Sham, P., Murray, R.M., and Frangou, S. (2004). Meta-analysis of the P300 and P50 waveforms in schizophrenia. *Schizophrenia Research*, **70**, 315–329.

Braun, C.M.J., Dumont, M., Duval, J., Hamel-Hébert, I., and Godbout, L. (2003). Brain modules of hallucination: An analysis of multiple patients with brain lesions. *Journal of Psychiatry and Neuroscience*, **28**, 432–439.

Brébion, G., Amador, X., David, A., Malaspina, D., Sharif, Z., and Gorman, J.M. (2000). Positive symptomatology and source-monitoring failure in schizophrenia—an analysis of symptom specific effects. *Psychiatry Research*, **95**, 119–131.

Bredesen, D.E. (1995). Neural apoptosis. *Annals of Neurology*, **38**, 839–851.

Breier, A., Alder, C.M., Weisenfeld, N., Su, T-P., Elman, I., Picken, L., Malhotra, A.K., and Pickar, D. (1998). Effects of dopamine release in healthy subjects: Application of a novel PET approach. *Synapse*, **29**, 142–147.

Breier, A., Buchanan, R.W., Elkashef, A., Munson, R.C., Kirkpatrick, B., and Gellad, F. (1992). Brain morphology and schizophrenia: A magnetic resonance imaging study of limbic, prefrontal cortex, and caudate structures. *Archives of General Psychiatry*, **49**, 921–926.

Breier, A., Malhotra, A.K., Pinals, D.A., Weisenfeld, N.I., and Pickar, D. (1997a). Association of ketamine-induced psychosis with focal activation of the prefrontal cortex in healthy volunteers. *American Journal of Psychiatry*, **154**, 805–811.

Breier, A., Su, T.P., Saunders, R., Carson, R.E., Kolachana, B.S., De Bartolomeis, A., Weinberger, D.R., Weisenfeld, N., Malholtra, A.K., Eckelman, W.C., and Pickar, D. (1997b). Schizophrenia is associated with elevated amphetamine-induced synaptic dopamine concentrations: Evidence from a novel positron emission tomography method. *Proceedings of the National Academy of Sciences of the United States of America*, **94**, 2569–2574.

Bremner, J.D., Randall, P., Scott, T.M., Bronen, R.A., Seibyl, J.P., Southwick, S.M., Delaney, R.C., McCarthy, G., Charney, D.S., and Innis, R.B. (1995). MRI-based measurement of hippocampal volume in patients with combat-related posttraumatic stress disorder. *American Journal of Psychiatry*, **152**, 973–981.

Bremner, J.D., Staib, L.H., Kaloupek, D., Southwick, S.M., Soufer, R., and Charney, D.S. (1999). Neural correlates of exposure to traumatic pictures and sound in Vietnam combat veterans with and without posttraumatic stress disorder: A positron emission tomography study. *Biological Psychiatry*, **45**, 806–816.

Brewer, W.J., Pantelis, C., Anderson, V., Velakoulis, D., Singh, B., Copolov, D.L., and McGorry, P.D. (2001). Stability of olfactory identification deficits in neuroleptic-naïve patients with first-episode psychosis. *American Journal of Psychiatry*, **158**, 107–115.

Brown, A., Susser, E., Lin, S., Neugebauer, R., and Gorman, J. (1995) In-

creased risk of affective disorders in males after second trimester prenatal exposure to the Dutch Hunger Winter of 1944–45. *British Journal
of Psychiatry*, **166**, 601–606.

Bruno, V., Battaglia, G., Copani, A., D'Onofrio, M., Di Iorio, P., De Blasi,
A., Melchiorri, D., Flor, P.J., and Nicoletti, F. (2001). Metabotropic glu-
tamate receptor subtypes as targets for neuroprotective drugs. *Journal of
Cerebral Blood Flow and Metabolism*, **21**, 1013–1033.

Buchanan, R.W., Strauss, M.E., Kirkpatrick, B., Holstein, C., Breier, A., and
Carpenter, W.T. (1994). Neuropsychological impairments in deficit vs.
nondeficit forms of schizophrenia. *Archives of General Psychiatry*, **51**,
804–811.

Buchsbaum, M.S., Haier, R.J., Potkin, S.G., Neuchterlein, K., Bracha, H.S.,
Katz, M., Lohr, J., Wu, J., Lottenberg, S., Jerabek, P.A., Trenary, M.,
Tafalla, R., Reynolds, C., and Bunney, W.E. (1992). Frontostiatal disor-
der of cerebral metabolism never-medicated schizophrenics. *Archives of
General Psychiatry*, **49**, 935–942.

Buchsbaum, M.S. and Hazlett, E.A. (1998). Positron emission tomography
studies of abnormal glucose metabolism in schizophrenia. *Schizophrenia
Bulletin*, **24**, 343–364.

Buchsbaum, M.S., Someya, T., Teng, C.Y., Abel, L., Chin, S., Najafi, A., Haier,
R.J., Wu, J., and Bunney, W.E. (1996). PET and MRI of the thalamus in
never-medicated patients with schizophrenia. *American Journal of Psychiatry*, **153**, 191–199.

Buchsbaum, M.S., Tang, C.Y., Peled, S., Gudbjartsson, H., Lu, D., Hazlett,
E.A., Downhill, J., Haznedar, M., Fallon, J.H., and Atlas, S.W. (1998).
MRI white matter diffusion anisotropy and PET metabolic rate in schizo-
phrenia. *Neuroreport*, **9**, 425–430.

Buckley, P.F., Moore, C., Long, H., Larkin, C., Thompson, P., Mulvany-
Redmond, O., Stack, J.P., Ennis, J.T., and Waddington, J.L. (1994).
[1]H-magnetic resonance spectroscopy of the left temporal and frontal
lobes in schizophrenia: Clinical, neurodevelopmental and cognitive correlates. *Biological Psychiatry*, **36**, 792–800.

Buka, S.L. and Fan, A.P. (1999). Association of prenatal and perinatal complications with subsequent bipolar disorder and schizophrenia. *Schizophrenia Research*, **39**, 113–119.

Buka, S.L., Tsuang, M.T., Torrey, E.F., Klebanoff, M.A., Bernstein, D., and
Yolken, R.H. (2001) Maternal infections and subsequent psychosis
among offspring. *Archives of General Psychiatry*, **58**, 1032–1037.

Bullmore, E., Brammer, M., Harvey, I., Murray, R., and Ron, M. (1995).
Cerebral hemispheric asymmetry revisited: Effects of handedness, gender and schizophrenia measured by radius of gyration in magnetic resonance images. *Psychological Medicine*, **25**, 349–363.

Bullmore, E.T., Frangou, S., and Murray, R.M. (1997). The dysplastic net
hypothesis: An integration of developmental and dysconnectivity theories of schizophrenia. *Schizophrenia Research*, **28**, 143–156.

Bunney, W.E. and Bunney, B.G. (2000). Evidence for a compromised dorsolateral prefrontal cortical parallel circuit in schizophrenia. *Brain Research Reviews*, **31**, 138–146.

Burgess, P.W., Scott, S.K., and Frith, C.D. (2003). The role of the rostral frontal cortex (and 10) in prospective memory: A lateral versus medial dissociation. *Neuropsychologia*, **41**, 906–918.

Burnett, P.W., Eastwood, S.L., and Harrison, P.J. (1996). 5HT1A and 5HT2A receptor mRNAs and binding sites densities are differentially altered in schizophrenia. *Neuropsychopharmacology*, **15**, 442–455.

Burns, J., Job, D., Bastin, M.E., Whalley, H., MacGillivray, T., Johnstone, E.C., and Lawrie, S.M. (2003). Structural disconnectivity in schizophrenia: A diffusion tensor magnetic resonance imaging study. *British Journal of Psychiatry*, **182**, 439–443.

Busatto, G.F., David, A.S., Costa, D.C., Ell, P.J., Pilowsky, L.S., Lucey, J.V., and Kerwin, R.W. (1995). Schizophrenic auditory hallucinations are associated with increased regional cerebral blood flow during verbal memory activation in a study using single photon emission computed tomography. *Psychiatry Research: Neuroimaging*, **61**, 255–264.

Busatto, G.F., Pilowsky, L.S., Costa, D.C., Ell, P.J., David, A.S., Lucey, J.V., and Kerwin, R.W. (1997). Correlation between reduced in vivo benzodiazepine receptor binding and severity of psychotic symptoms in schizophrenia. *American Journal of Psychiatry*, **154**, 56–63.

Bustillo, J.R., Lauriello, J., Rowland, L.M., Thomson, L.M., Petropoulos, H., Hammond, R., Hart, B., and Brooks, W.M. (2002). Longitudinal follow-up of neurochemical changes during the first year of antipsychotic treatment in schizophrenia patients with minimal previous medication exposure. *Schizophrenia Research*, **58**, 313–321.

Byne, W., Buchsbaum, M.S., Kemether, E., Hazlett, E.A., Shinwari, A., Mitropoulou, V., and Siever, L.J. (2001). Magnetic resonance imaging of the thalamic mediodorsal nucleus and pulvinar in schizophrenia and schizotypal personality disorder. *Archives of General Psychiatry*, **58**, 133–140.

Byne, W., Buchsbaum, M.S., Mattiace, L.A., Hazlett, E.A., Kemether, E., Elhakem, S.L., Purohit, D.P., Haroutunian, V., and Jones, L. (2002). Postmortem assessment of thalamic nuclear volumes in subjects with schizophrenia. *American Journal of Psychiatry*, **159**, 59–65.

Cahn, W., Hulshoff, H.E., Lems, E.B.T.E., van Haren, N.E.M., Schnack, H.G., van der Linden, J.A., Schothorst, P.F., van Engeland, H., and Kahn, R.S. (2002). Brain volume changes in first-episode schizophrenia: A 1-year follow-up study. *Archives of General Psychiatry*, **59**, 1002–1010.

Calabrese, G., Deicken, R.F., Fein, P.. Merrin, E.L., Schoenfeld, F., and Weiner, M.W. (1992). [31]Phosphorus magnetic resonance spectroscopy of the temporal lobes in schizophrenia. *Biological Psychiatry*, **32**, 26–32.

Calarge, C., Andreasen, N.C., and O'Leary, D.S. (2003). Visualizing how one brain understands another: A PET study of theory of mind. *American Journal of Psychiatry*, **160**, 1954–1964.

Calhoun, V.D., Kiehl, K.A., Liddle, P.F., and Pearlson, G.D. (2004). Aberrant localization of synchronous hemodynamic activity in auditory cortex reliably characterizes schizophrenia. *Biological Psychiatry*, **55**, 842–849.

Callicott, J.H., Bertolino, A., Egan, M.F., Mattay, V.S., Langheim, F.J.P., and Weinberger, D.R. (2000). Selective relationship between prefrontal N-acetylaspartate measures and negative symptoms. *American Journal of Psychiatry*, **157**, 1646–1651.

Callicott, J.H., Mattay, V.S., Marenco, S., Egan, M.F., and Weinberger, D.R. (2003). Complexity of prefrontal cortical dysfunction in schizophrenia: More than up or down. *American Journal of Psychiatry*, **160**, 2209–2215.

Campbell, S., Marriott, M., Nahmias, C., and MacQueen, G.M. (2004). Lower hippocampal volume in patients suffering from depression: A meta-analysis. *American Journal of Psychiatry*, **161**, 598–607.

Cannon, M., Jones, P.B., and Murray, R.M. (2002). Obstetric complications and schizophrenia: Historical and meta-analytic review. *American Journal of Psychiatry*, **159**, 1080–1092.

Cannon, T.D., van Erp, T.G.M., Huttunen, M., lonnqvist, J., Salonen, O., Valanne, L., Poutanen, V.-P., Standertskjold-Nordenstam, C.-G., Gur, R.E., and Yan, M. (1998). Regional gray matter, white matter, and cerebrospinal fluid distributions in schizophrenic patients, their siblings, and controls. *Archives of General Psychiatry*, **55**, 1084–1091.

Cantor-Graae, E., McNeil, T.F., Rickler, K.C., Sjostrom, K., Rawlings, R., Higgins, E.S., and Hyde, T.M. (1994a). Are neurological abnormalities in well discordant monozygotic co-twins of schizophrenic subjects the result of perinatal trauma? *American Journal of Psychiatry*, **151**, 1194–1199.

Cantor-Graae, E., McNeil, T.F., Torrey, E.F., Quinn, P., Bowler, A., Sjostrom, K., and Rawlings, R. (1994b). Link between pregnancy complications and minor physical anomalies in monozygotic twins discordant for schizophrenia. *American Journal of Psychiatry*, **151**, 1188–1193.

Cantor-Graae, E., Warkentin, S., Franzen, G., Risberg, J., and Ingvar, D.H. (1991). Aspects of stability of regional cerebral blood flow in chronic schizophrenia: An 18-year follow-up study. *Psychiatry Research*, **40**, 253–266.

Cardno, A.G. and Gottesman, I.I. (2000) Twin studies of schizophrenia: From bow-and-arrow concordances to Star Wars Mx and functional genomics. *American Journal of Medical Genetics*, **97**, 12–17.

Carlsson, A. (1988). The current status of the dopamine hypothesis of schizophrenia. *Neuropsychopharmacology*, **1**, 179–186.

Carlsson, A., Hansson, L.O., Waters, N., and Carlsson, M.L. (1999). A glutamatergic deficiency model of schizophrenia. *British Journal of Psychiatry*, **174** (Suppl. 37), 2–6.

Carlsson, A., Waters, N., Waters, S., and Carlsson, M.L. (2000). Network interactions in schizophrenia—therapeutic implications. *Brain Research Reviews*, **31**, 342–349.

Carlsson, M. and Carlsson, A. (1990). Schizophrenia: A subcortical neurotransmitter imbalance syndrome? *Schizophrenia Bulletin*, **16**, 425–432.

Carpenter W.T., Heinrichs, D.W., and Alphs, L.D. (1988). Deficit and non-deficit forms of schizophrenia: The concept. *American Journal of Psychiatry*, **145**, 578–583.

Carter, C.S., MacDonald, A.W., Ross, L.L., and Stenger, V.A. (2001). Anterior cingulate cortex activity and impaired self-monitoring of performance in patients with schizophrenia: An event-related fMRI study. *American Journal of Psychiatry*, **158**, 1423–1428.

Carter, C.S., Mintum, M., Nichols, T., and Cohen, J.D. (1997). Anterior cingulate gyrus dysfunction and selective attention deficits in schizophrenia: [^{15}O]H$_2$O PET study during single-trial Stroop Task performance. *American Journal of Psychiatry*, **154**, 1670–1675.

Carter, C.S., Perlstein, W., Ganguli, R., Brar, J., Mintun, M., and Cohen JD (1998). Functional hypofrontality and working memory dysfunction in schizophrenia. *American Journal of Psychiatry*, **155**, 1285–1287.

Carter, J.R. and Neufeld, R.W.J. (1999). Cognitive processing of multidimensional stimuli in schizophrenia: Formal modeling of judgment speed and content. *Journal of Abnormal Psychology*, **108**, 633–654.

Cascella, N.G., Macciardi, F., Cavallini, C., and Smeraldi, E. (1994). d-Cycloserine adjuvant therapy to conventional neuroleptic treatment in schizophrenia: An open-label study. *Journal of Neural Transmission*, **95**, 105–111.

Casey, D., Daniel, D.G., Wassef, A.A., Tracy, K.A., Wozniak, P., and Sommerville, K.W. (2003). Effects of divalproex combined with olanzapine or risperidone in patients with acute exacerbation of schizophrenia. *Neuropsychopharmacology*, **28**, 182–192.

Castner, S.A. and Goldman-Rakic, P.S. (2003). Amphetamine sensitization of hallucinatory-like behaviours is dependent on prefrontal cortex in nonhuman primates. *Biological Psychiatry*, **54**, 105–110.

Castner, S.A., Williams, G.V., and Goldman-Rakic, P.S. (2000). Reversal of antipsychotic-induced working memory deficits by short-term dopamine D1 receptor stimulation. *Science*, **287**, 2020–2022.

Cecil, K.M., Lenkinski, R.E., Gur, R.E., and Gur, R.C. (1999). Proton magnetic resonance spectroscopy in the frontal and temporal lobes of neuroleptic naïve patients with schizophrenia. *Neuropsychopharmacology*, **20**, 131–140.

Cendes, F., Andermann, F., Dubeau, F., Matthews, P.M., and Arnold, D.L. (1997). Normalization of neuronal metabolic dysfunction after surgery for temporal lobe epilepsy. *Neurology*, **49**, 1525–1533.

Chalfonte, B.L. and Johnson, M.K. (1996). Feature memory and binding in young and older adults. *Memory and Cognition*, **24**, 403–416.

Chalmers, D.J. (1996). *The conscious mind: In search of a fundamental theory.* New York, Oxford University Press.

Chapple, B., Grech, A., Sham, P., Toulopoulo, T., Walshe, M., Schulze, K., Morgan, K., Murray, R.M., and McDonald, C. (2004). Normal cerebral asymmetry in familial and non-familial schizophrenic probands and their unaffected relatives. *Schizophrenia Research*, **67**, 33–40.

Chen, R., Classen, J., Gerloff, C., Celnik, P., Wassermann, E.M., Hallett, M., and Cohen, L.G. (1997). Depression of motor cortex excitability by low-frequency transcranial magnetic stimulation. *Neurology*, **48**, 1398–1403.

Choe, B.-Y., Kim, K.-T., Suh, T.-S., Lee, C., Palk, I.-H., Bahk, Y.-W., Shinn, K.-S., and Lenkinoki, R.E. (1994). [1]H magnetic resonance spectroscopy characterization of neuronal dysfunction in drug-naïve, chronic schizophrenia. *Academic Radiology*, **1**, 211–216.

Chong, S.-A., Tan, C.-H., Lee, E.-L. and Liow, P.-H. (1998). Augmentation of risperidone with valproic acid. *Journal of Clinical Psychiatry*, **59**, 430.

Chowdari, K.V., Mirnics, K., Semwal, P., Wood, J., Lawrence, E., Bhatia, T., Deshpande, S.N., Thelma, B.K., Ferrell, R.E., Middleton. F.A., Devlin, B., Levitt, P., Lewis, D.A., and Nimgaonkar, V.L. (2002). Association and linkage analysis of *RGS4* polymorphisms in schizophrenia. *Human Molecular Genetics*, **11**, 1373–1380.

Chua, S.E. and McKenna, P.J. (1995). Schizophrenia—a brain disease? A critical review of structural and functional cerebral abnormality in the disorder. *British Journal of Psychiatry*, **166**, 563–582.

Chua, S.E., Wright, I.C., Poline, J-B., Liddle, P.F., Murray, R.M., Frackowiack, R.S.J., Friston, K.J., and McGuire, P.K. (1997). Grey matter correlates of syndromes in schizophrenia: A semi-automated analysis of structural magnetic resonance images. *British Journal of Psychiatry*, **170**, 406–410.

Churchland, P.S. (2002). Self-representation in nervous systems. *Science*, **296**, 308–310.

Ciompi, L. (1980). The natural history of schizophrenia in the long term. *British Journal of Psychiatry*, **136**, 413–420.

Cirillo, M.A. and Seidman, L.J. (2003). Verbal declarative memory dysfunction in schizophrenia: From clinical assessment to genetics and brain mechanisms. *Neuropsychology Review*, **13**, 43–77.

Citrome, L., Levine, J., and Allingham, B. (2000). Changes in the use of valproate and other mood stabilizers for patients with schizophrenia from 1994 to 1998. *Psychiatry Services*, **51**, 634–638.

Clark, C., Kopala, L., Li, D.K., and Hurwitz,T. (2001). Regional cerebral glucose metabolism in never-medicated patients with schizophrenia. *Canadian Journal of Psychiatry*, **46**, 340–345.

Clark, J.B. (1998). *N*-acetyl aspartate: A marker for neuronal loss or mitochondrial dysfunction. *Developmental Neuroscience*, **20**, 271–276.

Cleeremans, A. (2003). *The unity of consciousness: Binding, integration, and dissociation.* New York, Oxford University Press.

Cleghorn, J.M., Franco, S., Szechman, B., Kaplan, R.D., Szechman, H., Brown, G.M., Nahmias, C., and Garnett, E.S. (1992). Toward a brain map of auditory hallucinations. *American Journal of Psychiatry*, **149**, 1062–1069.

Cleghorn, J.M., Garnett, E.S., Nahmias, C., Firnau, G., Brown, G.M., Kaplan, R., Szechtman, H., and Szechtman, B. (1989). Increased frontal and reduced parietal glucose metabolism in acute untreated schizophrenia. *Psychiatry Research*, **28**, 119–133.

Cohen, R.M., Nordahl, T.E., Semple, W.E., Andreasen, P., Litman, R.E., and Pickar, D. (1997). The brain metabolic patterns of clozapine- and fluphenazine-treated patients with schizophrenia during a continuous performance task. *Archives of General Psychiatry*, **54**, 481–486.

Conn, P.J. and Pin, J.-P. (1997). Pharmacology and functions of metabotropic glutamate receptors. *Annual Review of Pharmacology and Toxicology*, **37**, 207–237.

Constantinidis, C., Williams, G.V., and Goldman-Rakic, P.S. (2002). A role for inhibition in shaping the temporal flow of information in prefrontal cortex. *Nature Neuroscience*, **5**, 175–180

Copolov, D.L., Seal, M.L., Maruff, P., Ulusoy, R., Wong, M.T.H., Tochon-Danguy, H.J., and Egan, G.F. (2003). Cortical activation associated with the experience of auditory hallucinations and perception of human speech in schizophrenia: A PET correlation study. *Psychiatry Research: Neuroimaging*, **122**, 139–152.

Cornblatt, B.A. and Keilp, J.G. (1994). Impaired attention, genetics, and the pathophysiology of schizophrenia. *Schizophrenia Bulletin*, **20**, 31–46.

Costa, J., Khaled, E., Sramek, J., Bunney, W., and Potkin, S.G, (1990). An open trial of glycine as an adjunct to neuroleptics in chronic treatment-refractory schizophrenics. *Journal of Clinical Psychopharmacology*, **10**, 71–72.

Coyle, J.T. (1996). The glutamatergic dysfunction hypothesis for schizophrenia. *Harvard Review of Psychiatry*, **3**, 241–253.

Craik, F.I.M., Moroz, T.M., Moscovitch, M., Stuss, D.T., Winocur, G., Tulving, E., and Kapur, S. (1999). In search of the self: A positron emission tomography study. *Psychological Science*, **10**, 26–34.

Crawford, J.R., Obonsawin, M.C., and Bremner, M. (1993). Frontal lobe impairment in schizophrenia: Relationship to intellectual functioning. *Psychological Medicine*, **23**, 787–790.

Crespo-Facorro, B., Paradiso, S., Andreasen, N.C., O'Leary, D.S., Watkins, G.L., Boles Ponto, L.L., and Hichwa, R.D. (1999). Recalling word lists reveals "cognitive dysmetria" in schizophrenia: A positron emission tomography study. *American Journal of Psychiatry*, **156**, 386–392.

Crick, F. (1984). Function of the thalamic reticular complex: The searchlight hypothesis. *Proceedings of the National Academy of Sciences of the United States of America*, **81**, 4586–4590.

Crismon, M.L., DeLeon, A., and Miller, A.L. (2003). Aripiprazole: Does partial dopaminergic agonism translate into clinical benefits? *Annals of Pharmacotherapy*, **37**, 738–740.

Crow, T.J. (1980). Molecular pathology in schizophrenia: More than one disease process? *British Medical Journal*, **28**, 66–68.

Crow, T.J. (1989) A current view of the type II syndrome: age of onset, intellectual impairment, and the meaning of structural changes in the brain. *British Journal of Psychiatry*, **155**, 15–20.

Crow, T.J. (1990a). The continuum of psychosis and its genetic origins: The sixty-fifth Maudsley lecture. *British Journal of Psychiatry*, **156**, 788–797.

Crow, T.J. (1990b). Temporal lobe asymmetries as the key to the etiology of schizophrenia. *Schizophrenia Bulletin*, **16**, 433–443.

Crow, T.J. (1995). A Darwinian approach to the origins of psychosis. *British Journal of Psychiatry*, **167**, 12–25.

Crow, T.J. (1997a) Schizophrenia as failure of hemispheric dominance for language. *Trends in Neuroscience*, **20**, 339–343.

Crow, T.J. (1997b). Is schizophrenia the price that *homo sapiens* pays for language? *Schizophrenia Research*, **28**, 127–141.

Crow, T.J. (1998). Schizophrenia as a transcallosal misconnection syndrome. *Schizophrenia Research*, **30**, 111–114.

Crow, T.J. (1999). Twin studies of psychosis and the genetics of cerebral asymmetry. *British Journal of Psychiatry*, **175**, 399–401.

Crow, T.J. (2000). Invited commentary on: functional anatomy of verbal fluency in people with schizophrenia and those at genetic risk. The genetics of asymmetry and psychosis. *British Journal of Psychiatry*, **176**, 61–63.

Csernansky, J.G., Csernansky, C.A., Kogelman, L., Montgomery, E.-M., and Bardgett, M.E. (1998) Progressive neurodegeneration after intracerebroventricular kainic acid administration in rats: Implications for schizophrenia. *Biological Psychiatry*, **44**, 1143–1150.

Cummings, J.L. (1986). Subcortical dementia: neuropsychology, neuropsychiatry, and pathophysiology. *British Journal of Psychiatry*, **149**, 682–697.

Curtis, V.A., Bullmore, E.T., Brammer, M.J., Wright, I.C., Williams, S.C.R., Morris, R.G., Sharma, T.S., Murray, R.M., and McGuire, P.K. (1998). Attenuated frontal activation during verbal fluency task in patients with schizophrenia. *American Journal of Psychiatry*, **155**, 1056–1063.

da Costa, D. A. (1997). The role of psychosurgery in the treatment of selected cases of refractory schizophrenia: A reappraisal. *Schizophrenia Research*, **28**, 223–230.

d'Alfonso, A.A.L., Aleman, A., Kessels, R.P.C., Schouten, E.A., Postma, A., van der Linden, J.A., Cahn, W., Greene, Y., de Haan, E.H.F., and Kahn, R.S. (2002). Transcranial magnetic stimulation of left auditory cortex in patients with schizophrenia: Effects on hallucinations and neurocognition. *Journal of Neuropsychiatry and Clinical Neurosciences*, **14**, 77–79.

Damasio, A. (1999). *The feeling of what happens: Body and emotion in the making of consciousness*. New York, Harcourt Brace and Company.

Damasio, A.R., Tranel, D., and Damasio, H. (1990). Individuals with sociopathic behaviour caused by frontal damage fail to respond autonomically to social stimuli. *Behavioural Brain Research*, **41**, 81–94.

Dandy, W.E. (1919). Roentgenography of the brain after the injection of air into the spinal cord. *Annals of Surgery*, **70**, 397–403.

Danion, J.M., Rizzo, L., and Bruant, A. (1999). Functional mechanisms underlying impaired recognition memory and conscious awareness in patients with schizophrenia. *Archives of General Psychiatry*, **56**, 639–644.

Danos, P., Baumann, B., Bernstein, H.-G., Stauch, R., Krell, D., Falkai, P., and Bogerts, B. (2002). The ventral lateral posterior nucleus of the thalamus in schizophrenia: A post-mortem study. *Psychiatry Research*, **144**, 1–9.

Danos, P., Baumann, B., Krämer, A., Bernstein, H.-G., Stauch, R. Krell, D., Falkai, P., and Bogerts, B. (2003). Volumes of association thalamic nuclei in schizophrenia: A post-mortem study. *Schizophrenia Research*, **60**, 141–155.

Dao-Castellana, M.H., Paillère-Martinot, M.L., Hantraye, P., Attar-Lévy, D., Rémy, P., Crouzel, C., Artiges, E., Féline, A., Syrota, A., and Martinot, J.L. (1997). Presynaptic dopaminergic function in the striatum of schizophrenic patients. *Schizophrenia Research*, **23**, 167–174.

Daprati, E., Franck, N., Georgieff, N., Proust, J., Pacherie, E., Dalery, J., and Jeannerod, M. (1997). Looking for agent: An investigation into consciousness of action and self-consciousness in schizophrenic patients. *Cognition*, **65**, 71–86.

David, A.S. (1994) Schizophrenia and the corpus callosum. Developmental, structural and functional relationships. *Behavioural Brain Research*, **64**, 203–211.

Davidson, L.L. and Heinrichs, R.W. (2003). Quantification of frontal and temporal lobe brain-imaging findings in schizophrenia: A meta-analysis. *Psychiatry Research: Neuroimaging*, **122**, 69–87.

Davidson, M., Reichenberg, A., Rabinwitz, J., Weiser, M., Kaplan, Z., and Mark, M. (1999a) Behavioural and intellectual markers for schizophrenia in apparently healthy male adolescents. *American Journal of Psychiatry*, **156**, 1328–1335.

Davidson, R.J., Abercrombie, H., Nitschke, J.B., and Putnam, K. (1999b). Regional brain function, emotion and disorders of emotion. *Current Opinion in Neurobiology*, **9**, 228–234.

Davis, K.L., Kahn, R.S., Ko, G., and Davidson, M. (1991). Dopamine in schizophrenia: A review and reconceptualization. *American Journal of Psychiatry*, **148**, 1474–1486.

Davis, K.L., Stewart, D.G., Friedman, J.I., Buchsbaum, M., Harvey, P.D., Hof, P.R., Buxbaum, J., and Haroutunian, V. (2003). White matter changes in schizophrenia: evidence for myelin-related dysfunction. *Archives of General Psychiatry*, **60**, 443–456.

Deakin, J.F.W., Slater, P., Simpson, M.D.C., Gilchrist, A.C., Skan, W.J., Royston, M.C., Reynolds, G.P., and Cross, A.J. (1989). Frontal cortical and left temporal glutamatergic dysfunction in schizophrenia. *Journal of Neurochemistry*, **52**, 1781–1786.

de Chaldée, M., Laurent, C., Thibault, F., Martinez, M., Samolyk, D., Petit, M., Campion, D., and Mallet, J. (1999). Linkage disequilibrium on the COMT gene in French schizophrenics and controls. *American Journal of Medical Genetics*, **88**, 452–457.

Deicken, R.F., Calabrese, G., Merris, E.L., Meyerhoff, D.J., Dillon, W.P., Weiner, M.W., and Fein, G. (1994). [31]Phosphorus magnetic resonance spectroscopy of the frontal and parietal lobes in chronic schizophrenia. *Biological Psychiatry*, **36**, 503–510.

Deicken, R.F., Eliaz, Y., Chosiad, L., Feiwell, R., and Rogers, L. (2002). Magnetic resonance imaging of the thalamus in male patients with schizophrenia. *Schizophrenia Research*, **58**, 135–144.

Deicken, R.F., Eliaz, Y., Feiwell, R., and Schuff, N. (2001a). Increased thalamic N-acetylaspartate in male patients with familial bipolar I disorder. *Psychiatry Research: Neuroimaging*, **106**, 35–45.

Deicken, R.F., Feiwell, R., Schuff, N., and Soher, B. (2001b). Evidence for altered cerebellar vermis neuronal integrity in schizophrenia. *Psychiatry Research: Neuroimaging*, **107**, 125–134.

Deicken, R.F., Johnson, C., Eliaz, Y., and Schuff, N. (2000). Reduced concentrations of thalamic N-acetylaspartate in male patients with schizophrenia. *American Journal of Psychiatry*, **157**, 644–647.

Deicken, R.F., Pegues, M., and Amend, D. (1999). Reduced hippocampal N-acetylaspartate without volume loss in schizophrenia. *Schizophrenia Research*, **37**, 217–223.

Deicken, R.F., Pegues, M.P., Anzalone, S., Feiwell, R., and Soher, B. (2003). Lower concentration of hippocampal N-acetylaspartate in familial bipolar I disorder. *American Journal of Psychiatry*, **160**, 873–882.

Deicken, R.F., Zhou, L., Schuff, N., Fein, G., and Weiner, M.W. (1998). Hippocampal neuronal dysfunction in schizophrenia as measured by proton magnetic resonance spectroscopy. *Biological Psychiatry*, **43**, 483–488.

Deicken, R.F., Zhou, L., Schuff, N., and Weiner, M.W. (1997). Proton magnetic resonance spectroscopy of the anterior cingulate region in schizophrenia. *Schizophrenia Research*, **27**, 65–71.

Delamillieure, P., Constans, J.-M., Fernandez, J., Brazo, P., Benali, K., Courthéoux, P., Thibaut, F., Petit, M., and Dollfus, S. (2002). Proton magnetic resonance spectroscopy (¹H MRS) in schizophrenia: Investigation of the right and left hippocampus, thalamus, and prefrontal cortex. *Schizophrenia Bulletin*, **28**, 329–339.

Delamillieure, P., Constans, J.M., Fernandez, J., Brazo, P., and Dollfus, S. (2000a). Proton magnetic resonance spectroscopy (¹H-MRS) of the thalamus in schizophrenia. *European Psychiatry*, **15**, 489–491.

Delamillieure, P., Fernandez, J., Coustans, J-M., Brazo, P., Benalo, K., Abadie, P., Vasse, T., Thibaut, F., Courtleoux, P., Petit, M., and Dollfus, S. (2000b). Proton magnetic resonance spectroscopy of the medial prefrontal cortex in patients with deficit schizophrenia: Preliminary report. *American Journal of Psychiatry*, **157**, 641–643.

DeLisi, L.E., Sakuma, M., Ge, S., and Kushner, M. (1998). Association of brain structural change with the heterogeneous course of schizophrenia from early childhood through five years subsequent to a first hospitalization. *Psychiatry Research: Neuroimaging*, **84**, 75–88.

DeLisi, L.E., Sakuma, M., Kushner, M., Finer, D.L., Hoff, A.L., and Crow, T.J. (1997a). Anomalous cerebral asymmetry and language processing in schizophrenia. *Schizophrenia Bulletin*, **23**, 255–271.

DeLisi, L.E., Sakuma, M., Maurizio, A.M., Relja, M., and Hoff, A.L. (2004).

Cerebral ventricular change over the first 10 years after the onset of schizophrenia. *Psychiatry Research: Neuroimaging,* **130**, 57–70.

DeLisi, L.E., Sakuma, M., Tew, W., Kushner, M., Hoff, A.L., and Grimson R (1997b). Schizophrenia as a chronic active brain process: A study of progressive brain change subsequent to the onset of schizophrenia. *Psychiatry Research: Neuroimaging,* **74**, 129–140.

DeLisi, L.E., Stritzke, P., Riordan, H., Holan, V., Boccio, A., Kushner, M., McClelland, J., Van Eyl, O., and Anand, A. (1992). The timing of brain morphological changes in schizophrenia and their relationship to clinical outcome. *Biological Psychiatry,* **31**, 241–254.

DeLisi, L.E., Tew, W., Xie, S., Hoff, A.L., Sakuma, M., Kushner, M., Lee, G., Shedlack, K., Smith, A.M., and Grimson, R. (1995). A prospective follow-up study of brain morphology and cognition in first-episode schizophrenic patients: Preliminary findings. *Biological Psychiatry,* **38**, 349–360.

Deutch, A.Y. (1993). Prefrontal cortical dopamine systems and the elaboration of functional corticostriatal circuits: Implications for schizophrenia and Parkinson's disease. *Journal of Neural Transmission,* **91**, 197–221.

Deutsch, S.I., Rosse, R.B., Billingslea, E.N., Bellack, A.S., and Mastropaolo, J. (2002). Topiramate antagonizes MK-801 in an animal model of schizophrenia. *European Journal of Pharmacology,* **449**, 121–125.

Deutsch, S.I., Rosse, R.B., Schwartz, B.L., and Mastropaolo, J. (2001). A revised excitotoxic hypothesis of schizophrenia: Therapeutic implications. *Clinical Neuropharmacology,* **24**, 43–49.

Deutsch, S.I., Schwartz, B.L., Rosse, R.B., Mastropaolo, J., Marvel, C.L., and Drapalski, A.L. (2003). Adjuvant topiramate administration: A pharmacological strategy for addressing NMDA receptor hypofunction in schizophrenia. *Clinical Neuropharmacology,* **26**, 199–206.

Devinsky, O. and Luciano, D. (1993). The contributions of the anterior cingulate cortex to human behaviour. In B.A. Vogt and M. Gabriel (Eds.), *Neurobiology of the cortex and limbic thalamus* (pp. 527–556). Boston, Birkhauser.

Dewey, S.L., Smith, G.S., Logan, J., Alexoff, D., Ding, Y.S., King, P., Pappas, N., Brodie, J., and Ashley, C.R. (1995). Serotonergic modulation of striatal dopamine measured with positron emission tomography (PET) and in vivo microdialysis. *Journal of Neuroscience,* **15**, 821–829.

Dickey, C.C., McCarley, R.W., and Shenton, M.E. (2002). The brain in schizotypal personality disorder: A review of structural MRI and CT findings. *Harvard Review of Psychiatry,* **10**, 1–15.

Diefendorf, A.R. and Dodge, R. (1908). An experimental study of the ocular reactions of the insane from photographic records. *Brain,* **31**, 451–489.

Dierks, T., Linden, D.E.J., Jandl, M., Formisano, E., Goebel, R., Lanfermann, H., and Singer, W. (1999). Activation of Heschl's gyrus during auditory hallucinations. *Neuron,* **22**, 615–621.

Dolan, R.J., Fletcher, P., Frith, C.D., Friston, K.J., Frackowiak, R.S.J., and

Grasby, P.M. (1995). Dopaminergic modulation of impaired cognitive activation in the anterior cingulate cortex in schizophrenia. *Nature*, **378**, 180–182.

Dolan, R.J., Fletcher, P.C., McKenna, P., Friston K.J., and Frith C.D. (1999). Abnormal neural integration related to cognition in schizophrenia. *Acta Psychiatrica Scandinavica*, **99** (Suppl. 395), 58–67.

Dose, M., Hellweg, R., Yassouridis, A., Theisen, M., and Emrich, H.M. (1998). Combined treatment of schizophrenic psychoses with haloperidol and valproate. *Pharmacopsychiatry*, **31**, 122–125.

Drapalski, A.L., Rosse, R.B., Peebles, R.R., Schwartz, B.L., Marvel, C.L., and Deutsch, S.I. (2001). Topiramate improves deficit symptoms in a patient with schizophrenia when added to a stable regimen of antipsychotic medication. *Clinical Neuropharmacology*, **24**, 290–294.

Drevets, W.C. (1998). Functional neuroimaging studies of depression: The anatomy of melancholy. *Annual Review of Medicine*, **49**, 341–361.

Drevets, W.C. (2000). Neuroimaging studies of mood disorders. *Biological Psychiatry*, **48**, 813–829.

Drevets, W.C. and Raichle, M.E. (1992). Neuroanatomical circuits in depression: Implications for treatment mechanisms. *Psychopharmacology Bulletin*, **28**, 261–274.

Dror, V., Shamir, E., Ghanshani, S., Kimhi, R., Swartz Barak, Y., Weizman, R., Avivi, L., Litmanovitch, T., Fantino, E., Kalman, K., Jones, E.G., Chandy, K.G., Gargus, J.J., Gutman, G.A., and Navon, R. (1999). hKCa3/KCNN3 potassium channel gene: Association of longer CAG repeats with schizophrenia in Israeli Ashkenazi Jews, expression in human tissues and localization to chromosome 1q21. *Molecular Psychiatry*, **4**, 254–260.

D'Souza, D.C., Charney, D., and Krystal, J. (1995). Glycine site agonists of the NMDA receptor: A review. *CNS Drug Reviews*, **1**, 227–260.

Dursun, S.M. and Deakin, J.F.W. (2001). Augmenting antipsychotic treatment with lamotrigine or topiramate in patients with treatment-resistant schizophrenia: A naturalistic case-series outcome study. *Journal of Psychopharmacology*, **15**, 297–301.

Dursun, S.M., McIntosh, D., and Milliken, H. (1999). Clozapine plus lamotrigine in treatment-resistant schizophrenia. *Archives of General Psychiatry*, **56**, 950.

Dye, S.M., Spence, S.A., Bench, C.J., Hirsch, S.R., Stefan, M.D., Sharma, T., and Grasby, P.M. (1999). No evidence for left superior temporal dysfunction in asymptomatic schizophrenia and bipolar disorder: PET study of verbal fluency. *British Journal of Psychiatry*, **175**, 367–374.

Ebmeier, K.P., Blackwood, D.H.R., Murray, C., Souza, V., Walker, S.M., Dougall, N., Moffoot, A.P.R., O'Carroll, R.E., and Goodwin, G.M. (1993). Single-photon emission computed tomography with ^{99m}Tc-Exametazime in unmedicated schizophrenic patients. *Biological Psychiatry*, **33**, 487–495.

Egan, M.F., Goldberg, T.E., Kolachana, B.S., Callicott, J.H., Mazzanti, C.M., Straub, R.E., Goldman, D., and Weinberger, D.R. (2001). Effect of

COMT Val[108/158] *Met* genotype on frontal lobe function and risk for schizophrenia. *Proceedings of the National Academy of Sciences of the United States of America*, **98**, 6917–6922.

Egan, M.F., Straub, R.E., Goldberg, T.E., Yakub, I., Callicott, J.H., Hariri, A.R., Mattay, V.S., Bertolino, A., Hyde, T.M., Shannon-Weickert, C., Akil, M., Crook, J., Vakkalanka, R.K., Balkissoon, R., Gibbs, R.A., Kleinman, J.E., and Weinberger, D.R. (2004). Variation in *GRM3* affects cognition, prefrontal glutamate, and risk for schizophrenia. *Proceedings of the National Academy of Sciences of the United States of America*, **101**, 12604–12609.

Eisen, A., Stewart, H., Schulzer, M., and Cameron, D. (1993). Anti-glutamate therapy in amyotrophic lateral sclerosis: A trial using lamotrigine. *Canadian Journal of Neurological Science*, **20**, 297–301.

Elkashef, A.M., Doudet, D., Bryant, T., Cohen, R.M., Li, S.H., and Wyatt, R.J. (2000). 6-(18)F-DOPA PET study in patients with schizophrenia: Positron emission tomography. *Psychiatry Research*, **100**, 1–11.

Elkis, H., Friedman, L., Wise, A., and Meltzer, H.Y. (1995). Meat-analysis of studies of ventricular enlargement and cortical sulcal prominence in mood disorders: Comparisons with controls or patients with schizophrenia. *Archives of General Psychiatry*, **52**, 735–746.

Elliott, R. and Sahakian, B.J. (1995). The neuropsychology of schizophrenia: Relations with clinical and neurobiological dimensions. *Psychological Medicine*, **25**, 581–594.

Eluri, R., Paul, C., Roemer, R., and Boyko, O. (1998). Single-voxel proton magnetic resonance spectroscopy of the pons and cerebellum in patients with schizophrenia. *Psychiatry Research: Neuroimaging*, **84**, 17–26.

Ende, G., Braus, D.F., Walter, S., and Henn, F.A. (2001a). Lower concentration of the thalamic *N*-acetylaspartate in patients with schizophrenia: A replication study. *American Journal of Psychiatry*, **158**, 1314–1316.

Ende, G., Braus, D.F., Walter, S., Weber-Fahr, W., Soher, B., Maudsley, A.A., and Henn, F.A. (2001b). Effects of age, medication, and illness duration on the *N*-acetylaspartate signal of the anterior cingulate region in schizophrenia. *Schizophrenia Research*, **41**, 389–395.

Epstein, J., Stern, E., and Silbersweig, D. (1999). Mesolimbic activity associated with psychosis in schizophrenia: Symptom-specific PET studies. *Annals of the New York Academy of Sciences*, **877**, 562–574.

Erecinska, M. and Silver, I.A. (1990). Metabolism and role of glutamate in mammalian brain. *Progress in Neurobiology*, **35**, 245–296.

Ettinger, U., Chitnis, X.A., Kumari, V., Fannon, D.G., Sumich, A.L., O'Ceallaigh, S., Doku, V.C., and Sharma, T. (2001). Magnetic resonance imaging of the thalamus in first-episode psychosis. *American Journal of Psychiatry*, **158**, 116–118.

Evans, C.L., McGuire, P.K., and David, A.S. (2000). Is auditory imagery defective in patients with auditory hallucinations? *Psychological Medicine*, **30**, 137–148.

Evins, A.E., Amico, E., Posever, T.A., Toker, R., and Goff, D.C. (2002).

D-cycloserine added to risperidone in patients with primary negative symptoms of schizophrenia. *Schizophrenia Research*, **56**, 19–23.

Falkai, P. and Bogerts, B. (1986) Cell loss in the hippocampus of schizophrenics. *European Archives of Psychiatry and Neurological Sciences*, **236**, 154–161.

Falkai, P. and Bogerts, B. (1993) Cytoarchitectonic and developmental studies in schizophrenia. In R. Kerwin (Ed.), *Neurobiology and Psychiatry*, Vol. 2 (pp. 43–70). Cambridge, UK, Cambridge University Press.

Fannon, D., Simmons, A., Tennakoon, L., O'Céallaigh, S., Sumich, A., Doku, V., Shew, C., and Sharma, T. (2003). Selective deficit of hippocampal *N*-acetylaspartate in antipsychotic-naïve patients with schizophrenia. *Biological Psychiatry*, **54**, 587–598.

Farber, N.B., Price, M.T., Labruyere, J., Nemnich, J., St. Peter, H., Wozniak, D.F., and Olney, J.W. (1993). Antipsychotic drugs block phencyclidine receptor-mediated neurotoxicity. *Biological Psychiatry*, **34**, 199–121.

Farde, L., Wiesel, F.A., Stone-Elander, S., Halldin, C., Nordstrom, A.L., Hall, H., and Sedvall, G. (1990). D2 dopamine receptors in neuroleptic-naïve schizophrenic patients. A positron emission tomography study with [11C] raclopride. *Archives of General Psychiatry*, **47**, 213–219.

Farrer, C., Franck, N., Frith, C.D., Decety, J., Georgieff, N., d'Amato, T., and Jeannerod, M. (2004). Neural correlates of action attribution in schizophrenia. *Psychiatry Research: Neuroimaging*,**131**, 31–44.

Farrer, C., Franck, N., Georgieff, N., Frith, C.D., Decety, J., and Jeannerod, M. (2003). Modulating the experience of agency: A positron emission tomography study. *Neuroimage*, **18**, 324–333.

Feenstra, M.G.P., Botterblom, M.H.A., and van Uum, J.F.M. (1998). Local activation of metabotropic glutamate receptors inhibits the handling-induced increased release of dopamine in the nucleus accumbens but not that of dopamine or noradrenaline in the prefrontal cortex: Comparison with inhibition of ionotropic receptors. *Journal of Neurochemistry*, **70**, 1106–1113.

Feinberg, I. (1982/1983). Schizophrenia: Caused by a fault in programmed synaptic elimination during adolescence? *Journal of Schizophrenia Research*, **17**, 319–334.

Feinberg, I. and Guazzelli, M. (1999). Schizophrenia—a disorder of the corollary discharge systems that integrate the motor systems of thought with the sensory systems of consciousness. *British Journal of Psychiatry*, **174**, 196–204.

Fitzgerald, K.D., Moore, G.J., Paulson, L.A., Stewart, C.M., and Rosenberg, G.R. (2000) Proton spectroscopic imaging of the thalamus in treatment-naïve pediatric obsessive-compulsive disorder. *Biological Psychiatry*, **47**, 174–182.

Flagstad, P., Mørk, A., Glenthø, B.Y., van Beek, J., Michael-Titus, A.T., and Didriksen, M. (2004). Disruption of neurogenesis on gestational day 17 in the rat causes behavioural changes relevant to positive and negative schizophrenia symptoms and alters amphetamine-induced dopamine release in the nucleus accumbens. *Neuropsychopharmacology*, **29**, 2052–2064.

Flaum, M., O'Leary, D.S., Swayze, V.W., Miller, D.D., Arndt, S., and Andreasen, N.C. (1995a). Symptom dimensions and brain morphology in schizophrenia and related psychotic disorders. *Journal of Psychiatry Research*, **29**, 261–276.

Flaum, M., Swayze, V.W., O'Leary, D.S., Yuh, W.T.C., Ehrhardt, J.C., Arndt, S.V., and Andreasen, N.C. (1995b). Effects of diagnosis, laterality, and gender on brain morphology in schizophrenia. *American Journal of Psychiatry*, **152**, 704–714.

Fletcher, P., McKenna, P.J., Friston, K.J., Frith C.D., and Dolan, R.J. (1999). Abnormal cingulate modulation of fronto-temporal connectivity in schizophrenia. *NeuroImage*, **9**, 337–342.

Fletcher, P.C., McKenna, P.J., Frith, C.D., Grasby, P.M., Friston, K.J., and Dolan, R.J. (1998). Brain activations in schizophrenia during a graded memory task studied with functional neuroimaging. *Archives of General Psychiatry*, **55**, 1001–1008.

Flor-Henry, P. (1969). Psychosis and temporal lobe epilepsy: A controlled investigation. *Epilepsia*, **10**, 363–395.

Fossati, P., Hevenor, S.J., Graham, S.J., Grady, C., Keightley, M., Craik F., and Mayberg, H. (2003). In search of the emotional self: An fMRI study using positive and negative emotional words. *American Journal of Psychiatry*, **160**, 1938–1945.

Franck, N., Farrer, C., Georgieff, N., Marie-Cardine, M., Daléry, J., d'Amato, T., and Jeannerod, M. (2001). Defective recognition of one's own actions in patients with schizophrenia. *American Journal of Psychiatry*, **158**, 454–459.

Frankle, W.G., Lerma, J., and Laruelle, M. (2003). The synaptic hypothesis of schizophrenia. *Neuron*, **39**, 205–216.

Freedman, R., Adler, L.E., Gerhardt, G.A., Waldo, M., Baker, N., Rose, G.M., Drebing, C., Nagamoto, H., Bickford-Wimer, P., and Franks, R. (1987). Neurobiological studies of sensory gating in schizophrenia. *Schizophrenia Bulletin*, **13**, 667–678.

Friedman, D. and Squires-Wheeler, E. (1994). Event-related potentials (ERPs) as indicators of risk for schizophrenia. *Schizophrenia Bulletin*, **20**, 63–74.

Friston, K.J. (1998). The disconnection hypothesis. *Schizophrenia Research*, **30**, 115–125.

Friston, K.J. (1999). Schizophrenia and the disconnection hypothesis. *Acta Psychiatrica Scandinavica*, **99** (Suppl. 395), 68–79.

Friston, K.J. and Frith, C.D. (1995). Schizophrenia: A disconnection syndrome? *Clinical Neuroscience*, **3**, 89–97.

Frith, C.D. (1987). The positive and negative symptoms of schizophrenia reflect impairments in the perception and initiation of action. *Psychological Medicine*, **17**, 631–648.

Frith, C. (1995). Functional imaging and cognitive abnormalities. *Lancet*, **346**, 615–20.

Frith, C.D., Blakemore, S.-J., and Wolpert, D.M. (2000). Explaining the symptoms of schizophrenia: Abnormalities in the awareness of action. *Brain Research Reviews*, **31**, 357–363.

Frith, C. and Dolan, R. (1996). The role of the prefrontal cortex in higher cognitive functions. *Cognitive Brain Research*, **5**, 175–181.

Frith, C.D. and Done, D.J. (1988). Towards a neuropsychology of schizophrenia. *British Journal of Psychiatry*, **153**, 437–443.

Frith, C.D., Friston, K.J., Herold, S., Silbersweig, D., Fletcher, P., Cahill, C., Dolan, R.J., Frackowiak, R.S.J., and Liddle, P.F. (1995). Regional brain activity in chronic schizophrenic patients during the performance of a verbal fluency task. *British Journal of Psychiatry*, **167**, 343–349.

Frith, C.D. and Frith, U. (1999). Interacting minds—a biological basis. *Science*, **286**, 1692–1695.

Frith, C.D., Leary, J., Cahill, C., and Johnstone, E.C. (1991). IV. Performance on psychological tests: Demographic and clinical correlates of the results of these tests. *British Journal of Psychiatry*, **159** (Suppl. 13), 26–29.

Fudge, J.L., Powers, J.M., Haber, S.N., and Caine, E.D. (1998). Considering the role of the amygdala in psychotic illness: A clinicopathological correlation. *Journal of Neuropsychiatry and Clinical Neuroscience*, **10**, 383– 394.

Fujimoto, T., Nakano, T., Takano, T., Hokazono, Y., Asakura, T., and Tsuji, T. (1992). Study of chronic schizophrenics using ^{31}P magnetic resonance chemical shift imaging. *Acta Psychiatrica Scandinavica*, **86**, 455–462.

Fukuzako, H., Fukuzako, T., Hashiguchi, T., Kodaura, S., Takigawa, M., and Fujimoto, T. (1999a). Changes in levels of phosphorous metabolites in temporal lobes of drug-naïve schizophrenic patients. *American Journal of Psychiatry*, **156**, 1205–1208.

Fukuzako, H., Kodama, S., Fukuzako, T., Yamada, K., Doi, W., Sato, D., and Takigawa, M. (1999b). Subtype-associated metabolite differences in the temporal lobe in schizophrenia detected by proton magnetic resonance spectroscopy. *Psychiatry Research: Neuroimaging*, **92**, 45–56.

Fukuzako, H., Takeuchi, K., Hozazano, Y., Fugako, T., Yamada, K., Hashiguchi, T., Obo, Y., Ueyama, K., Takigawa, M., and Fujimoto, T. (1995). Proton magnetic resonance spectroscopy of the left medial temporal and frontal lobes in chronic schizophrenia: Preliminary report. *Psychiatry Research: Neuroimaging*, **61**, 193–200.

Fuller, R., Nopoulos, P., Arndt, S., O'Leary, D., Beng-Choon, H., and Andreasen, N.C. (2002). Longitudinal assessment of premorbid cognitive functioning in patients with schizophrenia through examination of standardized scholastic test performance. *American Journal of Psychiatry*, **159**, 1183–1189.

Fuster, J.M. (Ed.) (1998). *The prefrontal cortex: Anatomy, physiology, and neuropsychology of the frontal lobes, second edition*. New York, Raven Press.

Gabriel, S.M., Haroutunian, V., Powchik, P., Honer, W.G., Davidson, M.,

Davidson, M., Davies, P., and Davis, K.L. (1997). Increased concentrations of presynaptic proteins in the cingulate cortex of subjects with schizophrenia. *Archives of General Psychiatry*, **54**, 559–566.

Ganguli, R., Carter, C., Mintun, M., Brar, J., Becker, J., Sarma, R., Nichols, T., and Bennington, E. (1997). PET brain mapping study of auditory verbal supraspan memory versus visual fixation in schizophrenia. *Biological Psychiatry*, **41**, 33–42.

Gao, X-M., Sakai, K., Roberts, R.C., Conley, R.R., Dean, B., and Tamminga, C.A. (2000). Ionotropic glutamate receptors and expression of *N*-methyl-D-aspartate receptor subunits in subregions of human hippocampus: Effects of schizophrenia. *American Journal of Psychiatry*, **157**, 1141–1149.

Garver, D.L., Nair, T.R., Christensen, J.D., Holcomb, J.A., and Kingsbury, S.J. (2000). Brain and ventricle instability during psychotic episodes of the schizophrenias. *Schizophrenia Research*, **44**, 11–22.

Gaser, C., Nenadic, I., Buchsbaum, B.R., Hazlett, E.A., and Buchsbaum, M.S. (2004). Ventricular enlargement in schizophrenia related to volume reduction of the thalamus, striatum, and superior temporal cortex. *American Journal of Psychiatry*, **161**, 154–156.

Geddes, J.R. and Lawrie, S.M. (1995). Obstetric complications and schizophrenia: A meta-analysis. *British Journal of Psychiatry*, **167**, 786–793.

Georgieff, N. and Jeannerod, M. (1998). Beyond consciousness of external reality: A 'who' system for consciousness of action and self-consciousness. *Consciousness and Cognition*, **7**, 465–477.

Gerber, D.J., Hall, D., Miyakawa, T., Demars, S., Gogos, J.A., Karayiorgou, M., and Tonegawa, S. (2003). Evidence for association of schizophrenia with genetic variation in the 8p21.3 gene, *PPP3CC*, encoding the calcineurin gamma subunit. *Proceedings of the National Academy of Sciences of the United States of America*, **100**, 8993–8998.

Gilbert, A.R., Rosenberg, D.R., Harenski, K., Spencer, S., Sweeney, J.A., and Keshavan, M.S. (2001). Thalamic volumes in patients with first-episode schizophrenia. *American Journal of Psychiatry*, **158**, 618–624.

Gilmore, J.H., Jarskog, L.F., Vadlamudi, S., and Lauder, J.M. (2004). Prenatal infection and risk for schizophrenia: IL-Iβ, IL-6, and TNF-α inhibit cortical neuron dendrite development. *Neuropsychopharmacology*, **29**, 1221–1229.

Glantz, L.A. and Lewis, D.A. (1997). Reduction of synaptophysin immunoreactivity in the prefrontal cortex of subjects with schizophrenia. *Archives of General Psychiatry*, **54**, 660–669.

Glantz, L.A. and Lewis, D.A. (2000). Decreased dendritic spine density on prefrontal cortical pyramidal neurons in schizophrenia. *Archives of General Psychiatry*, **57**, 65–73.

Glatt, S.J., Faraone, S.V., and Tsuang, M.T. (2003). Association between a functional catechol O-methyltransferase gene polymorphism and schizophrenia: Meta-analysis of case–control and family-based studies. *American Journal of Psychiatry*, **160**, 469–476.

Gluck, M.R., Thomas, R.G., Davis, K.L., and Haroutunian, V. (2002). Implications for altered glutamate and GABA metabolism in dorsolateral prefrontal cortex of aged schizophrenic patients. *American Journal of Psychiatry*, **159**, 1165–1173.

Goff, D.C., Tsai, G., Levitt, J., Amico, E., Manoach, D., Schoenfeld, D.A., Hayden, D.L., McCarley, R., and Coyle, J.T. (1999). A placebo-controlled trial of D-cycloserine added to conventional neuroleptics in patients with schizophrenia. *Archives of General Psychiatry*, **56**, 21–27.

Goff, D.C., Tsai, G., Manoach, D.S., and Coyle, J.T. (1995). Dose-finding trial of D-cycloserine added to neuroleptics for negative symptoms in schizophrenia. *American Journal of Psychiatry*, **152**, 1213–1215.

Goff, D.C., Tsai, G., Manoach, D.S., Flood, J., Darby, D.G., and Coyle, J.T. (1996). D-cycloserine added to clozapine for patients with schizophrenia. *American Journal of Psychiatry*, **153**, 1628–1630.

Goff, D.C. and Wine, L. (1997). Glutamate in schizophrenia: Clinical and research implications. *Schizophrenia Research*, **27**, 157–168.

Gogtay, N., Giedd, J.N., Lusk, L., Hayashi, K.M., Greenstein, D., Vaituzis, A.C., Nugent, T.F., Herman, D.H., Clasen, L.S., Toga, A.W., Rapoport, J.L., and Thompson, P.M. (2004a). Dynamic mapping of human cortical development during childhood through early adulthood. *Proceedings of the National Academy of Sciences of the United States of America*, **101**, 8174–8179.

Gogtay, N., Sporn, A., Clasen, L.S., Nugent, T.F., Greenstein, D., Nicolson, R., Giedd, J.N., Lenane, M., Gochman, P., Evans, A., and Rapaport, J.L. (2004b). Comparison of progressive cortical gray matter loss in childhood-onset schizophrenia with that in childhood-onset atypical psychoses. *Archives of General Psychiatry*, **61**, 17–22.

Gold, J.M., Carpenter, C., Randolf, C., Goldberg, T.E., and Weinberger, D.R. (1997). Auditory working memory and Wisconsin Card Sorting Test performance in schizophrenia. *Archives of General Psychiatry*, **54**, 159–165.

Gold, S., Arndt, S., Nopoulis, P., O'Leary, D.S., and Andreasen, N.C. (1999). Longitudinal study of cognitive function in first-episode and recent-onset schizophrenia. *American Journal of Psychiatry*, **156**, 1342–1348.

Goldberg, T.E., Egan, M.F., Gscheidle, T., Coppola, R., Weickert, T., Kolachana, B.S., Goldman, D., and Weinberger, D.R. (2003). Executive subprocesses in working memory: Relationship to catechol-O-methyltransferase Val158Met genotype and schizophrenia. *Archives of General Psychiatry*, **60**, 889–896.

Goldberg, T.E., Saint-Cyr, J.A., and Weinberger, D.R. (1990). Assessment of procedural learning and problem solving in schizophrenic patients by Tower of Hanoi type tasks. *Journal of Neuropsychiatry and Clinical Neuroscience*, **2**, 165–173.

Goldberg, T.E., Torrey, E.F., Berman, K.F., and Weinberger, D.R. (1994). Relations between neuropsychological performance and brain morphology and physiological measures in monozygotic twins discordant for schizophrenia. *Psychiatry Research: Neuroimaging*, **55**, 51–61.

Golden, C.J., Moses, J.A., Zelazowski, R., Graber, B., Zatz, L.M., Horvath, T.B., and Berger, P.A. (1980). Cerebral ventricular size and neuropsychological impairment in young chronic schizophrenics: Measurement by the standardized Luria-Nebraska neurophysiological battery. *Archives of General Psychiatry*, **37**, 619–623.

Goldman-Rakic, P.S. (1994). Working memory dysfunction in schizophrenia. *Journal of Neuropsychiatry and Clinical Neuroscience*, **6**, 348–357.

Goldman-Rakic, P.S. (1999). The physiological approach: functional architecture of working memory and disordered cognition in schizophrenia. *Biological Psychiatry*, **46**, 650–661.

Good, K.P., Martzke, J.S., Milliken, H.I., Honer, W.G., and Kopala, L.C. (2002). Unirhinal olfactory identification deficits in young male patients with schizophrenia and related disorders: Association with memory impairment. *Schizophrenia Research*, **56**, 211–223.

Goodale, M. and Milner, D. (2004). *Sight unseen*. New York, Oxford University Press.

Grace, A.A. (1991). Phasic versus tonic dopamine release and the modulation of dopamine system responsivity: A hypothesis for the etiology of schizophrenia. *Neuroscience*, **41**, 1–24.

Grace, A.A. (1993). Cortcal regulation of subcortical systems and its possible relevance to schizophrenia. *Journal of Neural Transmission*, **1**, 111–134.

Grace, A.A. (2000). Gating of information flow within the limbic system and the pathophysiology of schizophrenia. *Brain Research Reviews*, **31**, 330–341.

Gray, J.A. (1995). The contents of consciousness: A neuropsychological conjecture. *Behavioral and Brain Sciences*, **18**, 659–722.

Gray, J.A. (1998). Integrating schizophrenia. *Schizophrenia Bulletin*, **24**, 249–266.

Gray, J.A. (2004). *Consciousness: Creeping up on the hard problem*. New York, Oxford University Press.

Gray, J.A., Feldon, J., Rawlins, J.N.P., Hemsley, D.R., and Smith, A.D. (1991) The neuropsychology of schizophrenia. *Behavioural and Brain Sciences*, **14**, 1–84.

Graybiel, A.M. (1995). Building action repertoires: Memory and learning functions of the basal ganglia. *Current Opinion in Biology*, **5**, 733–741.

Graybiel, A.M. (1997). The basal ganglia and cognitive pattern generators. *Schizophrenia Bulletin*, **23**, 459–469.

Green, M. and Walker, E. (1985). Neuropsychological performance and positive and negative symptoms in schizophrenia. *Journal of Abnormal Psychology*, **94**, 460–469.

Green, M.F. and Nuechterlein, K.H. (1999). Cortical oscillations and schizophrenia: Timing is of the essence. *Archives of General Psychiatry*, **56**, 1007–1008.

Greenamyre, J.T. and Porter, R.H.P. (1994). Anatomy and physiology of glutamate in the CNS. *Neurology*, **44**, S7–S13.

Grieve, K.L., Acuña, C., and Cudeiro, J. (2000). The primate pulvinar nuclei: Vision and action. *Trends in Neuroscience*, **23**, 35–39.

Grossberg, S. (2000a). The imbalanced brain: From normal behaviour to schizophrenia. *Biological Psychiatry*, **48**, 81–98.

Grossberg, S. (2000b). How hallucinations may arise from brain mechanisms of learning, attention, and volition. *Journal of the International Neuropsychological Society*, **6**, 583–592.

Gründer, G., Carlsson, A., and Wong, D.F. (2003a). Mechanism of new antipsychotic medications: Occupancy is not just antagonism. *Archives of General Psychiatry*, **60**, 974–977.

Gründer, G., Vernaleken, I., Müller, M.J., Davids, E., Heydari, N., Buchholz, H.G., Bartenstein, P., Munk, O.L., Stoeter, P., Wong, D.F., Gjedde, A., and Cumming, P. (2003b). Subchronic haloperidol downregulates dopamine synthesis capacity in the brain of schizophrenic patients in vivo. *Neuropsychopharmacology*, **28**, 787–794.

Grunwald, T., Boutros, N.N., Pezer, N., von Oertzen, J., Fernández, G., Schaller, C., and Elger, C.E. (2003). Neuronal substrates of sensory gating within the human brain. *Biological Psychiatry*, **53**, 511–519.

Grunze, H., Greene, R.W., Moller, H.J., Meyer, T., and Walden, J. (1998). Lamotrigine may limit pathological excitation in the hippocampus by modulating a transient potassium outward current. *Brain Research*, **791**, 330–334.

Gruzelier, J.H. (1984). Hemispheric imbalances in schizophrenia. *International Journal of Psychophysiology*, **1**, 227–240.

Gruzelier, J.H. (1999). Functional neuropsychophysiological asymmetry in schizophrenia: A review and reorientation. *Schizophrenia Bulletin*, **25**, 91–120.

Gruzelier, J.H. and Flor-Henry, P. (Eds.). (1979). *Hemispheric asymmetries of function in psychopathology*. Amsterdam, Elsevier.

Gruzelier, J., Seymour, K., Wilson, L., Jolley, A., and Hirsch, S. (1988). Impairments on neuropsychologic tests of temporohippocampal and frontohippoampal functions and word fluency in remitting schizophrenia and affective disorders. *Archives of General Psychiatry*, **45**, 623–629.

Gualtieri, C.T., Adams, A., Shen, C.D., and Loiselle, D. (1982). Minor physical anomalies in alcoholic and schizophrenic adults and hyperactive and autistic children. *American Journal of Psychiatry*, **139**, 640–643.

Guidotti, A., Auta, J., Davis, J.M., DiGiorgi Gerevini, V., Dwivedi, Y., Grayson, D.R., Impagnatiello, F., Pandey, G., Pesold, C., Sharma R., Uzunov, D., and Costa, E. (2000). Decrease in reelin and glutamic acid decarboxylase$_{67}$ (GAD$_{67}$) expression in schizophrenia and bipolar disorder: A postmortem brain study. *Archives of General Psychiatry*, **57**, 1061–1069.

Gupta, S., Andreasen, N.C., Arndt, S., Flaum, M., Schultz, S.K., Hubbard, W.C., and Smith, M. (1995). Neurological soft signs in neuroleptic-naïve and neuroleptic-treated schizophrenic patients and in normal comparison subjects. *American Journal of Psychiatry*, **152**, 191–196.

Gur, R.E., Cowell P., Turetsky, B.I., Gallacher, F., Cannon, T., Bilker, W., and Gur, R.C. (1998). A follow-up magnetic resonance imaging study of schizophrenia: Relationship of neuroanatomical changes to clinical and neurobehavioural measures. *Archives of General Psychiatry*, **55**, 145–152.

Gur, R.E., Jaggi, J.L., Shtasel D.L., Ragland, J.D., and Gur, R.C. (1994). Cerebral blood flow in schizophrenia: Effects of memory processing on regional activation. *Biological Psychiatry*, **35**, 3–15.

Gur, R.E., McGrath, C., Chan, R.M., Schroeder, L., Turetsky, B.I., Kohler, C., Alsop, D., Maldjian, J., Ragland, J.D., and Gur, R.C. (2002). An fMRI study of facial emotion processing in patients with schizophrenia. *American Journal of Psychiatry*, **159**, 1992–1999.

Gur, R.E., Mozley, D., Resnick, S.M., Mozley, L.H., Shtasel, D.L., Gallacher, F., Arnold, S.E., Karp, J.S., Alavi, A., Reivich, M., and Gur, R.C. (1995). Resting cerebral glucose metabolism in first-episode and previously treated patients with schizophrenia relates to clinical features. *Archives of General Psychiatry*, **52**, 657–667.

Gur, R.E., Turetsky, B.I., Bilker, W.B., and Gur, R.C. (1999). Reduced gray matter volume in schizophrenia. *Archives of General Psychiatry*, **56**, 905–911.

Gusnard, D.A., Akbudak, E., Shulman, G.L., and Raichle, M.E. (2001). Medial prefrontal cortex and self-referential mental activity: Relation to a default mode of brain function. *Proceedings of the National Academy of Sciences of the United States of America*, **98**, 4259–4264.

Haber, S. and Fudge, J.L. (1997). The interface between dopamine neurons and the amygdala: Implications for schizophrenia. *Schizophrenia Research*, **23**, 471–482.

Hanley, J., Rickles, W.R., Crandall, P.H., and Walter, R.D. (1972). Automatic recognition of EEG correlates of behavior in a chronic schizophrenic patient. *American Journal of Psychiatry*, **128**, 74–78.

Hare, E.H. (1974). The changing content of psychiatric illness. *Journal of Psychosomatic Research*, **18**, 283–289.

Harrison, P.J. (1999). The neuropathology of schizophrenia: A critical review of the data and their interpretation. *Brain*, **122**, 593–624.

Harrison, P.J. and Owen, M.J. (2003). Genes for schizophrenia? Recent findings and their pathophysiological implications. *Lancet*, **361**, 417–419.

Harrison, P.J. and Weinberger, D.R. (2005). Schizophrenia genes, gene expression, and neuropathology: on the matter of their convergence. *Molecular Psychiatry* **10**, 40–68.

Harsing, L. G., Gacsalyi, I., Szabo, G., Schmidt, E., Sziray, N., Sebban, C., Tesolin-Decros, B., Matyus, P., Egyed, A., Spedding, M., and Levay, G. (2003). The glycine transporter-1 inhibitors NFPS and Org 24461: A pharmacological study. *Pharmacology, Biochemistry and Behaviour*, **74**, 811–825.

Hartman, M., Steketee, M.C., Silva, S., Lanning, K., and Andersson, C. (2003). Wisconsin Card Sorting Test performance in schizophrenia: The role of working memory. *Schizophrenia Research*, **63**, 201–217.

Hashimoto, T., Nishino, N., Nakai, H., and Tanaka, G. (1991). Increase in serotonin 5-HT1A receptors in prefrontal and temporal cortices of brains from patients with chronic schizophrenia. *Life Sciences*, **48**, 355–363.

Haug, J. (1962). Pneumoencephalographic studies in mental disease. *Acta Psychiatrica Scandinavica*, **38** (Suppl. 165), 11–104.

Hazlett, E.A., Buchsbaum, M.S., Kemether, E., Bloom, R., Platholi, J., Brickman, A.M., Shihabuddin, L., Tang, C., and Byne, W. (2004). Abnormal glucose metabolism in the mediodorsal nucleus of the thalamus in schizophrenia. *American Journal Psychiatry*, **161**, 305–314.

Healy, D.J., Haroutunian, V., Powchik, P., Davidson, M., Davis, K.L., Watson, S.J., and Meador-Woodruff, J.H. (1998). AMPA receptor binding and subunit mRNA expression in prefrontal cortex and striatum of elderly schizophrenics. *Neuropsychopharmacology*, **19**, 278–286.

Heath, R.G. (1954). *Studies in schizophrenia: A multidisciplinary approach to mind–body relationships*. Cambridge, MA, Harvard University Press.

Heath, R.G., Franklin, D.E., and Shraberg, D. (1979). Gross pathology of the cerebellum in patients diagnosed and treated as functional psychiatric disorders. *Journal of Nervous and Mental Disease*, **167**, 585–592.

Heckers, S., Curran, T., Goff, D., Rauch, S.L., Fischman, A.J., Alpert, N.M., and Schacter, D.L. (2000). Abnormalities in the thalamus and prefrontal cortex during episodic object recognition in schizophrenia. *Biological Psychiatry*, **48**, 651–657.

Heckers, S., Goff, D., Schacter, D.L., Savage, C.R., Fischman, A.J., Alpert, N.M., and Rauch, S.L. (1999). Functional imaging of memory retrieval in deficit vs. nondeficit schizophrenia. *Archives of General Psychiatry*, **56**, 1117–1123.

Heckers, S., Rauch, S.L., Goff, D., Savage, C.R., Schacter, D.L., Fischman, A.J., and Alpert, N.M. (1998). Impaired recruitment of the hippocampus during conscious recollection in schizophrenia. *Nature Neuroscience*, **1**, 318–323.

Heim, S., Kissler, J., Elbert, T., and Rockstroh, B. (2004). Cerebral lateralization in schizophrenia and dyslexia: Neuromagnetic responses to auditory stimuli. *Neuropsychologia*, **42**, 692–697.

Heimberg, C., Kosmoroski, R.A,, Lawson, W.B., Cardwell, D., and Karson, C.N. (1998). Regional proton magnetic resonance spectroscopy in schizophrenia and exploration of drug effect. *Psychiatry Research: Neuroimaging*, **83**, 105–115.

Heimer, L. (2000). Basal forebrain in the context of schizophrenia. *Brain Research Reviews*, **31**, 205–235.

Heinrichs, R.W., and Zakzanis, K.K. (1998). Neurocognitive deficit in schizophrenia: A quantitative review of the evidence. *Neuropsychology*, **12**, 426–445.

Hemsley, D.R. (1987). An experimental psychological model for schizophrenia. In H. Häfner, W.F. Gattaz, and W. Janzarik (Eds.), *Search for the causes of schizophrenia* (pp. 179–188). New York, Springer-Verlag.

Henry, C., Guegant, G., Cador, M., Arnauld, E., Arsaut, J., Le Moal, M., and Demotes-Mainard, J. (1995). Prenatal stress in rats facilitates amphetamine-induced sensitization and induces long-lasting changes in dopamine receptors in the nucleus accumbens. *Brain Research*, **685**, 179–186.

Heresco-Levy, U. and Javitt, D.C. (2004). Comparative effects of glycine and D-cycloserine on persistent negative symptoms in schizophrenia: A retrospective analysis. *Schizophrenia Research*, **66**, 89–96.

Heresco-Levy, U., Javitt, D.C., Ermilov, M., Mordel, C., Horowitz, A., and Kelly, D. (1996). Double-blind, placebo-controlled, crossover trial of glycine adjuvant therapy for treatment-resistant schizophrenia. *British Journal of Psychiatry*, **169**, 610–617.

Heresco-Levy, U., Javitt, D.C., Ermilov, M., Mordel, C., Silipo, G., and Lichtenstein, M. (1999). Efficacy of high-dose glycine in the treatment of enduring negative symptoms of schizophrenia. *Archives of General Psychiatry*, **56**, 29–36.

Hesslinger, B., Normann, C., Langosch, J., Klose, P., Berger, M., and Walden, J. (1999). Effects of carbamazepine and valproate on haloperidol plasma levels and on psychopathological outcome in schizophrenic patients. *Journal of Clinical Psychopharmacology*, **19**, 310–315.

Heydebrand, G., Weiser, M., Rabinowitz, J., Hoff, A.L., DeLisi, L.E., and Csernansky, J.G. (2004). Correlates of cognitive deficits in first episode schizophrenia. *Schizophrenia Research*, **68**, 1–9.

Hietala, J., Syvälahti, E., Vilkman, H., Vuorio, K., Räakköläinen, V., Bergman, J., Haaparanta, M., Solin, O., Kuoppamäki, M., Eronen, E., Ruotsalainen, U., and Salokangas, R.G. (1999). Depressive symptoms and presynaptic dopamine function in neuroleptic-naïve schizophrenia. *Schizophrenia Research*, **35**, 41–50.

Hietala, J., Syvälahti, E., Vuorio, K., Räkköläinen, V., Bergman, J., Haaparanta, M., Solin, O., Kuoppamäki, M., Kirvelä, O., Ruotsalainen, U., and Salokangas, R.G. (1995). Presynaptic dopamine function in striatum of neuroleptic-naïve schizophrenic patients. *Lancet*, **346**, 1130–1131.

Hijman, R., Hulshoff, H.E., Sitskoorn, M.M., and Kahn, R.S. (2003). Global intellectual impairment does not accelerate with age in patients with schizophrenia: A cross-sectional analysis. *Schizophrenia Bulletin*, **29**, 509–517.

Hill, K., Mann, L., Laws, K.R., Stephenson, C.M.E., Nimmo-Smith, I., and McKenna, P.J. (2004a). Hypofrontality in schizophrenia: A meta-analysis of functional imaging studies. *Acta Psychiatrica Scandinavica*, **110**, 243–256.

Hill, S.K., Schuepbach, D., Herbener, E.S., Keshavan, M.S., and Sweeney, J.A. (2004b). Pretreatment and longitudinal studies of neuropsychological deficits in antipsychotic-naïve patients with schizophrenia. *Schizophrenia Research*, **68**, 49–63.

Hirayasu, Y., McCarley, R.W., Salisbury, D.F., Tanaka, S., Kwon, J.S., Frumin, M., Snyderman, D., Yurgelun-Todd, D., Kikinis, R., Jolesz, F.A., and Shenton, M.E. (2000). Planum temporale and Heschl gyrus volume reduction in schizophrenia: A magnetic resonance imaging study of first-episode patients. *Archives of General Psychiatry*, **57**, 692–699.

Ho, B-C., Alicata, D., Ward, J., Moser, D.J., O'Leary, D.S., Arndt, S., and Andereasen, N.C. (2003a). Untreated initial psychosis: Relation to cognitive deficits and brain morphology in first-episode schizophrenia. *American Journal of Psychiatry*, **160**, 142–148.

Ho, B-C., Andreasen, N.C., Flaum, M., Nopoulos, P., and Miller, D. (2000). Untreated initial psychosis: Its relation to quality of life and symptoms remission in first-episode schizophrenia. *American Journal of Psychiatry*, **157**, 808–815.

Ho, B-C., Andreasen, N.C., Nopoulos, P., Arndt, S., Magnotta, V., and Flaum, M. (2003b). Progressive structural brain abnormalities and their relationship to clinical outcome: A longitudinal magnetic resonance imaging study early in schizophrenia. *Archives of General Psychiatry*, **60**, 585–594.

Ho, B-C., Mola, C., and Andreasen, N.C. (2004). Cerebellar dysfunction in neuroleptic naïve schizophrenic patients: Clinical, cognitive, and neuroanatomical correlates of cerebellar neurologic signs. *Biological Psychiatry*, **55**, 1146–1153.

Hofer, A., Weiss, E.A., Golaszewski, S.M., Siedentopf, C.M., Brinkhoff, C., Kremser, C., Felber, S., and Fleischhacker, W.W. (2003). An fMRI study of episodic encoding and recognition of words in patients with schizophrenia in remission. *American Journal of Psychiatry*, **160**, 911–918.

Hoff, A.L., Sakuma, M., Razi, K., Heydebrand, G., Csernansky, J.G., and DeLisi, L.E. (2000). Lack of association between duration of untreated illness and severity of cognitive and structural brain deficits at first episode of schizophrenia. *American Journal of Psychiatry*, **157**, 1824–1828.

Hoff, A.L., Sakuma, M., Wieneke, M., Horon, R., Kushner, M., and DeLisi, L.E. (1999). Longitudinal neuropsychological follow-up study of patients with first-episode schizophrenia. *American Journal of Psychiatry*, **156**, 1336–1341.

Hoffman, R.E., Boutros, N.N., Berman, R.M., Roessler, E., Belger, A., Krystal, J.H., and Charney, D.S. (1999). Transcranial magnetic stimulation of the left temporoparietal cortex in three patients reporting hallucinated "voices". *Biological Psychiatry*, **46**, 130–132.

Hoffman, R.E., Boutros, N.N., Hu, S., Berman, R.M., Krystal, J.H., and Charney, D.S. (2000). Transcranial magnetic stimulation and auditory hallucinations in schizophrenia. *Lancet*, **355**, 1073–1075.

Hoffman, R.E. and Cavus, I. (2002). Slow transcranial magnetic stimulation, long-term depotentiation, and brain hyperexcitability disorders. *American Journal of Psychiatry*, **159**, 1093–1102.

Hoffman, R.E., Hawkins, K.A., Gueorguieva, R., Boutros, N.N., Rachid, F., Carroll. K., and Krystal, J.H. (2003). Transcranial magnetic stimulation of left temporoparietal cortex and medication-resistant auditory hallucinations. *Archives of General Psychiatry*, **60**, 49–56.

Hoffman, R.E. and McGlashan, T.H. (1993). Parallel distributed processing and the emergence of schizophrenic symptoms. *Schizophrenia Bulletin*, **19**, 119–140.

Hogarty, G.E., Goldberg, S.C., and Schooler, N.R. (1974). Drug and sociotherapy in the aftercare of schizophrenic patients III. Adjustment of non-relapsed patients. *Archives of General Psychiatry*, **31**, 609–618.

Holcomb, H.H., Lahti, A.C., Medoff, D.R., Weiler, M., Dannals, R.F., and Tamminga, C.A. (2000). Brain activation patterns in schizophrenic and comparison volunteers during a matched-performance auditory recognition task. *American Journal of Psychiatry*, **157**, 1634–1645.

Holcomb, H.H., Lahti, A.C., Medoff, D.R., Weiler, M., and Tamminga, C.A. (2001). Sequential regional cerebral blood flow brain scans using PET with $H_2^{15}O$ demonstate ketamine actions in CNS dynamically. *Neuropsychopharmacology*, **25**, 165–172.

Holinger, D.P., Shenton, M.E., Wible, C.G., Donnino, R., Kikinis, R., Jolez, F.A., and McCarley, R.W. (1999). Superior temporal gyrus volume abnormalities and thought disorder in left-handed schizophrenic men. *American Journal of Psychiatry*, **156**, 1730–1735.

Holzman, P.S. (1987). Recent studies of psychophysiology in schizophrenia. *Schizophrenia Bulletin*, **13**, 49–75.

Holzman, P.S. (1996). On the trail of the genetics and pathophysiology of schizophrenia. *Psychiatry*, **59**, 117–127.

Holzman, P.S. (2000). Eye movements and the search for the essence of schizophrenia. *Brain Research Reviews*, **31**, 350–356.

Holzman, P.S., Proctor, L.R., and Hughes, D.W. (1973). Eye-tracking patterns in schizophrenia. *Science*, **181**, 179–181.

Hsiao, M.-C., Lin, K.-J., Liu, C.-Y., Tzen, K.-Y. and Yen, T.-C. (2003). Dopamine transpoter change in drug-naïve schizophrenia: An imaging study with ^{99m}Tc-TRODAT-1. *Schizophrenia Research*, **65**, 39–46.

Huber, G., Gross, G., Schüttler, R., and Linz, M. (1980). Longitudinal studies of schizophrenic patients. *Schizophrenia Bulletin*, **6**, 592–605.

Hubl, D., Koenig, T., Strik, W., Federspiel, A., Kreis, R., Boesch, C., Maier, S.E., Schroth, G., Lovblad, K., and Dierks, T. (2004). Pathways that make voices: White matter changes in auditory hallucinations. *Archives of General Psychiatry*, **61**, 658–668.

Hulshoff Pol, H.E., Schnack, H.G., Mandl, R.C.W., van Haren, N.E.M., Koning, H., Collins, L., Evans, A.C., and Kahn, R.S. (2001). Focal gray matter density changes in schizophrenia. *Archives of General Psychiatry*, 58, 1118–1125.

Hunter, R. and MacAlpine, I. (1982). *Three hundred years of psychiatry 1535–1860*. Hartsdale, NY, Carlisle Publishing, Inc.

Hurwitz, T., Kopala, L., Clark, C., and Jones, B. (1988). Olfactory deficits in schizophrenia. *Biological Psychiatry*, **23**, 123–128.

Huttenlocher, P.R. (1979). Synaptic density in human frontal cortex—developmental changes and effects of aging. *Brain Research*, **163**, 195–205.

Huttenlocher, P.R. and Dabholkar, A.S. (1997). Regional differences in synaptogenesis in the human cerebral cortex. *Journal of Comparative Neurology*, **387**, 167–178.

Hyde, T.M., Ziegler, J.C., and Weinberger, D.R. (1992). Psychiatric disturbances in metachromatic leukodystrophy: Insights into the neurobiology of psychosis. *Archives of Neurology*, **49**, 401–406.

Ichimiya, T., Okubo, Y., Suhara, T., and Sudo, Y. (2001). Reduced volume of the cerebellar vermis in neuroleptic-naïve schizophrenia. *Biological Psychiatry*, **49**, 20–27.

Illowsky, B.P., Juliano, D.M., Bigelow, L.B., and Weinberger, D.R. (1988). Stability of CT scan findings in schizophrenia: Results of an 8-year follow-up study. *Journal of Neurology, Neurosurgery, and Psychiatry*, **51**, 209–213.

Ingraham, L.J. and Kety, S.S. (2000). Adoption studies of schizophrenia. *American Journal of Medical Genetics*, **97**, 18–22.

Ingvar, D.H. and Franzen, G. (1974). Abnormalities of cerebral blood flow distribution in patients with chronic schizophrenia. *Acta Psychiatrica Scandinavica*, **50**, 425–462.

Ingvar, D.H. and Franzen, G. (1975). Absence of activation in frontal structures during psychological testing of chronic schizophrenics. *Journal of Neurology, Neurosurgery and Psychiatry*, **38**, 1027–1032.

Ishimaru, M., Kurumaji, A., and Toru, M. (1994). Increases in strychnine-insensitive glycine binding sites in cerebral cortex of chronic schizophrenics: Evidence for glutamate hypothesis. *Biological Psychiatry*, **35**, 84–95.

Jackson, M.E., Homayoun, H., and Moghaddam, B. (2004). NMDA receptor hypofunction produces concomitant firing rate potentiation and burst activity reduction in the prefrontal cortex. *Proceedings of the National Academy of Sciences of the United States of America*, **101**, 8467–8472.

Jacob, H. and Beckmann, H. (1986).Prenatal developmental disturbances in the limbic allocortex in schizophrenics. *Journal of Neural Transmission*, **65**, 303–326.

Jacobi, W. and Winkler, H. (1927). Encephalographische Studien an chronisch Schizophrenen. *Archiv für Psychiatrie und Nervenkrankheiten*, **81**, 299–332.

Jacobsen, L.K., Giedd, J.N., Castellanos, F.X., Vaituzis, A.C., Hamburger, S.D., Kumra, M.S.S., Lenane, M.C., and Rapaport, J.L. (1998). Progressive reduction of temporal lobe structures in childhood-onset schizophrenia. *American Journal of Psychiatry*, **155**, 678–685.

James, A.C.D., Javaloyes, A., James, S., and Smith, D.M. (2002). Evidence for non-progressive changes in adolescent-onset schizophrenia: Follow-up magnetic resonance imaging study. *British Journal of Psychiatry*, **180**, 339–344.

Javitt, D.C. (2004). Glutamate as a therapeutic target in psychiatric disorders. *Molecular Psychiatry*, **9**, 984–997.

Javitt, D.C., Balla, A., Burch, S., Suckow, R. Xie, S., Sershen, H. (2003). Reversal of phencyclidine-induced dopaminergic dysregulation by N-methyl-D-aspartate receptor/glycine-site agonists. *Neuropsychopharmacology*, **29**, 300–307.

Javitt, D.C., Doneshka, P., Zylberman, I., Ritter, W., and Vaughan, H.G. (1993). Impairment of early cortical processing in schizophrenia: An event-related potential confirmation study. *Biological Psychiatry*, **33**, 513–519.

Javitt, D.C., Silipo, G., Shelley, A-M., Bark, N., Park, M., Lindenmayer, J-P., Suckow, R., and Zukin, S.R. (2001). Adjunctive high-dose glycine in the treatment of schizophrenia. *International Journal of Neuropsychopharmacology*, **4**, 385–391.

Javitt, D.C., Zylberman, I., Zukin, S.R., Heresco-Levy, U., and Lindenmayer, J-P. (1994). Amelioration of negative symptoms in schizophrenia by glycine. *American Journal of Psychiatry*, **151**, 1234–1236.

Jaynes, J. (1977). *The origin of consciousness in the breakdown of the bicameral mind*. Boston, Houghton Mifflin Co.

Jeanmonod, D., Schulman, J., Ramirez, R., Cancro, R., Lanz, M., Morel, A., Magnin, M., Siegemund, M., Kronberg, E., Ribary, U., and Llinás, R. (2003). Neuropsychiatric thalamocortical dysrhythmia: Surgical implications. *Neurosurgery Clinics of North America*, **14**, 251–265.

Jensen, J.E., Al-Semaan, Y.M., Williamson, P.C., Neufeld, R.W.J., Menon, R.S., Schaefer, B., Densmore, M., and Drost, D.J. (2002). Region specific changes in phospholipids metabolism in chronic, medicated schizophrenia: ^{31}P-MRS study at 4.0 Tesla. *British Journal of Psychiatry*, **180**, 39–44.

Jensen, J.E., Miller, J., Williamson, P.C., Neufeld, R.W.J., Menon, R.S., Malla, A., Manchanda, R., Schaefer, B., Densmore, M., and Drost, D.J. (2004). Focal changes in brain energy and phosholipid metabolism in first episode schizophrenia: ^{31}P-MRS chemical shift imaging study at 4 Tesla. *British Journal of Psychiatry*, **184**, 409–415.

Jentsch, J.D. and Roth, R.H. (1999). The neuropsychopharmacology of phencyclidine: From NMDA receptor hypofunction to the dopamine hypothesis of schizophrenia. *Neuropsychopharmacology*, **20**, 201–225.

Jentsch, J.D., Taylor, J.R., and Roth, R.H. (1998). Subchronic phencyclidine administration increases mesolimbic dopamine system responsivity and augments stress- and amphetamine-induced hyperlocomotion. *Neuropsychopharmacology*, **19**, 105–113.

Jessen, F., Scheef, L., Germeshausen, L., Tawo, Y., Kockler, M., Kuhn, K-U., Maier, W., Schild, H.H., and Heun, R. (2003). Reduced hippocampal activation during encoding and recognition of words in schizophrenic patients. *American Journal of Psychiatry*, **160**, 1305–1312.

Jeste, D.V., Del Carmen, R., Lohr, J.B., and Wyatt, R.J. (1985). Did schizophrenia exist before the eighteenth century? *Comprehensive Psychiatry*, **26**, 493–503.

Johnson, S.C., Baxter, L.C., Wilder, L.S., Pipe, J.G., Heiserman, J.E., and Prigatano, G.P. (2002). Neural correlates of self-reflection. *Brain*, **125**, 1808–1814.

Johnstone, E.C., Crow, T.J., Frith, C.D., Husband, J., and Kreel, L. (1976). Cerebral ventricular size and cognitive impairment in chronic schizophrenia. *Lancet*, **2**, 924–926.

Jones, E.G. (1997). Cortical development and thalamic pathology in schizophrenia. *Schizophrenia Bulletin*, **23**, 483–501.

Jones, E.G. (2001). The thalamic matrix and thalamocortical synchrony. *Trends in Neurosciences*, **24**, 595–601.

Jones, H.M. and Pilowsky, L.S. (2002). Dopamine and antipsychotic drug action revisited. *British Journal of Psychiatry*, **181**, 271–275.

Jones, P.B., Guth, C., Lewis, S.M., and Murray, R.M. (1994). Low intelligence and poor educational achievement precede early onset schizophrenic psychosis. In A.S. David and J.C. Cutting (Eds.), *The Neuropsychology of Schizophrenia* (pp. 131–144). Hillsdale, NJ, Lawrence Erlbaum.

Josin, G.M. and Liddle, P.F. (2001). Neural network analysis of the pattern of functional connectivity between cerebral areas in schizophrenia. *Biological Cybernetics*, **84**, 117–122.

Joyce, J.N., Shane, A., Lexow, N., Winokur, A., Casanova, M.F., and Kleinman, J.E. (1993). Serotonin uptake sites and serotonin receptors are altered in the limbic system of schizophrenics. *Neuropsychopharmacology*, **8**, 315–336.

Kane, J.M. (1989). The current status of neuroleptic therapy. *Journal of Clinical Psychiatry*, **50**, 322–328.

Kane, J.M., Carson, W.H., Saha, A.R., McQuade, R.D., Ingenito, G.G., Zimbroff, D.L., and Ali, M.W. (2002). Efficacy and safety of aripiprazole and haloperidol versus placebo in patients with schizophrenia and schizoaffective disorder. *Journal of Clinical Psychiatry*, **63**, 763–771.

Kane, J., Honigfeld, G., Singer, J., and Meltzer, H. (1988). Clozapine for the treatment-resistant schizophrenic: A double-blind, comparison with chlorpromazine. *Archives of General Psychiatry*, **45**, 789–796.

Kaplan, R.D., Szechtman, H., Franco, S., Szechtman, B., Nahmias, C., Garnett, E.S., List, S., and Cleghorn, J.M. (1993). Three clinical syndromes of schizophrenia in untreated subjects: Relation to brain glucose activity measured by positron emission tomography (PET). *Schizophrenia Research*, **11**, 47–54.

Kapur, S. (2003). Psychosis as a state of aberrant salience: A framework linking biology, phenomenology, and pharmacology in schizophrenia. *American Journal of Psychiatry*, **160**, 13–23.

Kapur, S. and Remington, G. (1996). Serotonin–dopamine interaction and its relevance to schizophrenia. *American Journal of Psychiatry*, **153**, 466–476.

Kapur, S. and Seeman, P. (2001). Does fast dissociation from the dopamine D_2 receptor explain the action of atypical antipsychotics? A new hypothesis. *American Journal of Psychiatry*, **158**, 360–369.

Karlsson, P., Farde, L., Halldin, C., and Sedvall, G. (2002). PET study of D1 dopamine receptor binding in neuroleptic-naïve patients with schizophrenia. *American Journal of Psychiatry*, **159**, 761–767.

Kasai, K., Shenton, M.E., Salisbury, D.F., Hirayasu, Y., Lee, C-U., Ciszewski, A.A., Yurgelun-Todd, D., Kikinis, R., Jolesz, F.A., and McCarley, R.W. (2003a). Progressive decrease of left superior temporal gyrus gray matter volume in patients with first-episode schizophrenia. *American Journal of Psychiatry*, **160**, 156–164.

Kasai, K., Shenton, M.E., Salisbury, D.F., Hirayasu, Y., Onitsuka, T., Spencer, M.H., Yurgelun-Todd, D., Kikinis, R., Jolesz, F.A., and McCarley, R.W. (2003b). Progressive decrease of left Heschl gyrus and planum temporale gray matter volume in first-episode schizophrenia: A longitudinal magnetic resonance imaging study. *Archives of General Psychiatry*, **60**, 766–775.

Kasai, K., Yamada, H., Kamio, S., Nakagome, K., Iwanami, A., Fukuda, M., Yumoto, M., Itoh, K., Koshida, I., Abe, O., and Kato, N. (2002). Neuromagnetic correlates of impaired automatic categorical perception of speech sounds in schizophrenia. *Schizophrenia Research*, **59**, 159–172.

Kato, T., Shiori, T., Murashita, J., Hamakawa, H., Inubushi, T., and Takahashi, S. (1995). Lateralized abnormality of high-energy phosphate and bilateral reduction of phosphomonoester measured by phosphorus-31 magnetic resonance spectroscopy of the frontal lobes in schizophrenia. *Psychiatry Research: Neuroimaging*, **61**, 151–160.

Kato, K., Shishido, T., Ono, M., Shishido, K., Kobayashi, M., and Niwa, S. (2001). Glycine reduces novelty- and methamphetamine-induced locomotor activity in neonatal ventral hippocampal damaged rats. *Neuropsychopharmacology*, **24**, 330–332.

Kawasaki, Y., Maeda, Y., Sakai, N., Higashima, M., Yamaguchi, N., Koshino, Y., Hisada, K., Suzuki, M., and Matsuda, H. (1996). Regional cerebral blood flow in patients with schizophrenia: Relevance to symptom structures. *Psychiatry Research: Neuroimaging*, **67**, 49–58.

Kawasaki, Y., Maeda, Y., Suzuki, M., Urata, K., Higashima, M., Kiba, K., Yamaguchi, N., Matsuda, H., and Hisada, K. (1993). SPECT analysis of regional cerebral blood flow changes in patients with schizophrenia during the Wisconsin Card Sorting Test. *Schizophrenia Research*, **10**, 109–116.

Kay, S.R. (1991). *Positive and negative syndromes in schizophrenia: Assessment and research*. New York, Brunner/Mazel.

Ke, Y., Coyle, J.T., Simpson, N.S., Gruber, S.A., Renshaw, P.F., and Yurgelun-Todd, D.A. (2003). Frontal brain NAA T2 values are significantly lower in schizophrenia. *Schizophrenia Research*, **60** (Suppl.), 242.

Keefe, R.S.E. (2000). Working memory dysfunction and its relevance in schizophrenia. In T. Sharma and P.D. Harvey (Eds.), *Cognitive Functioning in Schizophrenia* (pp. 16–49). Oxford, Oxford University Press.

Kegeles, L.S., Abi-Dargham, A., Zea-Ponce, Y., Rodenhiser-Hill, J., Mann, J.J., Van Heertum, R.L., Cooper, T.B., Carlsson, A., and Laruelle, M. (2000a). Modulation of amphetamine-induced striatal dopamine release by ketamine in humans: Implications for schizophrenia. *Biological Psychiatry*, **48**, 627–640.

Kegeles, L.S., Martinez, D., Kochan, L.D., Hwang, D-R., Huang, Y., Mawlawi, O., Suckow, R.F., Van Heertum, R.L., and Laruelle, M. (2002). NMDA antagonist effects on striatal dopamine release: Positron emission tomography studies in humans. *Synapse*, **43**, 19–29.

Kegeles, L.S., Shungu, D.C., Anjilvel, S., Chan, S., Ellis, S.P., Xanthopoulos,

E., Malaspina, D., Gorman, J.M., Mann, J.J., Laruelle, M., and Kaufman, C.A. (2000b). Hippocampal pathology in schizophrenia: Magnetic resonance imaging and spectroscopy studies. *Psychiatry Research: Neuroimaging*, **98**, 163–175.

Kelley, W.M., Macrae, C.N., Wyland, C.L., Caglar, S., Inati, S., and Heatherton, T.F. (2002). Finding the self? An event-related fMRI study. *Journal of Cognitive Neuroscience*, **14**, 785–794.

Kemether, E.M., Buchsbaum, M.S., Byne, W., Hazlett, E.A., Haznedar, M., Brickman, A.M., Platholi, J., and Bloom, R. (2003). Magnetic resonance imaging of mediodorsal, pulvinar, and centromedian nuclei of the thalamus in patients with schizophrenia. *Archives of General Psychiatry*, **60**, 983–991.

Kendler, K.S., McGuire, M., Gruenberg, A.M., O'Hare, A., Spellman, M., and Walsh, D. (1993). The Roscommon Family Study. I. Methods, diagnosis of probands, and risk of schizophrenia in relatives. *Archives of General Psychiatry*, **50**, 527–540.

Kerr, S.L. and Neale, J.M. (1993). Emotion perception in schizophrenia: Specific deficit or further evidence of generalized poor performance? *Journal of Abnormal Psychology*, **102**, 312–318.

Keshavan, M.S. (1999). Development, disease and degeneration in schizophrenia: A unitary pathophysiological model. *Journal of Psychiatric Research*, **33**, 513–521.

Keshavan, M.S., Diwadkar, V.A., DeBellis, M., Dick, E., Kotwal, R., Rosenberg, D.R., Sweeney, J.A., Minshew, N., and Pettegrew, J.W. (2002a). Development of the corpus callosum in childhood, adolescence and early adulthood. *Life Sciences*, **70**, 109–1922.

Keshavan, M.S., Diwadkar, V.A., Harenski, K., Rosenberg, D.R., Sweeney, J.A., and Pettegrew, J.W. (2002b). Abnormalities of the corpus callosum in first-episode treatment-naïve schizophrenia. *Journal of Neurology, Neurosurgery and Psychiatry*, **72**, 757–760.

Keshavan, M.S., Haas, G.L., Kahn, C.E., Aguilar, E., Dick, E.L., Schooler, N.R., Sweeney, J.A., and Pettegrew, J.W. (1998). Superior temporal gyrus and the course of early schizophrenia: Progressive, static or reversible? *Journal of Psychiatry Research*, **32**, 161–167.

Keshavan, M.S., Stanley, J.H., and Pettegrew, J.W. (2000). Magnetic resonance spectroscopy in schizophrenia: Methodological issues and findings—part II. *Biological Psychiatry*, **48**, 369–380.

Kim, J.H. and Vezina, P. (1998). Metabotropic glutamate receptors are necessary for sensitization by amphetamine. *Neuroreport*, **9**, 403–406.

Kim, J.-J., Kwon, J.S., Park, H.J., Youn, T., Kang, D.H., Kim, M.S., Lee, D.S., and Lee, M.C. (2003). Functional disconnection between the prefrontal and parietal cortices during working memory processing in schizophrenia: A [^{15}O]H$_2$O PET study. *American Journal of Psychiatry*, **160**, 919–923.

Kim, J.-J., Mohamed, S., Andreasen, N.C., O'Leary, D.S., Watkins, G.L., Boles

Ponto, L.L., and Hichwa, R.D. (2000). Regional neural dysfunctions in chronic schizophrenia studied with positron emission tomography. *American Journal of Psychiatry*, **157**, 542–548.

Kinney, H.C., Brody, B.A., Kloman, A.S., and Gilles, F.H. (1988). Sequence of central nervous system myelination in human infancy II. Patterns of myelination in autopsied infants. *Journal of Neuropathology and Experimental Neurology*, **47**, 217–234.

Kircher, T.T.J., Liddle, P.F., Brammer, M.J., Williams, S.C.R., Murray, R.M., and McGuire, P.K. (2001) Neural correlates of formal thought disorder in schizophrenia. *Archives of General Psychiatry*, **58**, 769–774.

Kircher, T.T.J., Senior, C., Phillips, M.L., Rabe-Hesketh, S., Benson, P.J., Bullmore, E.T., Brammer, M., Simmons, A., Bartels, M., and David, A.S. (2000). Recognizing one's own face. *Cognition*, **78**, B1–B15.

Kirov, G., Jones, P., Harvey, I., Lewis, S.W., Toone, B., Rifkin, L., Sham, P., and Murray, R.M. (1996). Do obstetric complications cause the earlier age of onset in male than female schizophrenics? *Schizophrenia Research*, **20**, 117–123.

Kissler, J., Müller, M.M., Fehr, T., Rockstroh, B., and Elbert, T. (2000). MEG gamma band activity in schizophrenia patients and healthy subjects in a mental arithmetic task and at rest. *Clinical Neurophysiology*, **111**, 2079–2087.

Knoll, J.L., Garver, D.L., Ramberg, J.E., Kinsbury, S.J., Croissant, D., and McDermott, B. (1998). Heterogeneity of the psychoses: Is there a neurodegenerative psychosis? *Schizophrenia Bulletin*, **24**, 365–379.

Ko, G.N., Korpi, E.R., Freed, W.J., Zalcman, S.J., and Bigelow, L.B. (1985). Effect of valproic acid on behaviour and plasma amino acid concentrations in chronic schizophrenic patients. *Biological Psychiatry*, **20**, 209–215.

Kodama, S., Fukuzako, H., Kiura, T., Nozoe, S., Hashiguchi, T., Yamada, K., Takenouchi, K., Takigawa, M., Nakabeppu, Y., and Nakajo, M. (2001). Aberrant brain activation following motor skill learning in schizophrenic patients as shown by functional magnetic resonance imaging. *Psychological Medicine*, **31**, 1079–1088.

Kohler, C.G., Bilker, W., Hagendoorn, M., Gur, R.E., and Gur, R.C. (2000). Emotion recognition deficit in schizophrenia: Association with symptomatology and cognition. *Biological Psychiatry*, **48**, 127–136.

Kolb, B. and Whishaw, I.Q. (1983). Performance of schizophrenic patients on tests sensitive to left or right frontal temporal parietal function in neurologic patients. *Journal of Nervous and Mental Disease*, **171**, 435–443.

Konick, L.C. and Friedman, L. (2001). Meta-analysis of thalamic size in schizophrenia. *Biological Psychiatry*, **49**, 28–38.

Konradi, C. and Heckers, S. (2003). Molecular aspects of glutamate dysregulation: Implications for schizophrenia and its treatment. *Pharmacology and Therapeutics*, **97**, 153–179.

Kovelman, J.A. and Scheibel, A.B. (1984). A neurohistological correlate of schizophrenia. *Biological Psychiatry*, **19**, 1601–1621.

Kraepelin, E. (1919). *Dementia praecox and paraphrenia* (R.M. Barclay, Trans., G.M. Robertson, Ed.), special edition, 1989. Birmingham, AL, The Classics of Medicine Library.

Krasnow, B., Tamm, L., Greicius, M.D., Yang, T.T., Glover, G.H., Reiss, A.L., and Menon, V. (2003). Comparison of fMRI activation at 3 and 1.5 T during perceptual, cognitive, and affective processing. *NeuroImage*, **18**, 813–826.

Krause, M., Fogel, W., Mayer, P., Kloss, M., and Tronnier, V. (2004). Chronic inhibition of the subthalamic nucleus in Parkinson's disease. *Journal of the Neurological Sciences*, **219**, 119–124.

Krause, M., Hoffman, W.E., and Hajós, M. (2003). Auditory sensory gating in the hippocampus and reticular thalamic neurons in anesthetized rats. *Biological Psychiatry*, **53**, 244–253.

Krystal, J.H., Abi-Saab, W., Perry, E., D'Souza, D.C., Liu, N., McDougall, L., Belger, A., Levine, L., and Breier, A. (2003). Modulation of ketamine-induced working memory deficits in healthy human subjects by group II metabotropic agonist, LY354740. *Biological Psychiatry*, **53**, 111S.

Krystal, J.H., Belger, A., Abi-Saab, W., Moghaddam, B., Charney, D.S., Anand, A., Madonick, S., and D'Souza, D.C. (2000). Glutamatergic contributions to cognitive dysfunction in schizophrenia. In T. Sharma and P. Harvey (Eds.), *Cognition in schizophrenia: impairments, importance, and treatment strategies* (pp. 126–153). New York, Oxford University Press.

Krystal, J.H., Belger, A., D'Souza, D.C., Anand, A., Charney, D.S., Aghajanian, G.K., and Moghaddam, B. (1999). Therapeutic implications of hyperglutamatergic effects of NMDA antagonists. *Neuropsychopharmacology*, **22**, S123–S157.

Krystal, J.H., Karper, L.P., Seibyl, J.P., Freeman, G.K., Delaney, R., Bremner, J.D., Heninger, G.R., Bowers, M.B., and Charney, D.S. (1994). Subanesthetic effects of the noncompetitive NMDA antagonist, ketamine in humans: Psychomimetic, perceptual, cognitive, and neuroendocrine responses. *Archives of General Psychiatry*, **51**, 199–214.

Kubicki, M., Shenton, M.E., Salisbury, D.F., Hirayasu, Y., Kasai, K., Kikinis, R., Jolesz, F.A., and McCarley, R.W. (2002). Voxel-based morphometric analysis of gray matter in first episode schizophrenia. *NeuroImage*, **17**, 1711–1719.

Kubicki, M., Westin, C-F., Nestor, P.G., Wible, C.G., Frumin, M., Maier, S.E., Kikinis, R., Jolesz, F.A., McCarley, R.W., and Shenten, M.E. (2003). Cingulate fasciculus integrity disruption in schizophrenia: A magnetic resonance diffusion tensor imaging study. *Biological Psychiatry*, **54**, 1171–1180.

Kurachi, M., Kobayashi, K., Matsubara, R., Hiramatsu, H., Yomaguchi, N., Matsuda, H., Maeda, T., and Hisada, K. (1985). Regional cerebral blood flow in schizophrenic disorders. *European Neurology*, **24**, 176–181.

Kwon, J.S., Shenton, M.E., Hirayasu, Y., Salisbury, D.F., Fischer, I.A., Dickey, C.C., Yurgelun-Todd, D., Tohen, M., Kikinis, P.H.R., Jolesz, F.A., and

McCarley, R.W. (1998). MRI study of cavum septi pellucidi in schizophrenia, affective disorder, and schizotypal personality disorder. *American Journal of Psychiatry*, **155**, 509–515.

Laasko, A., Vilkman, H., Alakare, B., Haaparanta, M., bergman, J., Solin, O., Peurasaari, J., Räkköläinen, V., Syvälahti, E., and Hietala, J. (2000). Striatal dopamine transporter binding in neuroleptic-naïve patients with schizophrenia studied with positron emission tomography. *American Journal of Psychiatry*, **157**, 269–271.

Laberge, D.L. (1995). *Attentional processing: The brain's art of mindfulness*. Cambridge, MA, Harvard University Press.

Lahti, A.C., Holcomb, H.H., Medoff, D.R., and Tamminga, C.A. (1995a). Ketamine activates psychosis and alters limbic blood flow in schizophrenia. *Neuroreport*, **6**, 869–872.

Lahti, A.C., Holcomb, H.H., Medoff, D.R., Weiler, M.A., Tamminga, C.A., and Carpenter, W.T. (2001). Abnormal patterns of regional cerebral blood flow in schizophrenia with primary negative symptoms during an effortful auditory recognition task. *American Journal of Psychiatry*, **158**, 1797–1808.

Lahti, A.C., Holcomb, H.H., Weiler, M.A., Medoff, D.R., Frey, K.N., Hardin, M., and Tamminga, C.A. (2004). Clozapine not haloperidol re-establishes normal task-activated rCBF in schizophrenia within the anterior cingulate cortex. *Neuropsychopharmacology*, **29**, 171–178.

Lahti, A.C., Koffel, B., Laporte, D., and Tamminga, C.A. (1995b) Subanesthetic doses of ketamine stimulate psychosis in schizophrenia. *Neuropsychopharmacology*, **13**, 9–19.

Lampe, I.K., Hulshoff, H.E., Janssen, J., Schnack, H.G., Kahn, R.S., and Heeren, T.J. (2003). Association of depression duration with reduction of global cerebral gray matter volume in female patients with recurrent major depressive disorder. *American Journal of Psychiatry*, **160**, 2052–2054.

Laruelle, M. (1998). Imaging dopamine transmission in schizophrenia: A review and meta-analysis. *Quarterly Journal of Nuclear Medicine*, **42**, 211–221.

Laruelle, M. (2000). The role of endogenous sensitization in the pathophysiology of schizophrenia: Implications from recent brain imaging studies. *Brain Research Reviews*, **31**, 371–384.

Laruelle, M., Abi-Dargham, A., Gil, R., Kegeles, L., and Innis, R. (1999). Increased dopamine transmission in schizophrenia: Relationship to illness phases. *Biological Psychiatry*, **46**, 56–72.

Laruelle, M., Abi-Dargham, A., Van Dyck, C.H., Gil, R., DeSouza, C.D., Erdos, J., McCance, E., Rosenblatt, W., Fingado, C., Zoghbi, S.S., Baldwin, R.M., Seibyl, J.P., Krystal, J.H., Charney, D.S., and Innis, R.B. (1996). Single photon emission computerized tomography imaging of amphetamine-induced dopamine release in drug-free schizophrenic subjects. *Proceedings of the National Academy of Sciences of the United States of America*, **93**, 9235–9240.

Laruelle, M., Kegeles, L.S., and Abi-Dargham, A. (2003). Glutamate, dopamine, and schizophrenia from pathophysiology to treatment. *Annals of the New York Academy of Sciences*, **1003**, 138–158.

Lauer, M., Senitz, D., and Beckmann, H. (2001). Increased volume of the nucleus accumbens in schizophrenia. *Journal of Neural Transmission*, **108**, 645–660.

Lawrie, S.M. and Abukmeil, S. (1998). Brain abnormality in schizophrenia: A systematic and quatitative review of volumetric magnetic resonance imaging studies. *British Journal of Psychiatry*, **172**, 110–120.

Lawrie, S.M., Buechel, C., Whalley, H.C., Frith, C.D., Friston, K.J., and Johnstone, E.C. (2002). Reduced frontotemporal functional connectivity in schizophrenia associated with auditory hallucinations. *Biological Psychiatry*, **51**, 1008–1011.

Lawrie, S.M., Whalley, H., Kestelman, J.N., Abukmeil, S.S., Byrne, M., Hodges, A., Rimmington, J.E., Best, J.J.K., and Johnstone, E.C. (1999). Magnetic resonance imaging of the brain in people at high risk of developing schizophrenia. *Lancet*, **353**, 30–33.

Leach, M.J., Baxter, M.G., and Critchley, M.A. (1991). Neurochemical and behavioral aspects of lamotrigine. *Epilepsia*, **32** (Suppl. 2), S4–S8.

Leach, M.J., Swan, J.H., Eisenthal, D., Dopson, M., and Nobbs, M. (1993). BW619C89, a glutamate release inhibitor, protects against focal cerebral ischemic damage. *Stroke*, **24**, 1063–1067.

Leiderman, E., Zylberman, I., Zukin, S.R, Cooper, T.B., and Javitt, D.C. (1996). Preliminary investigation of high-dose oral glycine on serum levels and negative symptoms in schizophrenia: An open-label trial. *Biological Psychiatry*, **39**, 213–215.

Lennox, B.R., Park, S.B.G., Medley, I., Morris, P.G., and Jones, P.B. (2000). The functional anatomy of auditory hallucinations in schizophrenia. *Psychiatry Research: Neuroimaging*, **100**, 13–20.

Leonard, S., Gault, J., Hopkins, J., Logel, J., Vianzon, R., Short, M., Drebing, C., Berger, R., Venn, D., Sirota, P., Zerbe, G., Olincy, A., Ross, R.G., Adler, L., and Freedman, R. (2002). Association of promoter variants in the α7 nicotinic acetylcholine receptor subunit gene with inhibitory deficit found in schizophrenia. *Archives of General Psychiatry*, **59**, 1085–1096.

Le Pen, G., Kew, J., Alberrati, D., Borroni, E., Heitz, M.-P., and Moreau, J.-L. (2003). Prepulse inhibition deficits of the startle reflex in neonatal ventral hippocampal-lesioned rats: Reversal by glycine and a glycine transporter inhibitor. *Biological Psychiatry*, **54**, 1162–1170.

Levitan, C., Ward, P.B., and Catts, S.V. (1999). Superior temporal gyral volumes and laterality correlates of auditory hallucinations in schizophrenia. *Biological Psychiatry*, **46**, 955–962.

Levy, D.L., Holzman, P.S., Matthysse, S., and Mendell, N.R. (1994). Eye tracking and schizophrenia: A selective review. *Schizophrenia Bulletin*, **20**, 47–62.

Lewis, D.A. (1997). Development of the prefrontal cortex during adolescence: Insights into vulnerable neural circuits in schizophrenia. *Neuropsychopharmacology*, **16**, 385–398.

Lewis, D.A., Cruz, D.A., Melchitzky, D.S., and Pierri, J.N. (2001). Lamina-specific deficits in parvalbumin-immunoreactive varicosities in the prefrontal cortex of subjects with schizophrenia: Evidence for fewer projections from the thalamus. *American Journal of Psychiatry*, **158**, 1411–1422.

Lewis, R., Kapur, S., Jones, C., DaSilva, J., Brown, G.M., Wilson, A.A., Houle, S., and Zipursky, R.B. (1998). 5HT2 receptors in schizophrenia: A PET study using [18F]septoperone in neuroleptic-naïve patients and normal subjects. *American Journal of Psychiatry*, **156**, 72–78.

Lewis, S.W., Ford, R.A., Syed, G.M., Revely, A.M., and Toone, B.K. (1992). A controlled study of 99mTc-HMPAO single-photon emission imaging in chronic schizophrenia. *Psychological Medicine*, 22, 27–35.

Liddle, P.F. (1987) The symptoms of chronic schizophrenia: A re-examination of the positive-negative dichotomy. *British Journal of Psychiatry*, **151**, 145–151.

Liddle, P.F., Friston, K.J., Frith, C.D., Hirsch, S.R., Jones T., and Frackowiak, R.S.J (1992). Patterns of cerebral blood flow in schizophrenia. *British Journal of Psychiatry*, **160**, 179–186.

Liddle, P.F., Lane, C.J., and Ngan, E.T.C. (2000). Immediate effects of risperidone on cortico-striato-thalamic loops and the hippocampus. *British Journal of Psychiatry*, **177**, 402–407.

Liddle, P.F. and Morris, D.L. (1991). Schizophrenic syndromes and frontal lobe performance. *British Journal of Psychiatry*, **158**, 340–345.

Lidsky, T.I., Yablonsky-Alter, E., Zuck, L., and Banerjee, S.P. (1993). Antiglutamatergic effects of clozapine. *Neuroscience Letters*, **163**, 155–158.

Lieberman, J.A. (1999). Is schizophrenia a neurodegenerative disorder? A clinical and neurobiological perspective. *Biological Psychiatry*, **46**, 729–739.

Lieberman, J., Chakos, M., Wu, H., Alvir, J., Hoffman, E., Robinson, D., and Bilder, R. (2001). Longitudinal study of brain morphology in first episode schizophrenia. *Biological Psychiatry*, **49**, 487–499.

Lieberman, J.A., Kane, J.M., and Alvir, J. (1987). Provocative tests with psychostimulant drugs in schizophrenia. *Psychopharmacology*, **91**, 415–433.

Lieberman, J.A., Sheitman, B.B., and Kinon, B.J. (1997). Neurochemical sensitization in the pathophysiology of schizophrenia: Deficits and dysfunction in neuronal regulation and plasticity. *Neuropsychopharmacology*, **17**, 205–229.

Lillrank, S.M., Lipska, B.K., Bachus, S.E., Wood, G.K., and Weinberger, D.R. (1996). Amphetamine-induced c-fos in mRNA expression is altered in rats with neonatal ventral hippocampal damage. *Synapse*, **23**, 292–301.

Lim, K.O., Adalsteinsson, E., Spielman, D., Sullivan, E.V., Rosenbloom, M.J., and Pfefferbaum, A. (1998). Proton magnetic resonance spectroscopic imaging of cortical grey and white matter in schizophrenia. *Archives of General Psychiatry*, **55**, 346–352.

Lim, K.O., Hedehus, M., Moseley, M., de Crespigny, Y., Sullivan, E.V., and Pfefferbaum, A. (1999). Compromised white matter tract integrity in schizophrenia inferred from diffusion tensor imaging. *Archives of General Psychiatry*, **56**, 367–374.

Lim, K.O. and Helpern, J.A. (2002). Neuropsychiatric applications of DTI— a review. *NMR in Biomedicine*, **15**, 587–593.

Lindström, L.H., Gefvert, O., Hagberg, G., Lundberg, T., Bergström, M., Hartvig, P., and Långström, B. (1999). Increased dopamine synthesis rate in medial prefrontal cortex and striatum in schizophrenia indicated by L-(β-^{11}C) dopa and PET. *Biological Psychiatry*, **46**, 681–688.

Lipschitz, D.S., D'Souza, D.C., White, J.A., Charney, D.S., and Krystal, J.H. (1997). Clozapine blockade of ketamine effects in healthy subjects. *Biological Psychiatry*, **41**, 23S.

Lipska, B.K. (2004). Using animal models to test a neurodevelopmental hypothesis of schizophrenia. *Journal of Psychiatry and Neuroscience*, **29**, 282–286.

Lipska, B.K., Jaskiw, G.E., Chrapasta, S., Karoum, F., and Weinberger, D.R. (1992). Ibotemic acid lesion of the ventral hippocampus differentially affects dopamine and its metabolites in the nucleus accumbens and prefrontal cortex. *Brain Research*, **585**, 1–6.

Lipska, B.K., Swerdlow, N.R, Geyer, M.A., Jaskiw, G.E., Braff, D.L., and Weinberger, D.R. (1995). Neonatal excitotoxic hippocampal damage in rats causes post-pubertal changes in prepulse inhibition of startle and its disruption by apomorphine. *Psychopharmacology*, **122**, 35–43.

Lipska, B.K. and Weinberger, D.R. (1993). Delayed effects of neonatal hippocampal damage on haloperidol-induced catalepsy and apomorphine-induced stereotypic behaviours in the rat. *Developmental Brain Research*, **75**, 213–222.

Litman, R., Hommer, D., Clem, T., Ornsteen, M., Ollo, C., and Pickar, D. (1991). Correlation of Wisconsin Card Sorting Test performance with eye tracking in schizophrenia. *American Journal of Psychiatry*, **148**, 1580–1582.

Llinás, R.R. and Pare, D. (1991). Of dreaming and wakefulness. *Neuroscience*, **44**, 521–535.

Llinás, R., Ribary, U., Jeanmonod, D., Kronberg, E., and Mitra, P.P. (1999). Thalamocortical dysrhythmia: A neurological and neuropsychiatric syndrome characterized by magnetoencephalography. *Proceedings of the National Academy of Sciences of the United States of America*, **96**, 15222–15227.

Llinás, R., Ribary, U., Joliot, M., and Wang, X.-J. (1994). Content and context in temporal thalamocortical binding. In G. Buzáki, R. Llinás, W. Singer, A. Berthoz, and Y. Christen (Eds.), *Temporal coding in the brain* (pp. 251–272). Berlin, Springer-Verlag.

Loebel, A.D., Lieberman, J.A., Alvir, J.M.J., Mayerhoff, D.I., Geisler, S.H., and Szymanski, S.R. (1992). Duration of psychosis and outcome in first-episode schizophrenia. *American Journal of Psychiatry*, **149**, 1183–1188.

Loeber, R.T., Cintron, C.M.B., and Yurgelun-Todd, D.A. (2001). Morphometry of individual cerebellar lobules in schizophrenia. *American Journal of Psychiatry*, **158**, 952–954.

Longson, D., Simpson, M.D.C., and Deakin, J.F.W. (1994). Autoradiographic study of [³H]AMPA binding in frontal cortex in schizophrenia. *Schizophrenia Research*, **11**, 121.

Ludewig, K., Geye, M.A., Etzensberger, M., and Vollenweider, F.X. (2002). Stability of the acoustic startle reflex, prepulse inhibition, and habituation in schizophrenia. *Schizophrenia Research*, **55**, 129–137.

MacLean, P.D. (1978). Challenges of the Papez heritage. In K.E. Livingston and O. Hornykiewcz (Eds.), *Limbic mechanisms: The continuing evolution of the limbic system concept* (pp. 1–15). New York, Plenum Press.

MacQueen, G.M., Campbell, S., McEwen, B.S., Macdonald, K., Amano, S., Joffe, R.T., Nahmias, C., and Young, T. (2003). Course of illness, hippocampal function, and hippocampal volume in major depression. *Proceedings of the National Academy of Sciences of the United States of America*, **100**, 1387–1392.

Mahendra, B. (1981). Where have all the catatonics gone? *Psychological Medicine*, **11**, 669–671.

Maier, M., Ron, M.A., Barker, G.J., and Tofts, P.S. (1995). Proton magnetic resonance spectroscopy: An in vivo method of estimating hippocampal neuronal depletion in schizophrenia. *Psychological Medicine*, **25**, 1201–1209.

Maier, S.F. and Seligman, M.E.P. (1976). Learned helplessness: Theory and evidence. *Journal of Experimental Psychology General*, **105**, 3–46.

Malhotra, A.K., Adler, C.M., Kennison, S.D., Elman, I., Pickar, D., and Breier, A. (1997). Clozapine blunts N-methyl-D-aspartate antagonist-induced psychosis: A study with ketamine. *Biological Psychiatry*, **42**, 664–668.

Mann, K., Maier, W., Franke, P., Röschke, J., and Gänsicke, M. (1997). Inta- and interhemispheric electroencephalographram coherence in siblings discordant for schizophrenia and healthy volunteers. *Biological Psychiatry*, **42**, 655–663.

Manoach, D.S., Gollub, R.L., Benson, E.S., Searl, M.M., Goff, D.C., Halpern, E., Saper, C.B., and Rauch, S.L. (2000). Schizophrenic subjects show aberrant fMRI activation of dorsolateral prefrontal cortex and basal ganglia during working memory performance. *Biological Psychiatry*, **48**, 99–109.

Marcelis, M., Suckling, J., Woodruff, P., Hofman, P., Bullmore, E., and van Os, J. (2003). Searching for a structural endophenotype in psychosis using computational morphometry. *Psychiatry Research: Neuroimaging*, **122**, 153–167.

Margolis, R.L., Chuang, D.M., and Post, R.M. (1994). Programmed cell death: Implications for neuropsychiatric disorders. *Biological Psychiatry*, **46**, 946–956.

Martin, A., Wiggs, C.L., Ungerleider, L.G., and Haxby, J.V. (1996). Neural correlates of category-specific knowledge. *Nature*, **379**, 649–652.

Martinot, J.L., Peron-Magnan, P., Huret, J.D., Mazoyer, B., Baron, J.C., Boulenger, J.P., Loc'h, C., Maziere, B., Caillard, V., Loo, H., and Syrota, A. (1990). Striatal D_2 dopaminergic receptors assessed with positron emission tomography and [^{76}Br] bromospiperone in untreated schizophrenic patients. *American Journal of Psychiatry*, **147**, 44–50.

Mathalon, D.H., Pfefferbaum, A., Lim, K.O., Rosenbloom, M.J., and Sullivan, E.V. (2003). Compounded brain volume deficits in schizophrenia-alcoholism comorbidity. *Archives of General Psychiatry*, **60**, 245–252.

Mathalon, D.H., Sullivan, E.V., Lim, K.O., and Pfefferbaum, A. (2001). Progressive brain volume changes and the clinical course of schizophrenia in men: A longitudinal magnetic resonance imaging study. *Archives of General Psychiatry*, **58**, 148–157.

Mattay, V.S., Goldberg, T.E., Fera, F., Hariri, A.R., Tessitore, A., Egan, M.F., Kolachana, B., Callicott, J.H., and Weinberger, D.R. (2003). Catechol *O*-methyltransferase *val^{158}*-met genotype and individual variation in the brain response to amphetamine. *Proceedings of the National Academy of Sciences of the United States of America*, **100**, 6186–6191.

Mattson, M.P., Keller, J.N., and Begley, J.G. (1998). Evidence for synaptic apoptosis. *Experimental Neurology*, **153**, 35–48.

May, P.R.A., Tuma, A.H., and Dixon, W.J. (1981). Schizophrenia: A follow-up study of the results of five forms of treatment. *Archives of General Psychiatry*, **38**, 776–784.

Mayberg, H.S., Liotti, M., Brannan, S.K., McGinnis, S., Mahurin, R.K., Jerabek, P.A., Silva, J.A., Tekell, J.L., Martin, C.C., Lancaster, J.L., and Fox, P.T. (1999). Reciprocal libic-cortical function and negative mood: Converging PET findings in depression and normal sadness. *American Journal of Psychiatry*, **156**, 675–682.

McCarley, R.W., Salisbury, D.F., Hirayasu, Y., Yurgelun-Todd, D.A., Tohen, M., Zarate, C., Kikinis, R., Jolesz, F.A., and Shenton, M.E. (2002). Association between smaller left posterior superior temporal gyrus volume on magnetic resonance imaging and smaller left temporal P300 amplitude in first-episode schizophrenia. *Archives of General Psychiatry*, **59**, 321–331.

McEvoy, J.P., Schooler, N.R., and Wilson WH (1991). Predictors of therapeutic response to haloperidol in acute schizophrenia. *Psychopharmacology Bulletin*, **27**, 97–101.

McEwen, B.S. (1999). Stress and hippocampal plasticity. *Annual Review of Neuroscience*, **22**, 105–122.

McGhie, A. and Chapman, J. (1961). Disorders of attention and perception in early schizophrenia. *British Journal of Medical Psychology*, **34**, 103–116.

McGlashan, T.H. (1988). A selective review of recent North American long-term follow up studies of schizophrenia. *Schizophrenia Bulletin*, **14**, 515–542.

McGlashan, T.H. and Hoffman, R.E. (2000). Schizophrenia as a disorder of developmentally reduced synaptic connectivity. *Archives of General Psychiatry*, **57**, 637–648.

McGowan, S., Lawrence, A.D., Sales, T., Quested, D., and Grasby, P. (2004).

Presynaptic dopaminergic dysfunction in schizophrenia: A positron emission tomographic [^{18}F] fluorodopa study. *Archives of General Psychiatry*, **61**, 134–142.

McGuire, P.K., Shah, G.M.S., and Murray, R.M. (1993). Increased blood flow in Broca's area during auditory hallucinations in schizophrenia. *Lancet*, **342**, 703–706.

McGuire, P.K., Silbersweig, D.A., Wright, I., Murray, R.M., David, A.S., Frackowiak, R.S.J., and Frith, C.D. (1995). Abnormal monitoring of inner speech: A physiological basis for auditory hallucinations. *Lancet*, **346**, 596–600.

McIntosh, A.M., Semple, D., Tasker, K., Harrison, L.K., Owens, D.G.C., Johnstone E.C., and Ebmeier, K.P. (2004). Transcranial magnetic stimulation for auditory hallucinations in schizophrenia. *Psychiatry Research*, **127**, 9–17.

McNaughton, N.C., Leach, M.J., Hainsworth, A.H., and Randall, A.D. (1997). Inhibition of human N-type voltage-gated Ca^{2+} channels by the neuroprotective agent BW619C89. *Neuropsychopharmacology*, **36**, 1795–1798.

McNeil, T.F., Cantor-Graae, E., and Weinberger, D.R. (2000) Relationship of obstetrical complications and differences in size of brain structures in monozygotic twin pairs discordant for schizophrenia. *American Journal of Psychiatry*, **157**, 203–212.

Meador-Woodruff, J.H., Clinton, S.M., Beneyto, M., and McCullumsmith, R.E. (2003). Molecular abnormalities of the glutamate synapse in the thalamus in schizophrenia. *Annals of the New York Academy of Sciences*, **1003**, 75–93.

Meador-Woodruff, J.H. and Healy, D.J. (2000). Glutamate receptor expression in schizophrenic brain. *Brain Research Reviews*, **31**, 288–294.

Mednick, S.A., Huttunen, M.O., and Machon, R.A. (1994). Prenatal influenza infections and adult schizophrenia. *Schizophrenia Bulletin*, **20**, 263–267.

Mednick, S.A., Machon, R.A., Huttunen, M.O., and Bonett, D. (1988). Adult schizophrenia following prenatal exposure to an influenza epidemic. *Archives of General Psychiatry*, **45**, 189–192.

Meltzer, H.Y., Matsubara, S., and Lee, J.C. (1989). The ratios of serotonin and dopamine 2 affinities differentiate atypical and typical antipsychotic drugs. *Psychopharmacology Bulletin*, **25**, 390–397.

Mendrek, A., Laurens, K.R., Kiehl, K.A., Ngan, E.T.C., Stip, E., and Liddle, P.F. (2004). Changes in distributed neural circuitry function in patients with first-episode schizophrenia. *British Journal of Psychiatry*, **185**, 205–214.

Menon, V., Anagnoson, R.T., Glover, G.H., and Pfefferbaum, A. (2001a). Functional magnetic resonance imaging evidence for disrupted basal ganglia function in schizophrenia. *American Journal of Psychiatry*, **158**, 646–649.

Menon, V., Anagnoson, R.T., Mathalon, D.H., Glover, G.H., and Pfefferbaum, A. (2001b). Functional neuroanatomy of auditory working memory in schizophrenia: relation to positive and negative symptoms. *Neuroimage*, **13**, 433–446.

Mesulam, M.-M. (1990). Large-scale neurocognitive networks and distributed processing for attention, language, and memory. *Annals of Neurology*, **28**, 597–613.

Mesulam, M.-M. (2000). Behavioural neuroanatomy. In M.M. Mesulam (Ed.), *Principles of behavioural and cognitive neurology* (pp. 1–120). New York, Oxford University Press.

Mesulam, M.-M. (2002). The human frontal lobes: Transcending the default mode through contingent encoding. In D.T. Stuss, and R.T. Knight (Eds.), *Principles of frontal lobe function* (pp. 8–30). New York, Oxford University Press.

Metzinger, T. (Ed.) (2000). *Neural correlates of consciousness: Empirical and conceptual questions.* Cambridge, MA, The MIT Press.

Meyer-Lindenberg, A., Miletich, R.S., Kohn, P.D., Esposito, G., Carson, R.E., Quarantelli, M., Weinberger, D.R., and Berman, K.F. (2002). Reduced prefrontal activity predicts exaggerated striatal dopaminergic function in schizophrenia. *Nature Neuroscience*, **5**, 267–271.

Meyer-Lindenberg, A., Poline, J.-B., Kohn, P.D., Holt, J.L., Egan, M.F., Weinberger, D.R., and Berman, K.F. (2001). Evidence for abnormal cortical functional connectivity during working memory in schizophrenia. *American Journal of Psychiatry*, **15**, 1809–1817.

Middleton, F.A. and Strick, P.L. (2000). Basal ganglia and cerebellar loops: Motor and cognitive circuits. *Brain Research Reviews*, **31**, 236–250.

Middleton, F.A. and Strick, P.L. (2001). A revised neuroanatomy of frontal–subcortical circuits. In D.G. Lichter and J.L. Cummings (Eds.), *Frontal–subcortical circuits in psychiatric and neurological disorders* (pp. 44–58). New York, Guilford Press.

Miller, B.L (1991). A review of chemical issues in ^{1}H NMR spectroscopy: N-acetyl-L-aspartate, creatine and choline. *NMR in Biomedicine*, **4**, 47–52.

Miller, B.L., Seeley, W.W., Mychack, P., Rosen, J., Mena, I., and Boone, K. (2001a). Neuroanatomy of the self: Evidence from patients with frontotemporal dementia. *Neurology*, **57**, 817–821.

Miller, D.D., Andreasen, N.C., O'Leary, D.S., Watkins, G.L., Boles Ponto, L.L., and Hichwa, R.D. (2001b). Comparison of the effects of risperidone and haloperidol on regional cerebral blood flow in schizophrenia. *Biological Psychiatry*, **49**, 704–715.

Miller, R. (1989). Schizophrenia as a progressive disorder: Relations to EEG, CT, neuropathological and other evidence. *Progress in Neurobiology*, **33**, 17–44.

Millson, R.C., Owen, J.A., Lorberg, G.W., and Tackaberry, L. (2002). Topiramate for refractory depression. *American Journal of Psychiatry*, **159**, 675.

Mitelman, S.A., Shihabuddin, L., Brickman, A.M., Hazlett, E.A., and Buchsbaum, M.S. (2003). MRI assessment of gray and white matter distribution in Brodmann's areas of the cortex in patients with schizophrenia with good and poor outcomes. *American Journal of Psychiatry*, **160**, 2154–2168.

Miyamoto, S., Duncan, G.E., Marx, C.E., and Lieberman, J.A. (2005). Treatments for schizophrenia: A critical review of pharmacology and mechanisms of action of antipsychotic drugs. *Molecular Psychiatry*, **10**, 79–104.

Moberg, P.J., Agrin, R., Gur, R.E., Gur, R.C., Turetsky, B.I., and Doty, R.L. (1999). Olfactory dysfunction in schizophrenia: A qualitative and quantitative review. *Neuropsychopharmacology*, **21**, 325–340.

Mogenson, G.J., Jones, D.L., and Yim, C.Y. (1980). From motivation to action: Functional interface between limbic system and the motor system. *Progress in Neurobiology*, **14**, 69–97.

Moghaddam, B. (2002). Stress activation of glutamate neurotransmission in the prefrontal cortex: Implications for dopamine-associated psychiatric disorders. *Biological Psychiatry*, **51**, 775–787.

Moghaddam, B. (2003). Bringing order to the glutamate chaos in schizophrenia. *Neuron*, **40**, 881–884.

Moghaddam, B. and Adams, B.W. (1998). Reversal of phencyclidine effects by a group II metabotropic glutamate receptor agonist in rats. *Science*, **281**, 1349–1352.

Molina Rodriguez, V., Andreé, R.M., Castejón, M.J.P., Labrador, R.G., Navarrete, F.F., Delgado, J.L.C., and Vila, F.J.R. (1997). Cerebral perfusion correlates of negative symptomatology and parkinsonism in a sample of treatment-refractory schizophrenics: An exploratory 99mTc-HMPAO SPET study. *Schizophrenia Research*, **25**, 11–20.

Moore, H., West, A.R., and Grace, A.A. (1999). The regulation of forebrain dopamine transmission: Relevance to the pathophysiology and psychopathology of schizophrenia. *Biological Psychiatry*, **46**, 40–55.

Morice, E., Denis, C., Macario, A., Giros, B., and Nosten-Bertrand, M. (2005). Constitutive hyperdopaminergia is functionally associated with reduced behavioural lateralization. *Neuropsychopharmacology*, **30**, 575–581.

Moriñigo, A., Martin, J., Gonzalez, S., and Mateo, I. (1989). Treatment of resistant schizophrenia with valproate and neuroleptic drugs. *Hillside Journal of Clinical Psychiatry*, **11**, 199–207.

Morrison, A.P. and Haddock, G. (1997). Cognitive factors in source monitoring and auditory hallucinations. *Psychological Medicine*, **27**, 669–679.

Morrison, J.R. (1974). Changes in subtype diagnosis of schizophrenia: 1920–1966. *American Journal of Psychiatry*, **131**, 674–677.

Morrison-Stewart, S.L., Williamson, P.C., Corning, W.C., Kutcher, S.P., and Merskey, H. (1991). Coherence on electroencephalography and aberrant functional organization of the brain in schizophrenic patients during activation tasks. *British Journal of Psychiatry*, **159**, 636–644.

Morrison-Stewart, S.L., Williamson, P.C., Corning, W.C., Kutcher, S.P., Snow, W.G., and Merskey, H. (1992). Frontal and non-frontal lobe neuropsychological test performance and clinical symptoms of schizophrenia. *Psychological Medicine*, **22**, 353–359.

Munk-Jorgensen, P. (1995). Decreasing rates of incident schizophrenia cases in psychiatric service: A review of the literature. *European Psychiatry*, **10**, 129–141.

Murray, C.J.L. and Lopez, A.D. (Eds.) (1996). *The global burden of disease: A comprehensive assessment of mortality, and disability from diseases, injuries, and risk factors in 1990 and projected to 2020.* Cambridge, MA, Harvard University Press.

Nair, T.R., Christensen, J.D., Kingsbury, S.J., Kumar, N.G., Terry, W.M., and Garver, D.L. (1997). Progression of cerebroventricular enlargement and the subtyping of schizophrenia. *Psychiatry Research: Neuroimaging,* **74**, 141–150.

Nakanishi, S. (1992). Molecular diversity of glutamate receptors and implications for brain function. *Science,* **258**, 597–603.

Narr, K.L., Sharma, T., Woods, R.P., Thompson, P.M., Sowell, E.R., Rex, D., Kim, S., Asuncion, D., Jang, S., Mazziotta, J., and Toga, A.W. (2003). Increases in regional subarachnoid CSF without apparent cortical gray matter deficits in schizophrenia: Modulating effects of sex and age. *American Journal of Psychiatry,* **160**, 2169–2180.

Nasrallah, H.A. (1985). The unintegrated right cerebral hemispheric consciousness as alien intruder: A possible mechanism for Schneiderian delusions in schizophrenia. *Comprehensive Psychiatry,* **26**, 273–282.

Nasrallah, H.A. (1986). Cerebral hemispheric asymmetries and interhemispheric integration in schizophrenia. In H.A. Nasrallah and D.R. Weinberger (Eds.), *Handbook of schizophrenia, Vol. 1: The neurology of schizophrenia* (pp. 157–174). Elsevier, Amsterdam.

Nasrallah, H.A., Olson, S.C., McCalley-Whitters, M., Chapman, S., and Jacoby, C.G. (1986). Cerebral ventricular enlargement in schizophrenia. *Archives of General Psychiatry,* **43**, 157–159.

Nasrallah, H.A., Skinner, T.E., Schmalbrock, P., and Robitaille, P.M. (1994). In vivo proton magnetic resonance spectroscopy (H-1 MRS) of the hippocampal formation in schizophrenia: A pilot study. *British Journal of Psychiatry,* **165**, 481–485.

Nelson, M.D., Saykin, A.J., Flashman, L.A., and Riordan, H.J. (1998). Hippocampal volume reduction in schizophrenia as assessed by magnetic resonance imaging: A meta-analytic study. *Archives of General Psychiatry,* **55**, 433–440.

Nestor, P.G., Shenton, M.E., McCarley, R.W., Haimson, J., Smith, R.S., O'Donnell, B., Kimble, M., Kikinis, R., and Jolesz, F.A. (1993). Neuropsychological correlates of MRI temporal lobe abnormalities in schizophrenia. *American Journal of Psychiatry,* **150**, 1849–1855.

Neuchterlein, K.H., Dawson, M.E., and Green, M.F. (1994). Information processing abnormalities as neuropsychological vulnerability indicators for schizophrenia. *Acta Psychiatrica Scandinavica,* **90** (Suppl 384), 71–79.

Neuchterlein, K.H., Edell, W.S., Norris, M., and Dawson, M.E. (1986). Attentional vulnerability indicators, thought disorder, and negative symptoms. *Schizophrenia Bulletin,* **12**, 408–426.

Neufeld, R.W.J. and Williamson, P.C. (1996). Neuropsychological correlates of positive symptoms: Delusions and hallucinations. In C. Pantelis, H.E.

Nelson, and T.R.E. Barnes (Eds.), *Schizophrenia: A neuropsychological perspective* (pp. 205–235). London, John Wiley and Sons.

Newman, J. (1997a). Putting the puzzle together. Part I: Towards a general theory of the neural correlates of consciousness. *Journal of Consciousness Studies*, **4**, 47–66.

Newman, J. (1997b). Putting the puzzle together. Part II: Towards a general theory of the neural correlates of consciousness. *Journal of Consciousness Studies*, **4**, 100–121.

Newman, J. and Grace, A.A. (1999). Binding across time: The selective gating of frontal and hippocampal systems modulating working memory and attentional states. *Consciousness and Cognition*, **8**, 196–212.

Ninan, I. and Wang, R.Y. (2003). Modulation of the ability of clozapine to facilitate NMDA- and electrically evoked responses in the pyramidal cells of the rat medial prefrontal cortex by dopamine: Pharmacological evidence. *European Journal of Neuroscience*, **17**, 1306–1312.

Noga, J.T., Aylward, E., Barta, P.E., and Pearlson, G.D. (1995). Cingulate gyrus in schizophrenic patients and normal volunteers. *Psychiatry Research: Neuroimaging*, **61**, 201–208.

Nohara, S., Suzuki, M., Kurachi, M., Yamashita, I., Matsui, M., Seto, H., and Saitoh, O. (2000). Neural correlates of memory organization deficits in schizophrenia: A single photon emission computed tomography study with ^{99m}Tc-ethyl-cysteinate dimer during a verbal learning task. *Schizophrenia Research*, **42**, 209–222.

Nopoulis, P., Flashman, L., Flaum, M., Arndt, S., and Andreasen, N. (1994). Stability of cognitive functioning early in the course of schizophrenia. *Schizophrenia Research*, **14**, 29–37.

Nordahl, T.E., Carter, C.S., Salo, R.E., Kraft, L., Baldo, J., Salamat, S., Robertson, L., and Kusubov, N. (2001). Anterior cingulate metabolism correlates with Stroop errors in paranoid schizophrenia patients. *Neuropsychopharmacology*, **25**, 139–148.

Norman, R.M.G. and Malla, A.K. (1993). Stressful life events and schizophrenia I: A review of the research. *British Journal of Psychiatry*, **162**, 161–166.

Norman, R.M.G. and Malla, A.K. (2001). Duration of untreated psychosis: A critical examination of the concept and its importance. *Psychological Medicine*, **31**, 381–400.

Norman, R.M.G., Townsend, L., and Malla, A.K. (2001). Duration of untreated psychosis and cognitive functioning in first-episode patients. *British Journal of Psychiatry*, **179**, 340–345.

Nyberg, L., McIntosh, A.R., Cabeza, R., Habib, R., Houle, S., and Tulving, E. (1996). General and specific brain regions involved in encoding and retrieval of events: What, where and when. *Proceedings of the National Academy of Sciences of the United States of America*, **93**, 11280–11285.

O'Callaghan, E., Larkin, C., Kinsella, A., and Waddington, J.L. (1991a). Familial, obstetric and other clinical correlates of minor physical anomalies in schizophrenia. *American Journal of Psychiatry*, **148**, 479–483.

O'Callaghan, E., Redmond, O., Ennis, R., Stack, J., Kinsella, A., Ennis, J.T., Larkin, C., and Waddington, J.L. (1991b). Initial investigation of the left temporoparietal region in schizophrenia by ^{31}P magnetic resonance spectroscopy. *Biological Psychiatry,* **29**, 1149–1152.

O'Donnell, P. and Grace, A.A. (1998). Dysfunction in multiple interrelated systems as the neurobiological bases of schizophrenic symptom clusters. *Schizophrenia Bulletin,* **24**, 267–283.

O'Donnell, P., Greene, J., Pabello, N., Lewis, B.L., and Grace, A.A. (1999). Modulation of cell firing in the nucleus accumbens. *Annals New York Academy of Sciences,* **877**, 157–175.

Oertel, D. and Young, E.D. (2004). What's a cerebellar circuit doing in the auditory system? *Trends in Neurosciences,* **27**, 104–110.

Ogawa, S., Tank, D.W., Menon, R., Ellerman, J.M., Kim, S.-G., Merkle, H., and Ugurbil, K. (1992). Intrinsic signal changes accompanying sensory stimulation: Functional brain mapping with magnetic resonance imaging. *Proceedings of the National Academy of Science of the United States of America,* **89**, 5951–5955.

Okamura, N., Hashimoto, K., Shimizu, E., Koike, K., Ohgake, S., Koizumi, H., Kumakiri, C., Komatsu, N., and Iyo, M. (2003). Protective effects of LY379268, a selective group II metabotropic receptor agonist, on dizocilpine-induced neuropathological changes in rat retrosplenial cortex. *Brain Research,* **992**, 114–119.

O'Leary, D.D.M., Schlaggar, B.L., and Tuttle, R. (1994). Specification of neocortical areas and thalamocortical connections. *Annals of Neuroscience,* **17**, 419–439.

Olney, J.W. and Farber, N.B. (1995). Glutamate receptor dysfunction and schizophrenia. *Archives of General Psychiatry,* **52**, 998–1007.

Omori, M., Murata, T., Kimura, H., Koshimoto, Y., Kado, H., Ishimori, Y. Ito, H., and Wada, Y. (2000). Thalamic abnormalities in patients with schizophrenia revealed by proton magnetic resonance spectroscopy. *Psychiatry Research: Neuroimaging,* **98**, 155–162.

Orzack, M.H. and Kornetsky, C. (1966). Attention dysfunction in chronic schizophrenia. *Archives of General Psychiatry,* **14**, 323–326.

Ossowska, K., Pietraszek, M., Wardas, J., Nowak, G., and Wolfarth, S. (1999). Chronic haloperidol and clozapine administration increases the number of cortical NMDA receptors in rats. *Naunyn-Schmiedeberg's Archives of Pharmacology,* **359**, 280–287.

Overall, K.L. (2000). Natural animal models of human psychiatric conditions: Assessment of mechanisms and validity. *Progress Neuropsychopharmacology and Biological Psychiatry,* **24**, 727–776.

Owen, M.J., Williams, N.M., and O'Donovan, M.C. (2004). The molecular genetics of schizophrenia: New findings promise new insights. *Molecular Psychiatry,* **9**, 14–27.

Paillère-Martinot, M.-L., Caclun, A., Artiges, E., Poline, J.-B., Joliot, M., Mallet, L., Recasens, C., Attar-Lévy, D., and Martinot, J.-L. (2001). Cerebral gray matter and white matter reductions and clinical correlates in patients with early onset schizophrenia. *Schizophrenia Research*, **50**, 19–26.

Pakkenberg, B. (1990). Pronounced reduction of total neuron number in mediodorsal thalamic nucleus and nucleus accumbens in schizophrenics. *Archives of Gneral Psychiatry*, **47**, 1023–1028.

Pakkenberg, B. (1992). The volume of the mediodorsal thalamic nucleus in treated and untreated schizophrenics. *Schizophrenia Research*, **7**, 95–100.

Palmatier, M.A., Kang, A.M., and Kidd, K.K. (1999). Global variation in the frequencies of functionally different catechol-*O*-methyltransferase alleles. *Biological Psychiatry*, **46**, 557–567.

Pantelis, C., Barnes, T.R.E., and Nelson, H.E. (1992). Is the concept of fronto-subcortical dementia relevant to schizophrenia? *British Journal of Psychiatry*, **160**, 442–460.

Pantelis, C., Harvey, C.A., Plant, G., Fossey, E., Maruff, P., Stuart, G.W., Brewer, W.J., Nelson, H.E., Robbins, T.W., and Barnes, T.R.E. (2004). Relationship of behavioural and symptomatic syndromes in schizophrenia to spatial working memory and attentional set-shifting ability. *Psychological Medicine*, **34**, 693–703.

Pantelis, C., Velakoulis, D., McGorry, P.D., Wood, S.J., Suckling, J., Phillips, L.J., Yung, A.R., Bullmore, E.T., Brewer, W., Soulsby, B., Desmond, P., and McGuire, P.K. (2003). Neuroanatomical abnormalities before and after onset of psychosis: A cross-sectional and longitudinal MRI comparison. *Lancet*, **361**, 281–288.

Papez, J. W. (1937). A proposed mechanism of emotion. *Archives of Neurology*, **38**, 725–743.

Paradiso, S., Andreasen, N.C., Crespo-Facorro, B., O'Leary, D.S., Watkins, G.L., Boles Ponto, L.L., and Hichwa, R.D. (2003). Emotions in unmedicated patients with schizophrenia during evaluation with positron emission tomography. *American Journal of Psychiatry*, **160**, 1775–1783.

Park, S., Holzman, P.S., and Goldman-Rakic, P.S. (1995). Spatial working memory deficits in the relatives of schizophrenic patients. *Archives of General Psychiatry*, **52**, 821–828.

Pasamanick, B., Rogers, M.E., and Lilienfeld, A.M. (1956). Pregnancy experience and the development of behavior disorder in children. *American Journal of Psychiatry*, **112**, 613–618.

Pearlson, G.D. and Marsh, L. (1999). Structural brain imaging in schizophrenia: A selective review. *Biological Psychiatry*, **46**, 627–649.

Penn, A.A. (2001). Early brain wiring: Activity-dependent processes. *Schizophrenia Bulletin*, **27**, 337–347.

Perlman, W.R., Weikert, C.S., Akil, M., and Kleinman, J.E. (2004). Postmortem investigations of the pathophysiology of schizophrenia: The role of susceptibility genes. *Journal of Psychiatry and Neuroscience*, **29**, 287–293.

Perlstein, W.M., Carter, C.S., Noll, D.C., and Cohen, J.D. (2001). Relation of prefrontal cortex dysfunction to working memory and symptoms in schizophrenia. *American Journal of Psychiatry*, **158**, 1105–1113.

Perlstein, W.M., Dixit, N.K., Carter, C.S., Noll, D.C., and Cohen, J.D. (2003). Prefrontal cortex dysfunction mediates deficits in working memory and prepotent responding in schizophrenia. *Biological Psychiatry*, **53**, 25–38.

Peterson, B.S., Skudlarski, P., Gatenby, J.C., Zhang, H., Anderson, A.W., and Gore, J.C. (1999). An fMRI study of Stoop word-color interference: Evidence for cingulate subregions subserving multiple distributed attentional systems. *Biological Psychiatry*, **45**, 1237–1258.

Petralia, R.S., Wang, Y-X., Niedzielski, A.S., and Wenthold, R.J. (1996). The metabotropic glutamate receptors, MGLUR2 and MGLUR3, show unique postsynaptic, presynaptic and glial localizations. *Neuroscience*, **71**, 949–976.

Pettegrew, J.R., Keshavan, M., Panchalingam, K., Strychor, S., Kaplan, D.B., Tretta, M.G., and Allen, M. (1991). Alterations in brain high-energy phosphate and membrane phospholipid metabolism in first-episode, drug naïve schizophrenics: A pilot study of the dorsal prefrontal cortex by in vivo phosphorus 31 nuclear magnetic resonance spectroscopy. *Archives of General Psychiatry*, **48**, 563–568.

Pfefferbaum, A. and Zipursky, R.B. (1991). Neuroimaging studies of schizophrenia. *Schizophrenia Research*, **4**, 193.

Pilowsky, L.S., Costa, D.C., Ell, P.J., Murray, R.M., Verhoeff, N.P.L.G., and Kerwin, R.W. (1992). Clozapine, single photon emission tomography and the D2 dopamine receptor blockade hypothesis of schizophrenia. *Lancet*, **340**, 199–202.

Pilowsky, L.S., Costa, D.C., Ell, P.J., Verhoeff, N.P.L.G., Murray, R.M., and Kerwin, R.W. (1994). D_2 dopamine receptor binding in the basal ganglia of antipsychotic-free schizophrenic patients. An ^{123}I-IBZM single photon emission computerized tomography study. *British Journal of Psychiatry*, **164**, 16–26.

Popken, G.J., Bunney, W.E., Potkin, S.G., and Jones, E.G. (2000). Subnucleus-specific loss of neurons in medial thalamus of schizophrenics. *Proceedings of the National Academy of Sciences of the United States of America*, **97**, 9276–9280.

Portas, C.M., Goldstein, J.M., Shenton, M.E., Hokama, H.H., Wible, C.G., Fischer, I., Kikinis, R., Donnino, R., Jolsz, F.A., and McCarley, R.W. (1998). Volumetric evaluation of the thalamus in schizophrenic male patients using magnetic resonance imaging. *Biological Psychiatry*, **43**, 649–659.

Posner, M.I. (1994). Attention: The mechanisms of consciousness. *Proceedings of the National Academy of Sciences of the United States of America*, **91**, 7398–7403.

Potkin, S.G., Alva, G., Fleming, K., Anand, R., Keator, D., Carreon, D., Doo, M., Jin, Y., Wu, J.C., and Fallon, J.H. (2002). A PET study of the pathophysiology of negative symptoms in schizophrenia. *American Journal of Psychiatry*, **159**, 227–237.

Potkin, S.G., Buchsbaum, M.S., Jin, Y., Tang, C., Telford, J., Friedman, G., Lottenberg, S., Najafi, A., Gulasekaram, B., Costa, J., Richmond, G.H., and

Bunney, W.E. (1994). Clozapine effects on glucose metabolic rate in striatum and frontal cortex. *Journal of Clinical Psychiatry*, **55** (Suppl B), 63–66.

Potwarka, J., Drost, D.J., Williamson, P.C., Carr, T., Canaran, G., Rylett, R.J., and Neufeld, R.W.J. (1999) A ^{1}H decoupled ^{31}P chemical shift imaging study of medicated schizophrenic patients and healthy controls. *Biological Psychiatry*, **45**, 687–693.

Provencher, S.W. (1993). Estimation of metabolite concentrations from localized in vivo proton NMR spectra. *Magnetic Resonance in Medicine*, **30**, 672–679.

Pycock, C.J., Kerwin, R.W., and Carter, C.J. (1980). Effect of lesion of cortical dopamine terminals on subcortical dopamine receptors in rats. *Nature*, **286**, 74–77.

Rabiner, C.J., Wegner, J.T., and Kane, J.M. (1986). Outcome study of first-episode psychosis. I: Relapse rates after one year. *American Journal of Psychiatry*, **143**, 1155–1158.

Ragland, J.D., Goldberg, T.E., Wexler, B.E., Gold, J.M., Torrey, E.F., and Weinberger, D.R. (1992). Dichotic listening in monozygotic twins discordant and concordant for schizophrenia. *Schizophrenia Research*, **7**, 177–183.

Ragland, J.D., Gur, R.C., Glahn, D.C., Censits, D.M., Smith, R.J., Lazarev, M.G., Alavi, A., and Gur, R.E. (1998). Frontotemporal cerebral blood flow change during executive and declarative memory tasks in schizophrenia: A positron emission tomography study. *Neuropsychology*, **12**, 399–413.

Ragland, J.D., Gur, R.C., Raz, J., Schroeder, L., Kohler, C.G., Smith, R.J., Alavi, A., and Gur, R.E. (2001). Effect of schizophrenia on frontotemporal activity during word encoding and recognition: A PET cerebral blood flow study. *American Journal of Psychiatry*, **158**, 1114–1125.

Rajakumar, N., Leung, L.S., Rajakumar, B., and Rushlow, W. (2004). Altered neurotrophin receptor function in developing prefrontal cortex leads to adult-onset dopaminergic hyperresponsivity and impaired prepulse inhibition of acoustic startle. *Biological Psychiatry*, **55**, 797–803.

Rajakumar, N. and Rajakumar, B. (2003). An animal model showing adult-onset dopamine hyperactivity and neuropathological features of schizophrenia. *Schizophrenia Research*, **60**: 58.

Rapoport, J.L., Giedd, J., Kumra, S., Jacobsen, L., Smith, A., Nelson, J., and Hamburger, S. (1997). Childhood-onset schizophrenia: Progressive ventricular change during adolescence. *Archives of General Psychiatry*, **54**, 897–903.

Rapoport, M., van Reekum, R., and Mayberg, H. (2000). The role of the cerebellum in cognition and behaviour: A selective review. *Journal of Neuropsychiatry and Clinical Neuroscience*, **12**, 193–198.

Rauschecker, J.P. and Tian, B. (2000). Mechanisms and streams for processing of "what" and "where" in auditory cortex. *Proceedings of the National Academy of Sciences of the United States of America*, **97**, 11800–11806.

Raz, S. and Raz, N. (1990). Structural brain abnormalities in the major psychoses: A quantitative review of the evidence from computerized imaging. *Psychological Bulletin*, **108**, 93–108.

Reite, M., Teale, P., and Rojas, D.C. (1999). Magnetoencephalography: Applications in psychiatry. *Biological Psychiatry*, **45**, 1553–1563.

Reith, J., Benkelfat, C., Sherwin, A., Yasuhara, Y., Kuwabara, H., Andermann, F., Bachneff, S., Cumming, P., Diksic, M., Dyve, S.E., Etienne, P., Evans, A.C., Lal, S., Shevell, M., Savard, G., Wong, D.F., Chouinard, G., and Gjedde, A. (1994). Elevated dopa decarboxylase activity in living brain of patients with psychosis. *Proceeding of the National Academy of Sciences of the United States of America*, **91**, 11651–11654.

Renshaw, P.F., Yurgelun-Todd, D.A., Tohen, M., Gruber, S., and Cohen. B.M. (1995). Temporal lobe proton magnetic resonance spectroscopy of patients with first-episode psychosis. *American Journal Psychiatry*, **152**, 444–446.

Reveley, A.M., Reveley, M.A., Clifford, C.A., and Murray, R.M. (1982). Cerebral ventricular size in twins discordant for schizophrenia. *Lancet*, **1**(8271), 540–541.

Reynolds, G.P. (1983). Increased concentration and lateral asymmetry of amygdala dopamine in schizophrenia. *Nature*, **305**, 527–529.

Richardson-Burns, S.M., Haroutunian, V., Davis, K.L., Watson, S.J., and Meador-Woodruff, J.H. (1999). Metabotropic glutamate receptor mRNA expression in the schizophrenic thalamus. *Biological Psychiatry*, **47**, 22–28.

Rizzo, L., Danion, J.-M., Van der Linden, M., and Grangé, D. (1996). Patients with schizophrenia remember that an event has occurred, but not when. *British Journal of Psychiatry*, **168**, 427–431.

Robbins, T.W. (1990). The case for frontostriatal dysfunction in schizophrenia. *Schizophrenia Bulletin*, **16**, 391–402.

Robinson, T.E. and Becker, J.B. (1986). Enduring changes in brain and behaviour produced by chronic amphetamine administration: A review and evaluation of animal models of amphetamine psychosis. *Brain Research Reviews*, **11**, 157–198.

Rolls, E.T. (1999). The functions of the orbitofrontal cortex. *Neurocase*, **5**, 301–312.

Romito, I.M., Scerrati, M., Contarino, M.F., Iacoangeli, M., Bentivoglio, A.R., and Albanese, A. (2003). Bilateral high frequency subthalamic stimulation in Parkinson's disease: Long-term neurological follow-up. *Journal of Neurosurgical Sciences*, **47**, 119–128.

Ropohl, A., Sperling, W., Elstner, S., Tomandl, B., Reulbach, U., Kaltenhäuser, M., Kornhuber, J., and Maihöfner, C. (2004). Cortical activity associated with auditory hallucinations. *Neuroreport*, **15**, 523–526.

Rosse, R.B., Fay-McCarthy, M., Kendrick, K., Davis, R.E., and Deutsch, S.I. (1996). D-cycloserine adjuvant therapy to molindole in the treatment of schizophrenia. *Clinical Neuropharmacology*, **19**, 444–450.

Rosse, R.B., Theut, S.K., Banay, S.M., Banay-Schwartz, M., Leighton, M., Scarcella, E., Cohen, C.G., and Deutsch, S.I. (1989). Glycine adjuvant therapy to conventional neuroleptic treatment in schizophrenia: An open-label, pilot study. *Clinical Neuropharmacology*, **12**, 416–424.

Rossi, A., Serio, A., Stratta, P., Petruzzi, C., Schiazza, G., Mancini, F., and Casacchia, M. (1994). Planum temporale asymmetry and thought disorder in schizophrenia. *Schizophrenia Research*, **12**, 1–7.

Roth, R.M., Flashman, L.A., Saykin, A.J., McAllister, T.W., and Vidaver, R. (2004). Apathy in schizophrenia: Reduced frontal lobe and neuropsychological deficits. *American Journal of Psychiatry*, **161**, 157–159.

Rowe, A.D., Bullock, P.R., Polkey, C.E., and Morris, R.G. (2001). 'Theory of mind' impairments and their relationship to executive functioning following frontal lobe excisions. *Brain*, **124**, 600–616.

Rubenstein, J.L.R. and Rakic, P. (1999). Genetic control of cortical development. *Cerebral Cortex*, **9**, 521–523.

Rund, B.R. (1998). A review of longitudinal studies of cognitive functions in schizophrenic patients. *Schizophrenia Bulletin*, **24**, 425–435.

Russell, A.J., Munro, J.C., Jones, P.B., Hemsley, D.R., and Murray, R.M. (1997). Schizophrenia and the myth of intellectual decline. *American Journal of Psychiatry*, **15**, 635–639.

Sabri, O., Erkwoh, R., Schreckenberger, E.M., Cremerius, U., Schulz, G., Dickmann, C., Kaiser, E.M., Steinmeyer, E.M., Sass, H., and Buell, U. (1997). Regional cerebral blood flow and negative/positive symptoms in 24 drug-naïve schizophrenics. *Journal of Nuclear Medicine*, **38**, 181–188.

Sawa, A. and Snyder, S.H. (2002). Schizophrenia: diverse approaches to complex disease. *Science*, **296**, 692–695.

Schlaggar, B.L. and O'Leary, D.D.M, (1993). Patterning of the barrel field in somotosensory cortex with implications for the specification of neocortical areas. *Perspectives on Developmental Neurobiology*, **1**, 81–91.

Schoenfeldt-Lecuona, C., Herwig, U., Groen, G., Wunderlich, A.P., Walter, H., and Spitzer, M. (2001). fMRI guided neuronavigated transcranial magnetic stimulation in patients suffering from auditory hallucinations. *Schizophrenia Research*, **49** (Suppl. 1), 244–245.

Schröder, J., Buchsbaum, M.S., Siegel, B.V., Geider, F.J., Lohr, J., Tang, C., Wu, J., and Potkin, S.G. (1996). Cerebral metabolic activity correlates of subsyndromes in chronic schizophrenia. *Schizophrenia Research*, **19**, 41–53.

Schröder, J., Wenz, F., Schad, L.R., Baudendistel, K. and Knopp, M.V. (1995). Sensorimotor cortex and supplementary motor area changes in schizophrenia: A study with functional magnetic resonance imaging. *British Journal of Psychiatry*, **167**, 197–201.

Schwieler, L., Engberg, G., and Erhardt, S. (2004). Clozapine modulates midbrain dopamine neuron firing via interaction with the NMDA receptor complex. *Synapse*, **52**, 114–122.

Seckinger, R.A., Goudsmit, N., Coleman, E., Harkavy-Friedman, J., Yale, S., Rosenfield, P.J., and Malaspina, D. (2004). Olfactory identification and WAIS-R performance in deficit and nondeficit schizophrenia. *Schizophrenia Research*, **69**, 55–65.

Seeman, M.V. (1982). Gender differences in schizophrenia. *Canadian Journal of Psychiatry*, **27**, 107–112.

Seeman, P. (1987). Dopamine receptors and the dopamine hypothesis of schizophrenia. *Synapse*, **1**, 133–152.

Seidman, L.J., Faraone, S.V., Goldstein, J.M., Goodman, J.M., Kremen, W.S., Toomey, R., Tourville, J., Kennedy, D., Makris, N., Caviness, V.S., and Tsuang, M.T. (1999). Thalamic and amygdala-hippocampal volume reductions in first-degree relatives of patients with schizophrenia: An MRI-based morphometric analysis. *Biological Psychiatry*, **46**, 941–954.

Selemon, L.D. and Goldman-Rakic, P.S. (1999). The reduced neuropil hypothesis: A circuit based model of schizophrenia. *Biological Psychiatry*, **45**, 17–25.

Selemon, L.D., Kleinman, J.E., Herman, M.M., and Goldman-Rakic, P.S. (2002). Smaller frontal gray matter volume in postmortem schizophrenic brains. *American Journal of Psychiatry*, **159**, 1983–1991.

Selemon, L.D., Rajkowska, G., and Goldman-Rakic, P.S. (1995). Abnormally high neuronal density in the schizophrenia cortex. A morphometric analysis of prefrontal area 9 and occipital area 17. *Archives of General Psychiatry*, **52**, 805–818.

Selemon, L.D., Rajkowska, G., and Goldman-Rakic, P.S. (1998). Elevated neuronal density in prefrontal area 46 in brains from schizophrenia patients: Application of a three-dimensional, stereologic counting method. *Journal of Comprehensive Neurology*, **392**, 402–412.

Servan-Schreiber, D., Carter, C.S., Bruno, R.M., and Cohen, J.D. (1998). Dopamine and the mechanisms of cognition: Part II. D-amphetamine effects in human subjects performing a selective attention task. *Biological Psychiatry*, **43**, 723–729.

Servan-Schreiber, D., Cohen, J., and Steingard, S. (1996). Schizophrenic deficits in the processing of context: A test of a theoretical model. *Archives of General Psychiatry*, **53**, 1105–1112.

Shagass, C. (1991). EEG studies in schizophrenia. In S.R. Steinhauer, J.H. Gruzelier, and J. Zubin (Eds.), *Handbook of schizophrenia, Vol. 5: Neuropsychology, psychophysiology and information processing* (pp. 39–69). Amsterdam, Elsevier.

Shank, R.P., Gardocki, J.F., Streeter, A.J., and Marynoff, B.E. (2000). An overview of the preclinical aspects of topiramate: Pharmacology, pharmacokinetics, and mechanism of action. *Epilepsia*, **41** (Suppl. 1), S3–S9.

Shapleske, J., Rossell, S.L., Chitnis, X.A., Suckling, J., Simmons, A., Bullmore, E.T., Woodruff, P.W.R., and David, A.S. (2002). A computational morphometric MRI study of schizophrenia: Effects of hallucinations. *Cerebral Cortex*, **12**, 1331–1341.

Shapleske, J., Rossell, S.L., Woodruff, P.W.R., and David, A.S. (1999). The planum temporale: A systematic, quantitative review of its structural, functional and clinical significance. *Brain Research Reviews*, **29**, 26–49.

Sharma, T., Lancaster, E., Sigmundsson, T., Lewis, S., Takei, N., Gurling,

H., Barta, P., Pearlson, G., and Murray, R.M. (1999). Lack of normal pattern of cerebral asymmetry in familial schizophrenic patients and their relatives—the Maudsley family study. *Schizophrenia Research*, **40**, 111–120.

Sheline, Y.I. (2003). Neuroimaging studies of mood disorder effects on the brain. *Biological Psychiatry*, **54**, 338–352.

Shelton, R.C. and Weinberger, D.R. (1986). X-ray computerized tomography studies in schizophrenia: A review and synthesis. In S.R. Steinhauer, J.H. Gruzelier, and J. Zubin (Eds.), *Handbook of schizophrenia, Vol. 1: The neurology of schizophrenia* (pp. 207–250). Amsterdam, Elsevier.

Shenton, M.E., Dickey, C.C., Frumin, M., and McCarley, R.W. (2001). A review of MRI findings in schizophrenia. *Schizophrenia Research*, **49**, 1–52.

Shenton, M.E., Kikinis, R., Jolesz, F.A., Pollak, S.D., LeMay, M., Wible, C.G., Hokama, H., Martin, J., Metcalf, D., Coleman, M., and McCarley, R.W. (1992). Abnormalities of the left temporal lobe and thought disorder in schizophrenia: A quantitative magnetic resonance imaging study. *New England Journal of Medicine*, **327**, 604–612.

Shergill, S.S., Brammer, M.J., Williams, S.C.R., Murray, R.M., and McGuire, P.K. (2000a). Mapping auditory hallucinations in schizophrenia using functional magnetic resonance imaging. *Archives of General Psychiatry*, **57**, 1033–1038.

Shergill, S.S., Bullmore, E., Simmons, A., Murray, R.M., and McGuire, P.K. (2000b). Functional anatomy of auditory verbal imagery in schizophrenic patients with auditory hallucinations. *American Journal of Psychiatry*, **157**, 1691–1693.

Shergill, S.S., Murray, R.M., and McGuire, P.K. (1998). Auditory hallucinations: A review of psychological treatments. *Schizophrenia Research*, **32**, 137–150.

Shiori, T., Kato, T., Inubuski, T., Murashita, J., and Takahashi, S. (1994). Correlations of phosphomonoesterase measured by phosphorus-31 magnetic resonance spectroscopy in the frontal lobes and negative symptoms in schizophrenia. *Psychiatry Research: Neuroimaging*, **55**, 223–235.

Shorter, E. (1997). *A history of psychiatry*. Toronto, John Wiley and Sons.

Shulman, R.G. (2001). Functional imaging studies: Linking mind and basic neuroscience. *American Journal of Psychiatry*, **158**, 11–20.

Siever, L.J., Koenigsberg, H.W., Harvey, P., Mitropoulo, V., Laruelle, M., Abi-Dargham, A., Goodman, M., and Buchsbaum, M. (2002). Cognitive and brain function in schizotypal personality disorder. *Schizophrenia Research*, **54**, 157–167.

Sigmundsson, T., Suckling, J., Maier, M., Williams, S.C.R., Bullmore, E.T., Greenwood, K.E., Fukuda, R., Ron, M.A., and Toone, B.K. (2001). Structural abnormalities in frontal, temporal, and limbic regions and interconnecting white matter tracts in schizophrenic patients with prominent negative symptoms. *American Journal of Psychiatry*, **158**, 234–243.

Silbersweig, D.A., Stern, E., Frith, C., Cahill, C., Holmes, A., Gootoonk, S., Seaward, J., McKenna, P., Chua, S.E., Schnorr, L., Jones, T., and Frackowiak, R.S.J. (1995). A functional neuroanatomy of hallucinations in schizophrenia. *Nature*, **378**, 176–179.

Silver, H., Feldman, P., Bilker, W., and Gur, R.C. (2003). Working memory deficit as a core neuropsychological dysfunction in schizophrenia. *American Journal of Psychiatry*, **160**, 1809–1816.

Simpson, M.D., Lubman, D.I., Slater, P., and Deakin, J.F. (1996) Autoradiography with [^{3}H]8-OH-DPAT reveals increases in 5-HT(1A) receptors in ventral prefrontal cortex in schizophrenia. *Biological Psychiatry*, **39**, 919–928.

Slater, E. and Beard, A.W. (1963). The schizophrenia-like psychoses of epilepsy. Psychiatric aspects. *British Journal of Psychiatry*, **109**, 95–150.

Smith, G.S., Schloesser, R., Brodie, J.D., Dewey, S.L., Logan, J., Vitkun, S.A., Simkowitz, P., Hurley, A., Cooper, T., Volkow, N.D., and Cancro, R. (1998). Glutamate modulation of dopamine measured in vivo with positron emission tomography (PET) and 1C-raclopride in normal human subjects. *Neuropsychopharmacology*, **18**, 18–25.

Snyder, S.H. (2002). Forty years of neurotransmitters: A personal account. *Archives of General Psychiatry*, **59**, 983–994.

Soares, J.C. and Innis, R.B. (1999). Neurochemical brain imaging investigations of schizophrenia. *Biological Psychiatry*, **46**, 600–615.

Sommer, I.E.C, Ramsey, N.F., Mandl, R.C.W., van Oel, C.J., and Kahn, R.S. (2004). Language activation in monozygotic twins discordant for schizophrenia. *British Journal of Psychiatry*, **184**, 128–135.

Spence, S.A., Brooks, D.J., Hirsch, S.R., Liddle, P.F., Meehan, J., and Grasby, P.M. (1997). A PET study of voluntary movement in schizophrenic patients experiencing passivity phenomena (delusions of alien control). *Brain*, **120**, 1997–2011.

Spence, S.A., Liddle, P.F., Stefan, M.D., Hellewell, J.S.E., Sharma, T., Friston, K.J., Hirsch, S.R., Frith, C.D., Murray, R.M., Deakin, J.F.W., and Grasby, P.M. (2000). Functional anatomy of verbal fluency in people with schizophrenia and those at genetic risk: Focal dysfunction and distributed disconnectivity reappraised. *British Journal of Psychiatry*, **176**, 52–63.

Spencer, K.M., Nestor, P.G., Perlmutter, R., Niznikiewicz, M.A., Klump, M.C., Frumin, M., Shenton, M.E., and McCarley, R.W. (2004). Neural synchrony indexes disordered perception and cognition in schizophrenia. *Proceedings of the National Academy of Sciences of the United States of America*, **101**, 17288–17293.

Spencer, K.M., Nestor, P.G., Niznikiewicz, M.A., Salisbury, D.F., Shenton, M.E., and McCarley, R.W. (2003). Aberrant neural synchrony in schizophrenia. *Journal of Neuroscience*, **23**, 7407–7411.

Sporn, A.L., Greenstein, D.K., Gogtay, N., Jeffries, N.O., Lenane, M., Gochman, P., Clasen, L.S., Blumenthal, J., Giedd, J.N., and Rapaport, J.L. (2003). Progressive brain volume loss during adolescence in childhood-onset schizophrenia. *American Journal of Psychiatry*, **160**, 2181–2189.

Squire, L. (1992). Memory and the hippocampus: A sythesis of findings with rats, monkeys and humans. *Psychological Review,* **99**, 195–231.

Staal, W.G., Hulshoff, H.E., Schnack, H., Van der Schot, A.C., and Kahn, R.S. (1998). Partial volume decrease of the thalamus in relatives of patients with schizophrenia. *American Journal of Psychiatry,* **155**, 1784–1786.

Staal, W.G., Hulshoff, H.E., Shnack, H.G., van Haren, N.E.M., Seifert, N., and Kahn, R.S. (2001). Structural brain abnormalities in chronic schizophrenia at extremes of the outcome spectrum. *American Journal of Psychiatry,* **158**, 1140–1142.

Stanley, J.A., Drost, D.J., Williamson, P.C., and Thompson, R.T. (1995a). The use of a prior knowledge to quantify short echo in vivo ^{1}H MR spectra, *Magnetic Resonance in Medicine,* **34**, 17–24.

Stanley, J.A., Pettegrew, J.W., and Keshavan, M.S. (2000). Magnetic resonance spectroscopy in schizophrenia: Methodological issues and findings—part 1. *Biological Psychiatry,* **48**, 357–368.

Stanley, J.A., Williamson, P.C., Drost, D.J., Carr, T., Rylett, J., Malla, A., and Thompson, R.T. (1995b). In vivo prefrontal ^{31}P magnetic resonance spectroscopy in schizophrenic patients, *Archives of General Psychiatry,* **52**, 399–406.

Stanley, J.A., Williamson, P.C., Drost, D.J., Rylett, J., Carr, T., Malla, A., and Thompson, R.J. (1996). An in vivo proton magnetic resonance spectroscopy study of schizophrenic patients. *Schizophrenia Bulletin,* **22**, 597–609.

Stefanis, N., Frangou, S., Yakeley, J., Sharma, T., O'Connell, P., Morgan, K., Sigmudsson, T., Taylor, M., and Murray, R. (1999). Hippocampal volume reduction in schizophrenia: Effects of genetic risk and pregnancy and birth complications. *Biological Psychiatry,* **46**, 697–702.

Stefansson, H., Sigurdsson, E., Steinthorsdottir, V., Bjornsdottir, S., Sigmundsson, T., Ghosh, S., Brynjolfsson, J., Gunnarsdottir, S., Ivarsson, O., Chou, T.T., Hjaltason, O., Birgisdottir, B., Jonsson, H., Gudnadottir, V.G., Gudmundsdottir, E., Bjornsson, A., Ingvarsson, B., Ingason, A., Sigfusson, S., Hardardottir, H., Harvey, R.P., Lai, D., Zhou, M., Brunner, D., Mutel, V., Gonzalo, A., Lemke, G., Sainz, J., Johannesson, G., Andresson, T., Gudbjartsson, D., Manolescu, A., Frigge, M.L., Gurney, M.E., Kong, A., Gulcher, J.R., Petursson, H., and Stefansson, K. (2002). *Neuroregulin 1* and susceptibility to schizophrenia. *American Journal of Human Genetics,* **71**, 877–892.

Stein, D.J. (2000). Neurobiology of obsessive-compulsive spectrum disorders. *Biological Psychiatry,* **47**, 296–304.

Stein, D.J., Shoulberg, N., Helton, K., and Hollander, E. (1992). The neuroethological approach to obsessive-compulsive disorder. *Comprehensive Psychiatry,* **33**, 274–281.

Steriade, M., Gloor, P., Llinas, R.R., Lopes da Silva, F.H., and Mesulam, M.M. (1990). Basic mechanisms of cerebral rhythmic activities. *Electroencephalography and Clinical Neurophysiology,* **76**, 481–508.

Stevens, J.R. (1973). An anatomy of schizophrenia? *Archives of General Psychiatry*, **29**, 177–189.

Stevens, J.R. (1982). Neuropathology of schizophrenia. *Archives of General Psychiatry*, **39**, 1131–1139.

Straub, R.E., Jiang, Y., MacLean, C.J., Ma, Y., Webb, B.T., Myakishev, M.V., Harris-Kerr, C., Wormley, B., Sadek, H., Kadambi, N., Cesare, A.J., Gibberman, A., Wang, X., O'Neill, F.A., Walsh, D., and Kendler, K.S. (2002). Genetic variation in the 6p22.3 gene *DTNBP1*, the human ortholog of the mouse dysbindin gene, is associated with schizophrenia. *American Journal of Human Genetics*, **71**, 337–348.

Strauss, J.S., Carpenter, W.T., and Bartko, J.J. (1974). The diagnosis and understanding of schizophrenia. II: Speculations on the processes that underlie schizophrenic symptoms and signs. *Schizophrenia Bulletin*, **11**, 61–76.

Stuss, D.T., Gallup, G.G., Jr., and Alexander, M.P. (2001) The frontal lobes are necessary for 'theory of mind'. *Brain*, **124**, 279–286.

Stuss, D.T. and Knight, R.T. (ed.) (2002). *Principles of frontal lobe function*. New York, Oxford University Press.

Suddath, R.L., Christison, G.W., Torrey, E.F., Casanova, M.F., and Weinberger, D.R. (1990). Anatomical abnormalities in the brains of monozygotic twins discordant for schizophrenia. *New England Journal of Medicine*, **322**, 789–794.

Sur, C., Mallorga, P.J., Wittmann, M., Jacobson, M.A., Pascarella, D., Williams, J.B., Brandish, P.E., Pettibone, D.J., Scolnick, E.M., and Conn, P.J. (2003). N-desmethylclozapine, an allosteric agonist at muscarinic 1 receptor, potentiates N-methyl-D-aspartate receptor activity. *Proceedings of the National Academy of Sciences of the United States of America*, **100**, 13674–13679.

Susser, E.S. and Lin, S.P. (1992). Schizophrenia after prenatal exposure to the Dutch hunger winter of 1944–1945. *Archives of General Psychiatry*, **49**, 983–988.

Susser, E., Neugebauer, R., Hoek, H.W., Brown, A.S., Lin, S., Labovitz, D., and Gorman, J.M. (1996). Schizophrenia after prenatal famine: Further evidence. *Archives of General Psychiatry*, **53**, 25–31.

Suvisaari, J.M., Haukka, J., Tanskanen, A., and Lönnqvist, J.K. (1998). Age at onset and outcome in schizophrenia are related to the degree of familial loading. *British Journal of Psychiatry*, **173**, 494–500.

Suzuki, M., Nohara, S., Hagino, H., Kurokawa, K., Yotsutsuji, T., Kawasaki, Y., Takahashi, T., Matsui, M., Watanabe, N., Seto, H., and Kurachi, M. (2002). Regional changes in brain gray and white matter in patients with schizophrenia demonstrated with voxel-based analysis of MRI. *Schizophrenia Research*, **55**, 41–54.

Sweet, R.A., Bergen, S.E., Sun, Z., Sampson, A.R., Pierri, J.N., and Lewis, D.A. (2004). Pyramidal cell size reduction in schizophrenia: Evidence for involvement of auditory feed forward circuits. *Biological Psychiatry*, **55**, 1128–1137.

Swerdlow, N.R. and Geyer, M.A. (1998) Using an animal model of deficient sensorimotor gating to study the pathophysiology and new treatments of schizophrenia. *Schizophrenia Bulletin*, **24**, 285–301.

Swerdlow, N.R. and Koop, G.F. (1987). Dopamine, schizophrenia, mania, and depression: Toward a unified hypothesis of cortico-striato-pallido-thalamic function. *Behavioural and Brain Sciences*, **10**, 197–245.

Swerdlow, N.R., Martinez, Z.A., Hanlon, F.M., Platten, A., Farid, M., Auerbach, P., Braff, D.L., and Geyer, M. (2000). Toward understanding the biology of a complex phenotype: Rat strain and substrain differences in the sensorimotor gating-disruptive effects of dopamine agonists. *Journal of Neuroscience*, **20**, 4325–4336.

Szeszko, P.R., Goldberg, E., Gunduz-Bruce, H., Ashtari, M., Robinson, D., Malhotra, A.K., Lencz, T., Bates, J., Crandall, D.T., Kane, J.M., and Bilder, R.M. (2003). Smaller anterior hippocampal formation volume in antipsychotic-naïve patients with first-episode schizophrenia. *American Journal of Psychiatry*, **160**, 2190–2197.

Szeszko, P.R., Strous, R.D., Goldman, R.S., Ashtari, M., Knuth, K.H., Lieberman, J.A., and Bilder, R.M. (2002). Neuropsychological correlates of hippocampal volumes in patients experiencing a first episode of schizophrenia. *American Journal of Psychiatry*, **159**, 217–226.

Szymanski, S.R., Cannon, T.D., Gallacher, F., Erwin, R.I., and Gur, R.E. (1996). Course of treatment response in first-episode and chronic schizophrenia. *American Journal of Psychiatry*, **153**, 519–525.

Taber, M.T., Das, S., and Fibiger, H.C. (1995). Cortical regulation of subcortical dopamine release: Mediation via the tegmental area. *Journal of Neurochemistry*, **65**, 1407–1410.

Taber, M.T. and Fibiger, H.C. (1995). Electrical stimulation of the prefrontal cortex increases dopamine release in the nucleus accumbens of the rat: Modulation by metabotropic glutamate receptors. *Journal of Neuroscience*, **15**, 3896–3904.

Takahashi, T., Kawasaki, Y., Kurokawa, K., Hagino, H., Nohar, S., Yamashita, I., Nakamura, K., Murata, M., Matsui, M., Susuki, M., Seto, H., and Kurachi, M. (2002). Lack of normal structural asymmetry of the anterior cingulate gyrus in female patients with schizophrenia: A volumetric magnetic resonance imaging study. *Schizophrenia Research*, **55**, 69–81.

Tamminga, C.A. (1997). Gender and schizophrenia. *Journal of Clinical Psychiatry*, **58** (Suppl. 15), 33–37.

Tamminga, C. (1999). Glutamatergic aspects of schizophrenia. *British Journal of Psychiatry*, **174** (Suppl. 37), 12–15.

Tamminga, C.A., Thaker, G.K., Buchanen, R., Kirkpatrick, B., Alphs, L.D., Chase, T.N., and Carpenter, W.T. (1992) Limbic system abnormalities identified in schizophrenia using positron emission tomography with fluorodeoxyglucose and neocortical alterations with deficit syndrome. *Archives of General Psychiatry,* **49**, 522–530.

Tamminga, C.A., Vogel, M., Gao, X.M., Lahti, A.C., and Holcomb, H.H. (2000). The limbic cortex in schizophrenia: Focus on the anterior cingulate. *Brain Research Reviews,* **31**, 364–370.

Tauscher, J., Kapur, S., Verhoeff, P.L.G., Hussey, D.F., Daskalakis, Z.J., Tauscher-Wisniewski, S., Wilson, A.A., Houle, S., Kasper, S., and Zipursky, R.B. (2002). Brain serotonin 5-HT$_{1A}$ receptor binding in schizo-phrenia measured by positron emission tomography and [^{11}C]WAY-100635. *Archives of General Psychiatry,* **59**, 514–520.

Taylor, S.F., Liberzon, I., Decker, L.R., and Koeppe, R.A. (2002). A functional anatomic study of emotion in schizophrenia. *Schizophrenia Research,* **58**, 159–172.

Teale, P., Carlson, J., Rojas, D., and Reite, M. (2003). Reduced laterality of the source locations for generators of the auditory steady-state field in schizophrenia. *Biological Psychiatry,* **54**, 1149–1153.

Tekin, S., Ayut-Bingöl, C., Tanridağ, T., and Aktan, S. (1998). Antigluta-matergic therapy in Alzheimer's disease: Effects of lamotrigine. *Journal of Neural Transmission,* **105**, 295–303.

Tenn, C.C., Fletcher, P.J., and Kapur, S. (2003). Amphetamine-sensitized animals show a sensorimotor gating and neurochemical abnormality similar to that of schizophrenia. *Schizophrenia Research,* **64**, 103–114.

Théberge, J., Al-Semaan, Y., Williamson, P.C., Menon, R.S., Neufeld, R.W.J., Schaefer, B., Densmore, M., and Drost, D.J. (2003). Glutamate and glutamine in the anterior cingulate and thalamus of medicated patients with chronic schizophrenia and healthy comparison subjects measured with 4.0-T proton MRS. *American Journal of Psychiatry,* **160**, 2231–2233.

Théberge, J., Bartha, R., Drost, D.J., Menon, R.S., Malla, A., Takhar, J., Neufeld, R.W.J., Rogers, J., Pavlosky, W., Schaefer, B., Densmore, M., Al-Semaan, Y., and Williamson, P.C. (2002). Glutamate and glutamine measured with 4.0 T proton MRS in never-treated patients with schizophrenia and healthy volunteers. *American Journal of Psychiatry,* **159**, 1944–1946.

Thompson, P.M., Vidal, C., Giedd, J.N., Gochman, P., Blumenthal, J., Nicolson, R., Toga, A.W., and Rapoport, J.L. (2001). Mapping adolescent brain change reveals dynamic wave of accelerated gray matter loss in very early-onset schizophrenia. *Proceedings of the National Academy of Sciences of the United States of America,* **98**, 11650–11655.

Tibbo, P., Hanstock, C.C., Asghar, S., Silverstone, P., and Allen, P.S. (2000). Proton magnetic resonance spectroscopy (^{1}H-MRS) of the cerebellum in men with schizophrenia. *Journal of Psychiatry and Neuroscience,* **25**, 509–512.

Tibbo, P., Hanstock, C., Valiakalayil, A. and Allen, P. (2004). 3-T proton MRS investigation of glutamate and glutamine in adolescents at high genetic risk for schizophrenia. *American Journal of Psychiatry,* **161**, 1116–1118.

Tiihonen, J., Hallikainen, T., Ryynänen O-P., Repo-Tiihonen, E., Kotilainen,

I., Eronen, M., Toivonen, P., Wahlbeck, K., and Putkonen, A. (2003). Lamotrigine in treatment-resistant schizophrenia: a randomized placebo-controlled crossover trial. *Biological Psychiatry*, **54**, 1241–1248.

Tononi, G. and Edelman, G.M. (1998a). Consciousness and complexity. *Science*, **282**, 1846–1851.

Tononi, G. and Edelman, G.M. (1998b). Consciousness and the integration of information in the brain. In H.H. Jasper, L. Descarries, V.F. Castellucci, and S. Rossignol (Eds.), *Consciousness: At the frontiers of neuroscience* Philadelpiha, Lippincott-Raven. *Advances in Neurology*, **77**, 245–279.

Tononi, G. and Edelman, G.M. (2000). Schizophrenia and the mechanisms of conscious integration. *Brain Research Reviews*, **31**, 391–400.

Toone, B.K., Okocha, C.I., Sivakumar, K., and Syed, G.M. (2000). Changes in cerebral blood flow due to cognitive activation among patients with schizophrenia. *British Journal of Psychiatry*, **177**, 222–228.

Torres, I.J., O'Leary, D.S., and Andreasen, N.C. (2004). Symptoms and interference from memory in schizophrenia: Evaluation of Frith's model of willed action. *Schizophrenia Research*, **69**, 35–43.

Torrey, E.F. (2002). Studies of individuals with schizophrenia never treated with antipsychotic medications: A review. *Schizophrenia Research*, **58**, 101–115.

Torrey, E.F. and Kaufmann, C.A. (1986). Schizophrenia and neuroviruses. In H.A. Nasrallah and D.R. Weinberger (Eds.), *Handbook of schizophrenia, Vol. 1: The neurology of schizophrenia* (pp. 361–376). New York, Elsevier.

Toru, M., Watanabe, S., Shibuya, H., Nishikawa, T., Noda, K., Mitsushio, H., Ichikawa, H., Kurumaji, A., Takashima, M., Mataga, N., and Ogawa, A. (1988). Neurotransmitters, receptors and neuropeptides in post-mortem brains of schizophrenic patients. *Acta Psychiatrica Scandinavica*, **78**, 121–137.

Trichard, C., Paillère-Martinot, M.L., Attar-Levy, D., Blin, J., Feline, A., and Martinot, J.L. (1998). No serotonin 5HT2A receptor density abnormality in the cortex of schizophrenic patients studied with PET. *Schizophrenia Research*, **31**, 13–17.

Tsai, G. and Coyle, J.T. (2002). Glutamatergic mechanisms in schizophrenia. *Annual Reviews of Pharmacology and Toxicology*, **42**, 165–179.

Tsai, G., Hsien-Yuan, L., Yang, P., Chong, M.-Y., and Lange, N. (2004). Glycine transporter I inhibitor, N-methylglycine (Sarcosine), added to antipsychotics for the treatment of schizophrenia. *Biological Psychiatry*, **55**: 452–456.

Tsai, G., Passani, L.A., Slusher, B.S., Carter, R., Baer, L., Kleinman, J.E., and Coyle, J.T. (1995). Abnormal excitatory neurotransmitter metabolism in schizophrenic brains. *Archives of General Psychiatry*, **52**, 829–836.

Tsai, G., Yang, P., Chung, L.-C., Lange, N., and Coyle, J.T. (1998). D-serine added to antipsychotics for the treatment of schizophrenia. *Biological Psychiatry*, **44**, 1081–1089.

Tsuang, M.T., Woolson, R.F., and Fleming, J.A. (1979). Long-term outcome of the major psychoses I. Schizophrenia and affective disorders compared with psychiatrically symptom-free surgical conditions. *Archives of General Psychiatry*, **36**, 1295–1301.

Umbricht, D., Schmid, L., Koller, R., Vollenweider, F.X., Hell, D., and Javitt, D.C. (2000). Ketamine-induced deficits in auditory and visual context-dependent processing in healthy volunteers: Implications for models of cognitive deficits in schizophrenia. *Archives of General Psychiatry*, **57**, 1139–1147.

Urenjak, J., Williams, S.R., Gadian, D.G., and Noble, M. (1993). Proton nuclear magnetic resonance spectroscopy unambiguously identifies different neural cell types. *Journal of Neuroscience*, **13**, 981–989.

van Berckel, B.N.M., Hijman, R., van der Linden, J.A., Westenberg, H.G.M., van Ree, J.M., and Kahn, R.S. (1996). Efficacy and tolerance of D-cycloserine in drug-free schizophrenic patients. *Biological Psychiatry*, **40**, 1298–1300.

Van der Does, A.J.M. and Van den Bosch, R.J. (1992). What determines Wisconsin Card Sorting performance in schizophrenia? *Clinical Psychological Reviews*, **12**, 567–583.

Vanderschuren, L.J., Schmidt, E.D., De Varies, T.J., Van Moorsel, A.P., Tilders, F.J.H., and Schoffelmeer, A.N.M. (1999). A single exposure to amphetamine is sufficient to induce long-term behavioural, neuroendocrine, and sensitization in rats. *Journal of Neuroscience*, **19**, 9579–9586.

Van der Werf, Y.D., Witter, M.P., Uylings, H.B., and Jolles, J. (2000). Neuropsychology of infarctions in the thalamus: a review. *Neuropsychologia*, **38**, 613–627.

van Erp, T.G.M., Saleh, P.A., Huttunen, M., Lönnqvist, J., Kaprio, J., Salonen, O., Valanne. L., Poutanen, V.-P., Standertskjöld-Nordenstam, C.-G., and Cannon, T.D. (2004). Hippocampal volumes in schizophrenic twins. *Archives of General Psychiatry*, **61**, 346–353.

Veiel, H.O.F. (1997). A preliminary profile of neuropsychological deficits associated with major depression. *Journal of Clinical and Experimental Neuropsychology*, **19**, 587–603.

Verdoux, H., Geddes, J.R., Takei, N., Lawrie, S.M., Bovet, P., Eagles, J.M., Heun, R., McCreadie, R.G., McNeil, T.F., O'Callaghan, E., Stober, G., Willinger, M.U., Wright, P., and Murray, R.M. (1997). Obstetric complications and age at onset in schizophrenia: An international collaborative meta-analysis of individual patient data. *American Journal of Psychiatry*, **154**, 1220–1227.

Verma, A. and Moghaddam, B. (1998). Regulation of striatal dopamine release by metabotropic glutamate receptors. *Synapse*, **28**, 220–226.

Videbech, P. (2000). PET measurements of brain glucose metabolism and blood flow in major depressive disorder: A critical review. *Acta Psychiarica Scandinavica*, **101**, 11–20.

Vion-Dury, J., Salvan, A.M., Confort-Gouny, S., Dhiver, C., and Cozzone, P. (1995). Reversal of brain metabolic alterations with zidovudine detected by proton localised magnetic resonance spectroscopy. *Lancet*, **345**, 60–61.

Vita, A., Bressi, S., Perani, D., Invernizzi, G., Giobbio, G.M., Dieci, M., Garbarini, M., Del Sole, A., and Fazio, F. (1995). High-resolution SPECT study of regional cerebral blood flow in drug-free and drug-naïve schizophrenic patients. *American Journal of Psychiatry*, **152**, 876–882.

Vita, A., Sacchetti, E., Valvassori, G., and Cazzullo, C.L. (1988). Brain morphology in schizophrenia: A 2- to 5-year follow-up study. *Acta Psychiatrica Scandinavica*, **78**, 618–621.

Volk, D.W., Austin, M.C., Pierri, J.N., Sampson, A.R., and Lewis, D.A. (2000). Decreased glutamic acid decarboxylase$_{67}$ messenger RNA expression in a subset of prefrontal cortical γ-aminobutyric acid neurons in subjects with schizophrenia. *Archives of General Psychiatry*, **57**, 237–245.

Vollenweider, F.X., Leenders, K.L., Scharfetter, C., Antonin, A., Maguire, P., Missimer, J., and Angst, J. (1997). Metabolic hyperfrontality and psychopathology in the ketamine model of psychosis using positron emission tomography (PET) and [^{18}F]fluorodeoxyglucose (FDG). *European Neuropsychopharmacology*, **7**, 9–24.

Vollenweider, F.X., Vontobel, Oye, I., Hell, D., and Leenders, K.L. (2000). Effects of (S)-ketamine on striatal dopamine: a [11C]raclopride PET study of a model psychosis in humans. *Journal of Psychiatric Research*, **34**, 35–43.

Volz, H., Gaser, C., Hager, F., Rzanny, R., Ponisch, J., Mentzel, H., Kaiser, W.A., and Sauer, H. (1999). Decreased frontal activation in schizophrenics during stimulation with the continuous performance test—a functional magnetic resonance imaging study. *European Psychiatry*, **17**, 1–8.

Volz, H.-P., Gaser, C., and Sauer, H. (2000a). Supporting evidence for the model of cognitive dysmetria in schizophrenia—a structural magnetic resonance imaging study using deformation-based morphometry. *Schizophrenia Research*, **46**, 45–56.

Volz, H.-P., Riehemann, S., Maurer, I., Smesney, S., Sommer, M., Rzanny, R., Hostein, W., Czekalla, J., and Sauer, H. (2000b). Reduced phosphodiesters and high-energy phosphates in the frontal lobe of schizophrenic patients: A ^{31}P chemical shift spectroscopic imaging study. *Biological Psychiatry*, **47**, 954–961.

Volz, H.-P., Rzanny, R., May, S., Hegervald, H., Preufler, B., Hajek, M., Kaiser, W.A., and Sauer, H. (1997). ^{31}P magnetic resonance spectroscopy in the dorsolateral prefrontal cortex of schizophrenics with a volume selective technique—preliminary findings. *Biological Psychiatry*, **41**, 644–648.

Volz, H.-P., Rzanny, R., Rossger, G., Hubner, G., Kreitschmann-Andermahr, I., Kaiser, W.A., and Sauer, H. (1998). ^{31}P phosphorous magnetic resonance spectroscopy of the dorsolateral prefrontal region in schizophrenics—a study including 50 patients and 36 controls. *Biological Psychiatry*, **44**, 399–404.

Voorn, P., Vanderschuren, L.J.M.J., Groenewegen, H.J., Robbins, T., and Pennartz, C.M.A. (2004). Putting a spin on the dorsal–ventral divide of the striatum. *Trends in Neurosciences*, **27**, 468–474.

Waddington, J.L., Youssef, H.A., and Kinsella, A. (1995). Sequential cross-sectional and 10-year prospective study of severe negative symptoms in relation to duration of initially untreated psychosis in chronic schizophrenia. *Psychological Medicine*, **25**, 849–857.

Walker, E. and Lewine, R.J. (1990). Prediction of adult-onset schizophrenia from childhood home movies of the patients. *American Journal of Psychiatry*, **147**, 1052–1056.

Walker, E., McGuire, M., and Bettes, B. (1984). Recognition and identification of facial stimuli by schizophrenics and patients with affective disorders. *British Journal of Clinical Psychology*, **23**, 37–44.

Wang, F., Sun, Z., Cui, L., Du, X., Wang, X., Zhang, H., Cong, Z., Hong, N., and Zhang, D. (2004). Anterior cingulum abnormalities in male patients with schizophrenia determined through diffusion tensor imaging. *American Journal of Psychiatry*, **161**, 573–575.

Wang, Y. and Goldman-Rakic, P.S. (2004). D2 receptor regulation of synaptic burst firing in prefrontal cortical pyramidal neurons. *Proceedings of the National Academy of Sciences of the United States of America*, **101**, 5093–5098.

Ward, K.E., Friedman, L., Wise, A., and Schulz, S.C. (1996). Meta-analysis of brain and cranial size in schizophrenia. *Schizophrenia Research*, **22**, 197–213.

Wassef, A., Baker, J., and Kochan, L.D. (2003). GABA and schizophrenia: A review of basic science and clinical studies. *Journal of Clinical Psychopharmacology*, **23**, 601–640.

Wassef, A.A., Dott, S.G., Harris, A., Brown, A., O'Boyle, M., Meyer, W.J., and Rose, R.M. (1999). Critical review of GABA-ergic drugs in the treatment of schizophrenia. *Journal of Clinical Psychopharmacology*, **19**, 222–232.

Wassef, A.A., Dott, S.G., Harris, A., Brown, A., O'Boyle, M., Meyer, W.J., and Rose, R.M. (2000). Randomized, placebo-controlled pilot study of divalproex sodium in the treatment of acute exacerbations of chronic schizophrenia. *Journal of Clinical Psychopharmacology*, **20**, 357–361.

Wassef, A.A., Hafiz, N.G., Hampton, D., and Molloy, M. (2001). Divalproex sodium augmentation of haloperidol in hospitalized patients with schizophrenia: Clinical and economic implications. *Journal of Clinical Psychopharmacology*, **21**, 21–26.

Wassef, A., Watson, D.J., Morrison, P., Bryant, S., and Flack, J. (1989). Neuroleptic–valproic acid combination in the treatment of psychotic symptoms: A three-case report. *Journal of Clinical Psychopharmacology*, **9**, 45–48.

Waters, F.A.V., Maybery, M.T., Badcock, J.C., and Michie, P.T. (2004). Context memory and binding in schizophrenia. *Schizophrenia Research*, **68**, 119–125.

Waterworth, D.M., Bassett, A.S., and Brzustowicz, L.M. (2002). Recent advances in the genetics of schizophrenia. *Cellular and Molecular Life Sciences*, **59**, 331–348.

Waziri, R. (1988). Glycine therapy of schizophrenia. *Biological Psychiatry*, **23**, 209–214.

Weinberger, D.R. (1987). Implications of normal brain development for the pathogenesis of schizophrenia. *Archives of General Psychiatry*, **44**, 660–669.

Weinberger, D.R. (1991). Anteromedial temporal-prefrontal connectivity: A functional neuroanatomical system implicated in schizophrenia. In B.J. Carroll and J.E. Barnett (Eds.), *Psychopathology and the brain* (pp. 25–43). New York, Raven Press.

Weinberger, D.R. (1995). From neuropathology to neurodevelopment. *Lancet*, **346**, 552–557.

Weinberger, D.R., Berman, K.F., Suddath, R., and Torrey, E.F. (1992a). Evidence of dysfunction of a prefrontal–limbic network in schizophrenia: A magnetic resonance imaging and regional cerebral blood flow study of discordant monozygotic twins. *American Journal of Psychiatry*, **149**, 890–897.

Weinberger, D.R., Berman, K.F., and Zec, R.F. (1986). Physiological dysfunction of dorsolateral cortex in schizophrenia: I. Regional cerebral blood flow (rCBF) evidence. *Archives of General Psychiatry*, **43**, 114–124.

Weinberger, D.R., DeLisi, L.E., Neophytides, A.N., and Wyatt, R.J. (1981). Familial aspects of CT scan abnormalities in chronic schizophrenic patients. *Psychiatry Research*, **4**, 65–71.

Weinberger, D.R., Egan, M.F., Bertolino, A., Callicott, J.H., Mattay, V.S., Lipska, B.K., Berman, K.F., and Goldberg, T.E. (2001). Prefrontal neurons and the genetics of schizophrenia. *Biological Psychiatry*, **50**, 825–844.

Weinberger, D.R., Kleinman, J.E., Luchins, D.J., Bigelow, L.B., and Wyatt, R.J. (1980). Cerebellar pathology in schizophrenia: A post-mortem study. *American Journal of Psychiatry*, **137**, 359–361.

Weinberger, D.R. and McClure, R.K. (2002). Neurotoxicity, neuroplasticity, and magnetic resonance imaging morphometry: What is happening in the schizophrenic brain? *Archives of General Psychiatry*, **59**, 553–558.

Weinberger, D.R., Torrey, E.F., Neophytides, A.N., and Wyatt, R.J. (1979). Lateral ventricular enlargement in chronic schizophrenia. *Archives of General Psychiatry*, **36**, 735–739.

Weinberger, D.R., Zigun, J.R., Bartley, A.J., Jones, D.W., and Torrey, E.F (1992b). Anatomic abnormalities in the brains of monozygotic twins discordant and concordant for schizophrenia. *Clinical Neuropharmacology*, **15** (Suppl. 1), 122A–123A.

Wenz, F., Schad, L.R., Knopp, M.V., Baudendistel, K.T., Flömer, F., Shröder, J., and van Kaick, G. (1994). Functional magnetic resonance imaging at 1.5 T: Activation pattern in schizophrenic patients receiving neuroleptic medication. *Magnetic Resonance Imaging*, **12**, 975–982.

Wester, K., Irvine, D.R., and Hugdahl, K. (2001). Auditory laterality and attentional deficits after thalamic hemorrhage. *Journal of Neurology*, **248**, 676–683.

Wible, C.G., Anderson, J., Shenton, M.E., Kricun, A., Hirayasu, Y., Tanaka, S., Levitt, J.J., O'Donnell, B.F., Kikinis, R., Jolesz, F.A., and McCarley, R.W. (2001). Prefrontal cortex, negative symptoms, and schizophrenia: An MRI study. *Psychiatry Research: Neuroimaging*, **108**, 65–78.

Wible, C.G., Shenton, M.E., Hokama, H., Kikinis, R., Jolesz, F.A., Metcalf, D., and McCarley, R.W. (1995). Prefrontal cortex and schizophrenia: A quantitative magnetic resonance imaging study. *Archives of General Psychiatry*, **52**, 279–288.

Wilke, M., Kaufman, C., Grabner, A., Putz, B., Wetter, T.C., and Auer, D.P. (2001). Gray matter changes and correlates of disease severity in schizophrenia: A statistical parametric mapping study. *NeuroImage*, **13**, 814–824.

Williams, L.M., Das, P., Harris, A.W.F., Liddell, B.B., Brammer, M.J., Olivieri, G., Skerrett, D., Philips, M.L., David, A.S., Peduto, A., and Gordon, E. (2004). Dysregulation of arousal and amygdala–prefrontal systems in paranoid schizophrenia. *American Journal of Psychiatry*, **161**, 48–489.

Williams, S.M. and Goldman-Rakic, P.S. (1998). Widespread origin of the primate mesofrontal dopamine system. *Cerebral Cortex*, **8**, 321–345.

Williamson, P.C. and Drost, D.J. (2003). Brain phospholipid metabolism in schizophrenia: Assessment with ^{31}P magnetic resonance spectroscopy. In M. Peet, I. Glen, and D.F. Horrobin (Eds.), *Phosholipid spectrum disorders in psychiatry and neurology, second edition* (pp. 221–238). Carnforth, Lancashire, Marius Press.

Williamson, P., Drost, D., Stanley, J., Carr, T., Morrison, S., and Merskey, H. (1991a). Localized phosphorus 31 nuclear magnetic resonance spectroscopy in chronic schizophrenic patients and normal controls. *Archives of General Psychiatry*, **48**, 578.

Williamson, P., Pelz, D., Merskey, H., Morrison, S., and Conlon, P. (1991b). Correlation of negative symptoms in schizophrenia with frontal lobe parameters on magnetic resonance imaging. *British Journal of Psychiatry*, **159**, 130–134.

Williamson, P., Pelz, D., Merskey, H., Morrison, S., Karlik, S., Drost, D., Carr, T., and Conlon, P. (1992) Frontal, temporal, and striatal proton relaxation times in schizophrenic patients and normal comparison subjects. *American Journal of Psychiatry*, **149**, 549–551.

Winsberg, M.E., Sachs, N., Tate, D.L., Adalsteinsson, E., Spielman, D., and Ketter, T.A. (2000). Decreased dorsolateral prefrontal *N*-acetyl aspartate in bipolar disorder. *Biological Psychiatry*, **47**, 475–481.

Winterer, G., Coppola, R., Egan, M.F., Goldberg, T.E., and Weinberger, D.R. (2003). Functional and effective frontotemporal connectivity and genetic risk for schizophrenia. *Biological Psychiatry*, **54**, 1181–1192.

Winterer, G., Egan, M.F., Radler, T., Hyde, T., Coppola, R., and Weinberger, D.R. (2001). An association between reduced interhemisheric EEG coherence in the temporal lobe area and genetic risk for schizophrenia. *Schizophrenia Research*, **49**, 129–143.

Wise, S.P., Murray, E.A., and Gerfen, C.R. (1996). The frontal cortex–basal ganglia system in primates. *Critical Reviews in Neurobiology*, **10**, 317–356.

Wolkin, A., Choi, S.J., Szilagyi, S., Sanfilipo, M., Rotrosen, J.P., and Lim, K.O. (2003). Inferior frontal white matter anisotropy and negative symptoms of schizophrenia: A diffusion tensor imaging study. *American Journal of Psychiatry*, **160**, 572–574.

Wolkin, A. Sanfilipo, M., Wolf, A.P., Angrist, B., Brodie, J.D., and Rotrosen, J. (1992). Negative symptoms and hypofrontality in chronic schizophrenia. *Archives of General Psychiatry*, **49**, 959–965.

Wolkowitz, O.M. and Pickar, D. (1991). Benzodiazepines in the treatment of schizophrenia: A review and appraisal. *American Journal of Psychiatry*, **148**, 714–726.

Woo, T.-U.W., Walsh, J.P., and Benes, F.M. (2004). Density of glutamic acid decarboxylase 67 messenger RNA-containing neurons that express the N-methyl-D-aspartate receptor subunit NR_{2A} in the anterior cingulate cortex in schizophrenia and bipolar disorder. *Archives of General Psychiatry*, **61**, 649–657.

Wood, S.J., Velakoulis, D., Smith, D.J., Bond, D., Stuart, G.W., McGorry, P.D., Brewer, W.J., Bridle, N., Eritaia, J., Desmond, P., Singh, B., Copolov, D., and Pantelis, C. (2001). A longitudinal study of hippocampal volume in first episode psychosis and chronic schizophrenia. *Schizophrenia Research*, **52**, 37–46.

Woodruff, P.W.R., Mcmanus, I.C., and David, A.S. (1995). Meta-analysis of corpus callosum size in schizophrenia. *Journal of Neurology, Neurosurgery and Psychiatry*, **58**, 457–461.

Woodruff, P.W.R., Pearlson, G.D., Geer, M.J., Barta, P.E., and Chilcoat, H.D. (1993). A computerized magnetic resonance imaging study of corpus callosum morphology in schizophrenia. *Psychological Medicine*, **23**, 45–56.

Woodruff, P.W.R., Wright, I.C., Bullmore, E.T., Brammer, M., Howard, R.J., Williams, S.C.R., Shapleske, J., Rossell, S., David, A.S., McGuire, P.K., and Murray, R.M. (1997). Auditory hallucinations and the temporal cortical response to speech in schizophrenia: A functional magnetic resonance imaging study. *American Journal of Psychiatry*, **154**, 1676–1682.

Woods, B.T. (1998). Is schizophrenia a progressive neurodevelopmental disorder? Toward a unitary pathogenetic mechanism. *American Journal of Psychiatry*, **155**, 1661–1670.

Woods, B.T. and Yurgelin-Todd, D. (1991). Brain volume loss in schizophrenia: When does it occur and is it progressive? *Schizophrenia Research*, **5**, 202–204.

Woods, B.T., Yurgelin-Todd, D., Goldstein, J., Seidman, L.J., and Tsuang, M.T. (1996). MRI brain abnormalities in schizophrenia: One process or more? *Biological Psychiatry*, **40**, 585–596.

Wright, I.C., Ellison, Z.R., Sharma, T., Friston, K.J., Murray, R.M., and McGuire, P.K. (1999). Mapping of grey matter changes in schizophrenia. *Schizophrenia Research*, **35**, 1–14.

Wright, I.C., Rabe-Hesketh, S., Woodruff, P.W.R., David, A.S., Murray, R.M., and Bullmore, E.T. (2000). Meta-analysis of regional brain volumes in schizophrenia. *American Journal of Psychiatry*, **157**, 16–25.

Wyatt, R.J. (1991). Neuroleptics and the natural course of schizophrenia. *Schizophrenia Bulletin*, **17**, 325–351.

Wyatt, R.J. (1995). Early intervention for schizophrenia: Can the course of the illness be altered? *Biological Psychiatry*, **38**, 1–3.

Wyatt, R.J., Green, M.F., and Tuma, A.H. (1997). Long-term morbidity associated with delayed treatment of first admission schizophrenic patients: A re-analysis of the Camarillo State Hospital data. *Psychological Medicine*, **27**, 261–268.

Wyatt, R.J. and Hunter, I. (2001). Rationale for the study of early intervention. *Schizophrenia Research*, **51**, 69–76.

Yacubian, J., de Castro, C.C., Ometto, M., Barbosa, E., de Camargo, C.P., Tavares, H., Cerri, G.G., and Gattaz, W.F. (2002). ^{31}P-spectroscopy of frontal lobe in schizophrenia: Alterations in phospholipids and high-energy phosphate metabolism. *Schizophrenia Research*, **58**, 117–122.

Young, K.A., Manaye, K.F., Liang, C., Hicks, P.B., and German, D.C. (2000). Reduced number of mediodorsal and anterior thalamic neurons in schizophrenia. *Biological Psychiatry*, **47**, 944–953.

Yurgelun-Todd, D.A., Renshaw, P.F., Gruber, S.A., Ed, M., Waternaux, C., and Cohen, B.M. (1996a). Proton magnetic resonance spectroscopy of the temporal lobes in schizophrenics and normal controls. *Schizophrenia Research*, **19**, 55–59.

Yurgelun-Todd, D.A., Waternaux, C.M., Cohen, B.M., Gruber, S.A., English, C.D., and Renshaw, P.F. (1996b). Functional magnetic resonance imaging of schizophrenic patients and comparison subjects during word production. *American Journal of Psychiatry*, **153**, 200–205.

Zahn, T.P., Frith, C.D., and Steinhauer, S.R. (1991). Autonomic functioning in schizophrenia: electrodermal activity, heart rate, pupillography. In S.R. Steinhauer, J.H. Gruzelier, and J. Zubin (Eds.), *Handbook of schizophrenia, Vol. 5: Neuropsychology, psychophysiology and information processing* (pp. 185–224). Amsterdam, Elsevier.

Zakzanis, K.K. and Hansen, K.T. (1998). Dopamine D$_2$ densities and the schizophrenic brain. *Schizophrenia Research*, **32**, 201–206.

Zakzanis, K.K., Leach, L., and Kaplan, E. (1998). On the nature and pattern of neurocognitive function in major depressive disorder. *Neuropsychiatry, Neuropsychology and Behavioural Neurology*, **11**, 111–119.

Zakzanis, K.K., Poulin, P., Hansen, K.T., and Jolic, D. (2000). Searching the schizophrenic brain for temporal lobe deficits: A systematic review and meta-analysis. *Psychological Medicine*, **30**, 491–504.

Zalewski, C., Johnson-Selfridge, M.T., Ohriner, S., Zarella, K., and Seltzer, J.C. (1998). A review of neuropsychological differences between paranoid and nonparanoid schizophrenia patients. *Schizophrenia Bulletin*, **24**, 127–145.

Zipursky, R.B., Lambe, E.K., Kapur, S., and Mikulis, D.J. (1998). Cerebral gray matter volume deficits in first episode psychosis. *Archives of General Psychiatry*, **55**, 540–546.

Zipursky, R.B., Lim, K.O., Sullivan, E.V., Brown, B.W., and Pfefferbaum, A. (1992). Widespread cerebral gray matter volume deficits in schizophrenia. *Archives of General Psychiatry*, **49**, 195–205.

Zubin, J., Magaziner, J., and Steinhauser, S.R. (1983). The metamorphosis of schizophrenia: From chronicity to vulnerability. *Psychological Medicine*, **13**, 551–571.

Index

....

Note: Page numbers followed by *f* indicate figures.